The Essential Diabetes Cookbook

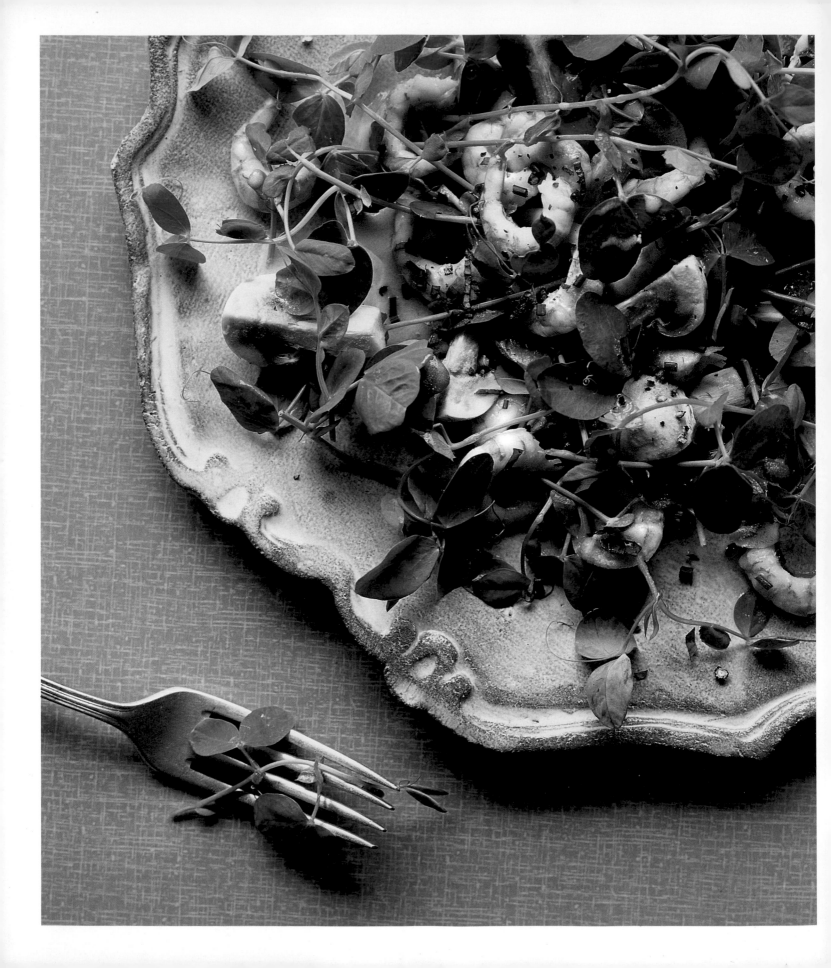

Antony Worrall Thompson

The Essential Diabetes Cookbook

GOOD HEALTHY EATING FROM AROUND THE WORLD

with Louise Blair BSc

Supported by

DiABETES UK

This edition published in 2016 by Kyle Books,
an imprint of Kyle Cathie Ltd.
192–198 Vauxhall Bridge Road
London SW1V 1DX
general.enquiries@kylebooks.com
www.kylecathie.co.uk

First published in Great Britain in 2010

10 9 8 7 6 5 4 3 2 1

ISBN 978 0 85783 379 2

Editor Judith Hannam
Editorial Assistant Vicki Murrell
Designer Jim Smith
Home Economist and Stylist Annie Nichols
Copyeditor Marion Moisy
Recipe Analyis Wendy Doyle
Production Kyle Cathie and Gemma John

A Cataloguing in Publication record for this title is available from the British Library.

Colour reproduction by Scanhouse
Printed and bound in China

Note about raw eggs and raw fish

It is recommended that eggs should not be eaten raw. Vulnerable people, such as pregnant or nursing mothers, babies, the young, the elderly and those with reduced immune efficiency, are advised to avoid eating raw or lightly cooked eggs. If you fall into these catagories you should also make sensible choices as to whether to eat raw fish.

Note about fat and saturated fat

The delicious recipes in this book have been written and adapted to make them healthier and use monounsaturated spreads and sunflower oils. Butter can be used in place of these but this will increase the saturated fat content of the dish.

If you are watching your weight, refer to the nutritional analysis at the bottom of each recipe. Where the fat content is high, these recipes are probably best kept for special occasions and not eaten every day.

Acknowledgements

Space is short but it's essential that I thank those that have helped in the making of this book, Kyle for having faith in realising that there is a real need for a comprehensive cookbook. To Diabetes UK who threw their considerable weight behind this idea. Thanks also go to Judith Hannam, my editor, who skilfully edited my work. A thank you to Jonathan Gregson who did justice to my recipes, with the stunning pictures. To David Wilby, Nicola Atherton, and Fiona Lindsay and the team at Limelight. I couldn't forget my wife, Jacinta and children, Toby and Billie for putting up with me. This book is dedicated to all those of those with diabetes; food can still be enjoyable.

Contents

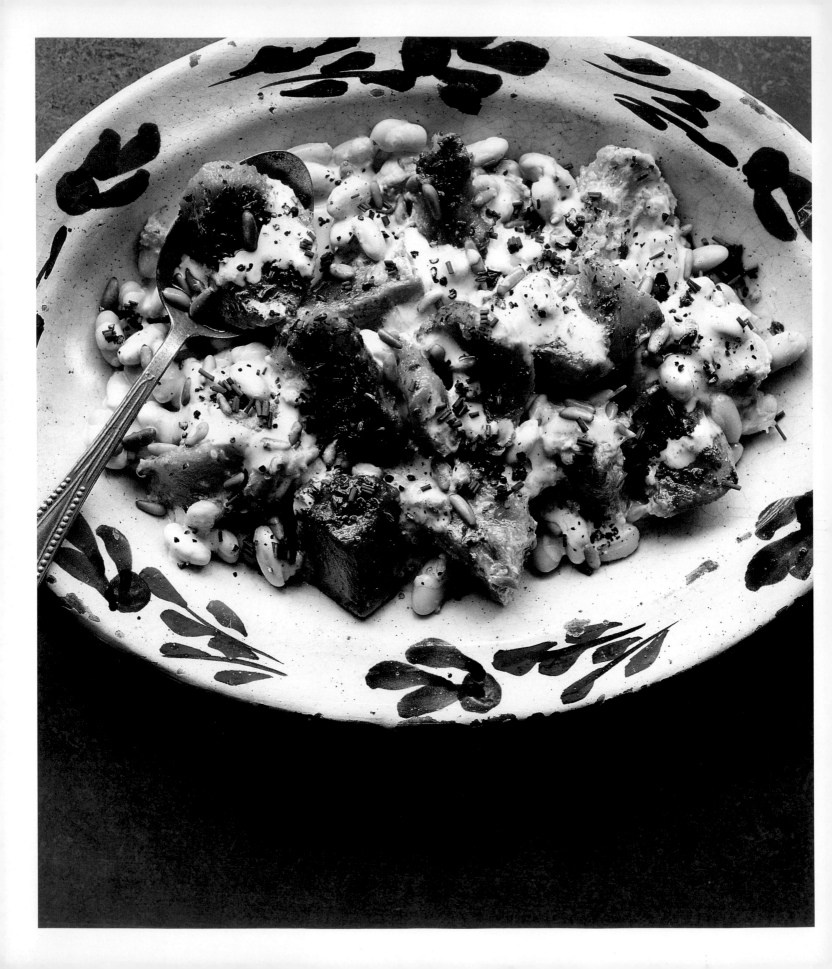

Foreword by Diabetes UK

I hope you enjoy *The Essential Diabetes Cookbook*.

Balancing your diet when you are living with diabetes can be a challenge, especially if you are recently diagnosed. Your food choices and eating habits are important in helping you manage your diabetes, but there is absolutely no reason you can't enjoy a wide variety of great food as part of your healthy balanced diet.

I hope you will find lots to enjoy from this collection of 185 exciting recipes, it's a great collection from all across the world.

A healthy balanced diet is not just important for people with diabetes – it is something we all should be aiming for. So these recipes are for everyone and anyone who wants to enjoy healthy, nutritious, great tasting dishes. I'm certainly looking forward to getting cooking.

Chris Askew
Chief Executive, Diabetes UK

DiABETES UK

is a charity registered in England and Wales (no.215199) and in Scotland (no.SC039136)

From AWT

I have now written four books designed specifically for people with diabetes, all of which have been well received. Many readers have written to me saying they have changed their life — some even that they've enabled them to come off insulin. This is very satisfying, especially as I'm neither a doctor nor a nutritionist. My main message has always been that you can still enjoy great food, it just requires small changes to your food and lifestyle, and keeping one word fixed firmly at the front of your mind: moderation.

If you have been diagnosed with Type 2 diabetes, recriminations are pointless. 'What if I had lost weight', 'I should have done more exercise', 'My sweet tooth has been my downfall' phrases like this inevitably spring to mind, but it doesn't do any good to look backwards, you need to look to the future. It's positive thinking you need; how am I going to enjoy my future and still have fun and pleasure at mealtimes?

'The fabulous recipes included here come from all over the world and prove that food for diabetes doesn't need to be boring.'

Don't get me wrong, you do need to make some lifestyle changes. Diet is one of the most important areas for people with diabetes to understand, as the correct diet will improve long-term glucose control. You must focus on food and its importance to you personally. For many with Type 2 Diabetes, it's all about losing weight and, more importantly, keeping it off. This a slow process, it won't just happen overnight, but losing 10 per cent of your body weight can improve the quality of your life enormously by lowering your blood pressure, reducing fasting blood glucose levels and improving blood fats.

I'm not, though, a fan of the word 'diet', as it implies loss and suffering. Having diabetes may mean lifestyle changes, but it doesn't mean having to give up foods you particularly love. It's that word moderation again, and making sensible choices. It's also about eating as wide a variety of foods as possible, about increasing the amount of fruit, vegetables, beans and lentils that you eat, as well as reducing the fat, salt and sugar too.

My aim with this book is to extend your knowledge of world foods. The fabulous recipes included here come from all the continents and prove that food for those with diabetes doesn't need to be boring. Our Western eating habits aren't always the easiest to adapt to diabetes requirements, whereas the everyday diet in some other cultures is much more in line with the diet for diabetes. Why not take our inspiration from there? Just think about all those wonderful vegetables from India and the Far East; lots of interesting spices give these dishes their flavour, without the need for too much animal fat or salt. Just cut out the ghee, add a delicious salad and you're there. Suddenly it's easy to eat six to eight portions of vegetables a day, plus you have the satisfaction of knowing that you're benefiting your body. World food offers so many ways of enjoying your new life with diabetes and it teaches you to think outside the box. With so many options, the world is your oyster.

Antony Worrall Thompson

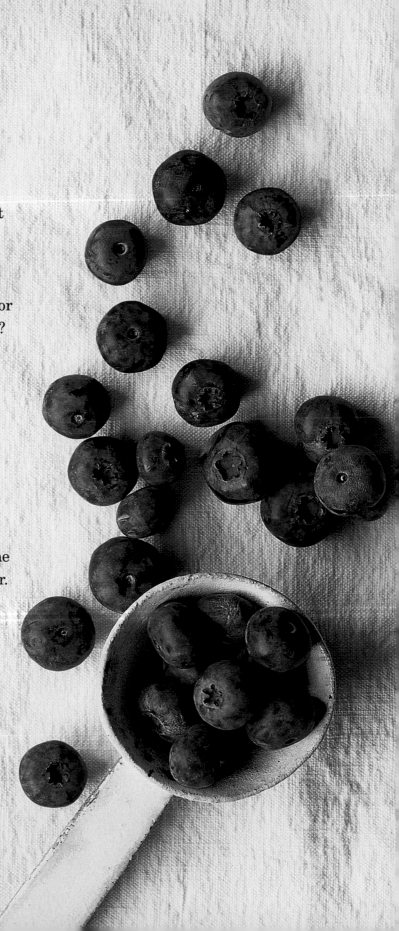

Introduction

With more than 4 million people in the UK diagnosed with diabetes and 549,000 predicted to have diabetes but remaining undiagnosed, diabetes is one of the major health issues of modern day UK and a huge problem worldwide. Numbers are increasing rapidly year on year. It is estimated that in 2015 diabetes affected some 450 million people aged 20–70 worldwide and according to estimates this figure is set to increase to 642 million by the year 2040, that's one in ten people. The predominant reasons for the huge number of Type 2 diabetes is obesity due to increasing sedentary lifestyles and poor diet.

Type 2 diabetes is finally being recognised as a global epidemic, with the potential to cause a worldwide healthcare crisis.

In the UK diabetes is costing the NHS an estimated £1 million per hour, equating to 10 per cent of its yearly budget. The total cost to the NHS to treat diabetes and its complications is a staggering 10 billion pounds a year.

What is diabetes?

Diabetes mellitus is a condition where the amount of glucose in the blood is too high, either because the body is not producing any or enough insulin, or the insulin it is producing is not effective enough. Glucose is released into the blood when you digest food and drinks containing carbohydrate. Insulin is essential to move the glucose out of the blood and into the cells in our body to be used for energy.

It also stops the liver from releasing glucose (we also get glucose from stores in our liver). If your body can't use insulin properly or produce enough, it can't use glucose to give you energy.

Diabetes types

There are two main types of diabetes. These are:

- Type 1 diabetes
- Type 2 diabetes

Type 1

Type 1 diabetes develops if the body is unable to produce any insulin. Type 1 diabetes is the least common of the two main types and accounts for one in ten of all people with diabetes. You cannot prevent Type 1 diabetes. It is treated by taking insulin several times a day and balancing it with food and activity.

Type 2

Type 2 diabetes develops when the body can still make some insulin, but not enough, or when the insulin that is produced does not work properly (known as insulin resistance). Type 2 diabetes is the most common of the two main types and accounts for one in nine of all people with diabetes. Type 2 diabetes is treated by healthy eating and being physically active. In addition to this medication, which may include insulin, is often required.

What are the signs and symptoms of diabetes?

- Going to the toilet a lot to pass urine
- Being really thirsty, drinking more and not

being able to quench your thirst
- Feeling more tired than usual
- Losing weight without trying to

You may also have noticed:
- Genital itching or regular episodes of thrush
- Cuts and wounds that took a long time to heal
- Blurred vision

People with undiagnosed Type 2 diabetes may have had no obvious symptoms at all.

The risk factors of Type 2 diabetes

Type 2 diabetes is caused by a combination of lifestyle and genes. Although we don't know exactly why it develops, certain factors do increase your risk, including:
- Age – being over 40 (or over 25 if you're South Asian).
- Weight – being overweight, especially if you have a large tummy.
- Ethnicity – being Black African, African Caribbean, South Asian or Chinese.
- Family link – having a parent, brother or sister with diabetes.
- Previous medical history – having high blood pressure, a history of heart attacks and stroke, gestational diabetes or severe mental illness treated with anti-psychotic medication.

Sometimes, though, there's nothing to explain why Type 2 diabetes develops. Not everyone who's overweight has it, while some people who are a healthy weight do have it.

'The more risk factors that apply to you, the greater your risk of having Type 2 diabetes'

If you've been told you have pre-diabetes impaired fasting glycaemia (IFG) or impaired glucose tolerance (IGT) it means the level of glucose (sugar) in your blood is higher than normal but you don't have diabetes. You should eat healthily, lose weight if you need to and be physically active to help reduce the risk of Type 2 diabetes. But make sure you're regularly tested for diabetes.

People from South Asian and Black communities who live in the UK are two to four times more likely to have Type 2 diabetes than the caucasian population.

What are the complications?

If diabetes is not well managed, complications can include heart attack, stroke, angina, foot and leg amputation, loss of vision and blindness, nerve pain or numbness in the hands, arms, feet and legs, impotence and sexual problems, gut problems, muscle weakness, wasting, twitching and cramps. Because Type 2 diabetes can remain undetected for 10 years or more before someone is diagnosed, by the time they are diagnosed half of those people will have begun to develop complications.

Around half of people with diabetes will die from 'cardiovascular complications' such as heart attack or stroke.

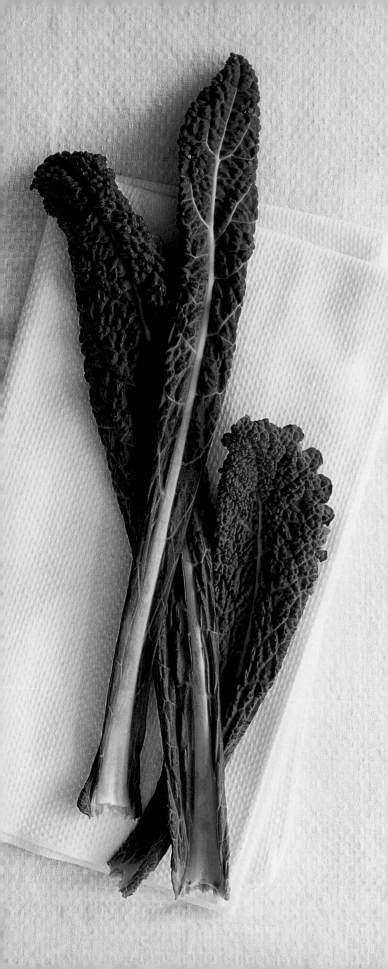

What now?

You and your diabetes team can help reduce your risk of complications by keeping to your personal health targets for:
- blood glucose levels (also called blood sugar levels)
- blood fat levels (cholesterol)
- blood pressure
- weight.

Weight Loss

I know we have all heard it before … 'you need to lose weight' … it sounds simple but the thought of dieting can make most of us groan. It's true, achieving and maintaining a healthy weight for your size boasts considerable health benefits. You probably don't need to lose as much as you think – losing between 5 and 10 per cent of your weight (that's 5–10kg if you are 100kg or about ¾ stone – 1½ stones if you are 15 stone) has health benefits such as lowering blood fats, blood pressure and blood glucose levels.

You don't have to reach an 'ideal' weight either – be realistic and aim to lose weight slowly over time (0.5–1.0 kg [1–2 lbs] a week).

Stick to it

The key to making changes is surely to make plans that are easy to stick to and are not too drastic. It may seem like a grand plan to cut out fat or goodies like sweet foods and pastries but after a while this can become really miserable and bingo, just one treat leads to two and before you know it you are back where you started!

So, keep it simple, make small changes that you are happy to stick to. Little changes such as using semi-skimmed milk instead of full-fat milk, trimming excess fat from meats before cooking, grilling or baking instead of deep frying, 1 biscuit instead of 2, a plain biscuit instead of a chocolate one or better still swapping the biscuits for a piece of fruit instead – these can all add up to significant calorie reductions over time and in turn weight loss and maybe a return to those clothes you grew out of!

Just because you are watching what you eat it doesn't mean that you need to cook separate meals from the rest of the family, a little healthy eating is good for everyone! Serve yourself a smaller portion and fill yourself up with vegetables or salad. A little bit of dessert on the odd occasion is fine, but generally it is better to have a piece of fruit or low-fat yoghurt.

Eat regular meals and healthy snacks, skipping meals means you are more likely to hunt out a quick fix and this can spell disaster.

Most importantly don't try to go it alone, a little bit of support will often give you the boost you need when you feel like giving up. Your local diabetes team are there to help, so ask for individual advice and support when needed.

Up the activity!

Get moving … it makes sense when you think about it. If you use up more energy (calories) than you take in then you are bound to lose weight. No-one is expecting you to take up marathon running if you haven't done exercise for some time. Set yourself a goal each week, then, as the weeks go by aim to try to do a little more and push yourself just a little further. The main thing is to take up something that you like, something that you want to go and do and most importantly something that you will keep up. Why not get together with a partner or friend and do something together – this means you are less likely to opt out as you will be letting them down as well as yourself.

It is recommended that adults should aim to be active daily. Over a week, activity should add up to at least 150 minutes (2½ hours) of moderate intensity activity in bouts of 10 minutes or more – one way to approach this is to do 30 minutes on at least 5 days a week. See if any of these inspire you to kick off the slippers and put on the trainers! You will really notice the difference in the way you feel and look as activity releases endorphins which boost your sense of happiness.

- See what classes your local gym, sports centre or leisure club offer, this could be yoga, pilates, aerobics. Book in for an appropriate level and try out something different.
- Take up bowling – not only are you exercising but you can probably fit in time for a chat with your friends.
- Try swimming or see if the pool does aqua aerobics. This is great as the water helps to

support your body but gives you a great work out at the same time. Swimming uses every muscle and is great for cardiovascular fitness.

- Walking require nothing but you and, best of all, it is free. Put on a pair of comfortable, well fitting shoes and join a local walking group or simply explore the area you live in. Walk to the shops or work instead of going by car/bus. Get off a few stops early if you have a long journey and walk the rest of the way.

- Get on your bike! Cycling gives you fresh air and a great look around your surrounding area and once you have the equipment then it is free to keep going. No excuses!

- If you are a little less mobile then don't worry, there are things you can do as well. Try some simple exercises at home to some music – stretching and lunging, maybe a little on-the-spot walking or jogging. Honestly, anything is better than nothing and you will still feel better for it.

- Before you start a new activity, check with your healthcare team about what impact it may have on your diabetes and any changes that may be needed to your medications.

What should I eat?

Making sensible food choices and adapting your eating habits will help you manage your diabetes and protect your long-term health. The good news is that you should still be able to enjoy a wide variety of food. The diet for diabetes isn't a special diet, there is nothing that you can't eat, it is just a case of applying some simple rules to your way of eating, trying to stick to them and getting the balance right.

Follow these steps to a healthy diet and you will be well on your way to a healthier you.

Eat regular meals each day

When blood sugar levels fall you feel hungry and may overeat, so keep your levels steady by eating regularly. Spacing your meals evenly can help you manage your hunger and stop you overeating. This can also help you lose weight as you're less likely to snack.

- Avoid skipping meals and space out your breakfast, lunch and evening meal throughout the day.

- If you need to have a snack between meals, remember to keep it healthy, a piece of fruit, a handful of nut and raisin mix, a low-fat yogurt or why not try some plain home-popped popcorn, which you could flavour with a little paprika or mixed spices.

- Start the day with a healthy breakfast – cereal with skimmed or semi-skimmed milk and a piece of fruit or muesli with some low-fat natural yogurt and sliced fruit, or a glass of juice and maybe some wholegrain toast with a little marmalade, jam or a topping of your choice.

- Lunch could be a healthy sandwich or stuffed pitta or something like a pasta, rice or pulse-based salad.

- For dinner have a form of carbohydrate like pasta, rice or potatoes and serve with some protein and plenty of vegetables or salad.

- Desserts – if you fancy something sweet after your meal, which let's face it, most of us do, then opt for low-fat yogurt, fruit or a fruit-based pudding which are healthier choices.

Include carbohydrate

Healthier sources of carbohydrate include wholegrain starchy foods, fruit and veg, pulses and some dairy foods. These are an important source of energy and provide fibre and essential vitamins. They all break down to glucose, so they will cause your blood sugar levels to be high if you eat large amounts. Find out more about carbohydrate portions to help you find the right portion size.

As well as how much, what is important is how quickly carbohydrates are broken down in your body and how quickly they are absorbed. I am sure you have heard of the term Glycaemic Index (GI). But what is it and how can it be of help or benefit to you? The glycaemic index (GI) tells you whether a food raises blood glucose levels quickly, moderately or slowly. Different carbohydrates are digested at different rates, and the GI is a ranking of how quickly each carbohydrate containing food and drink makes blood glucose levels rise after eating them.

The GI rating is between 1 and 100, depending on how slowly or quickly the food raises your blood glucose levels. The lower the number, the slower the carb is digested and absorbed as glucose in your bloodstream.

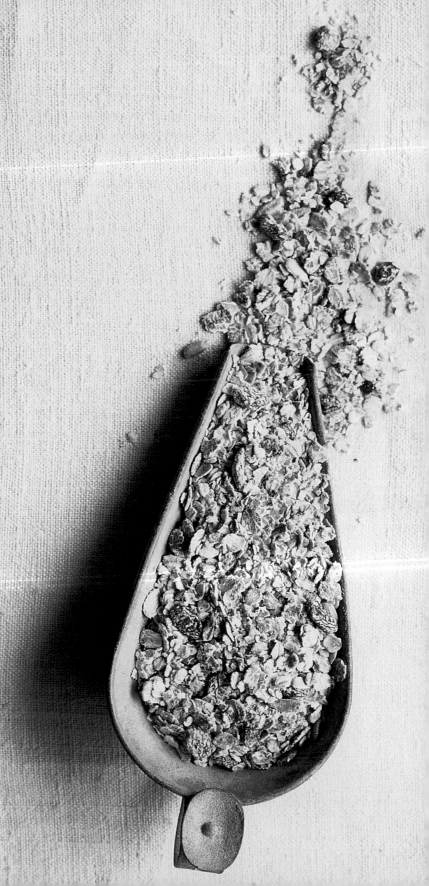

What are the benefts of slow acting carbohydrates?

Meals including low GI foods allow you to absorb carbohydrate at a slower rate. Research has shown that choosing these low-GI foods can help manage long-term blood glucose levels (HbA1c) in people with diabetes, especially in Type 2 diabetes. These foods are also better options for general health, whether or not you have diabetes.

Even for those without diabetes eating the low GI way may have a role in helping to prevent or reduce the risk of getting Type 2 diabetes in those at risk. One or two small changes can make all the difference.

GI lowdown

Individual foods can be categorised into low, medium and high GI (see the list opposite for a few examples of each). Generally, fruit and vegetables have a low to medium GI rating. They are digested slowly and can help reduce fluctuations in your blood glucose levels. Pulses like beans and lentils, basmati rice and whole grains are nourishing lower-GI foods.

LOW GI (0–55)
All bran
Rolled oats
New potatoes
Pearled barley
Nuts and raisins
Milk chocolate
Apple
Wholegrain bread
Broccoli

MEDIUM GI (56–69)
Shredded wheat
Nutrigrain
Baked potatoes
Couscous
Digestive biscuits
Muffins
Mangoes
White pitta
Beetroot

HIGH GI (70+)
Cornflakes
Weetabix
Mashed potato
Short-grain rice
Scones
Pretzels
Watermelon
French bread

So should I just choose low GI foods?

No. The amount of carbohydrate you eat still remains very important for controlling your blood sugar levels. Not all low-GI foods are healthy choices – chocolate, for example, has a low GI because of its fat content, which slows down the absorption of carbohydrate.

Other factors that can affect the GI rating include:

- Cooking methods: Frying, boiling and baking can alter the GI level. For example, the longer pasta is cooked, the higher the GI. That's why it's best to eat it al dente (firm to the bite) or reheated.

- Protein content: Like fat, protein slows down the absorption of carbohydrates, so milk and dairy products will have a low GI.

- Ripeness of fruit and vegetables: In general, the riper the fruit and some vegetables, the higher the GI.

- Fibre: This acts as a physical barrier that slows down the absorption of carbohydrate, so the more fibre in a food, the slower it's absorbed.

Eating to control your diabetes isn't just about GI ratings. Think of the bigger picture and choose foods low in saturated fat, salt and sugar as part of a healthy, balanced diet.

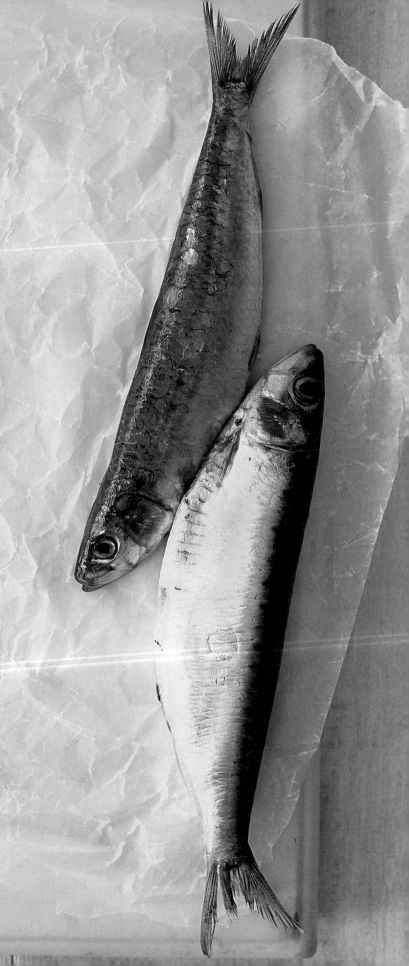

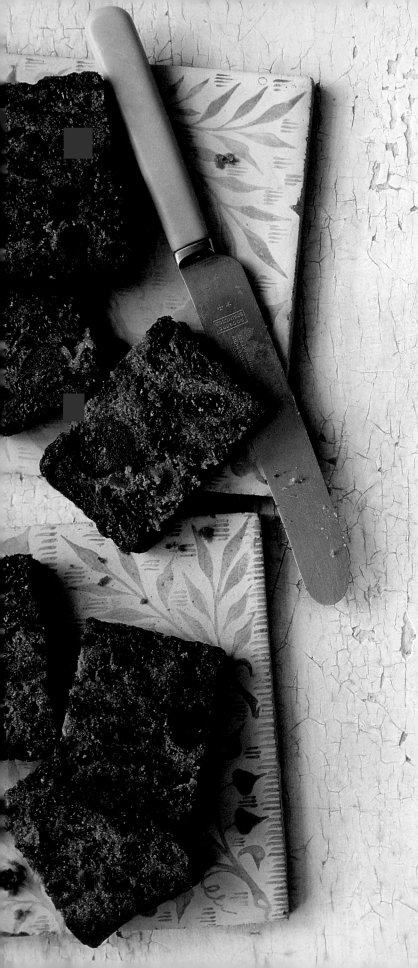

Putting GI into practice

- Kick start your day with a bowl of porridge and some chopped fruit.
- Snack on fruit or dried fruit or try some fruit loaf for something a little more substantial at snack time.
- Add lentils or pulses to casseroles or stews or even salads.
- Include more vegetables with your meals.
- Choose wholegrain foods.
- Choose basmati rice, pasta and sweet potato.

Read up on your fat facts

Fat contains more than twice the amount of calories as the same amount of carbohydrate or protein, so by cutting down on fat you will drastically reduce the amount of calories you consume and this in turn can aid weight loss. The type of fat you use can influence your heart health but remember all fat contains the same amount of calories.

- Cut down on saturated fats – these are hard fats like butter, lard, fat on meat and in dairy products. Saturated fats have a proven link with raised blood cholesterol and heart disease. Having too much harmful cholesterol in the blood increases the risk of coronary heart disease – the biggest killer in the UK.
- Trans fats or hydrogenated fats are chemically altered vegetable oils which change liquid oil into a solid fat. Trans fats have also been linked to high cholesterol and are found in cakes, biscuits and pastries. So it is a good idea to cut down on these too.
- Look out for unsaturated fats that are high in mono-unsaturates, like olive oil, rapeseed

oil and fats that come from some plant sources, these are a much better choice and can even have health benefits like lowering blood cholesterol.

- Omega-3 – research shows that eating a diet rich in long-chain Omega 3 fatty acids, which is found in oily fish like salmon, fresh tuna, herring and sardines, can help protect against heart disease, has anti-inflammatory properties and is good for joints. Omega 3 is essential to human health but cannot be manufactured by the body. For this reason Omega 3 fatty acids must be obtained from food. Aim to eat at least two portions of oily fish per week from sustainable sources.

Top tips to cut down on fat

- Finely grate strong cheese like cheddar or Parmesan as it has a strong flavour and you will need less, or use a reduced-fat version.
- Swap full-fat milk for semi or skimmed milk.
- Invest in an oil spray for light frying.
- Make sure the oil you use is really hot before you start cooking. Quickly cooking the outside will help reduce the amount of fat it will absorb.
- Remove all visible fat from food before and after cooking especially chicken skin which can cut the amount of saturated fat by at least one third.
- Choose low-fat spreads and salad dressings.

Go for 5 a day

We all know that the government recommends we eat at least five portions of fruit and vegetables a day, but how many of us can say that we actually do? It may seem like a lot but with a little planning you can improve your diet by including more fruit and vegetables.

- Have a sliced banana or other fruit on your cereal with a glass of juice – that's two portions before you've even stepped out of the door!
- A handful of dried fruit for a mid-morning snack.
- A piece of fruit with lunch.
- A large bowl of salad or vegetables with your evening meal and you will have managed to fit in at least 5 portions easily.
Remember though … go for a variety of fruit and vegetables in a range of colours to give you a good range of vitamins and anti-oxidants.

Cut down on sugar

You don't need to eliminate sweet foods and sugar from your diet but cut down and make sensible choices. Do you really need a biscuit or cake when you would be much better having a piece of fruit? There is no reason why you can't use ordinary sugar in baking and desserts, good blood glucose control can still be achieved when sugar and sugar-containing foods are eaten, just try to use less or have smaller portions.

Slash the salt

According to the Food Standards Agency, most of us are consuming up to twice as much as the recommended 6g or less of salt per day.

Evidence shows that a high salt intake is linked to many diseases including high blood pressure, heart disease and strokes. Sea salt, rock salt, garlic salt and natural salt are all forms of salt and contain sodium so try to cut down on all of these to improve your health.

If the nutritional label only gives the value of sodium (which is the part of salt associated with health risks) multiply that amount by two and a half to get the salt content, eg: 0.5g sodium x 2.5 = 1.25g salt.

Try the following:

- Cut back on processed foods, which account for 70 per cent of our salt intake.
- Flavour foods with herbs and spices instead of salt.
- Read food labels to choose 'low salt' and 'reduced salt' options.

Avoid diabetic foods

Foods labelled 'diabetic' or 'suitable for diabetics' are usually snacks and sweets that are high in fats and calories. These don't have special benefits for people with diabetes and are not recommended. They are often expensive and may lead to a stomach upset if you eat too much.

If you fancy a treat once in a while have a small amount of an ordinary treat.

Drink sensibly

If you drink alcohol, stick to the recommended daily alcohol limit, which is 2–3 units for women and 3–4 units for men.

Remember:

- 1 unit is a single measure (25ml) of spirits, ½ pint (284ml) of lager, beer or cider or ½ (175ml) glass of wine.
- Alcohol is high in calories. To lose weight, consider cutting back.
- Never drink on an empty stomach.

Shop clever

So, you now know the basics, but putting it all into practice can seem daunting and a little mind boggling. Try not to worry – all things new can seem hard when you first start out and something that has been so routine for so long like shopping, preparing food and eating may seem onerous. By following these tips you should find things easier.

Planning ahead

What I have always found is that a little planning makes the whole thing from shopping to cooking so much easier and cheaper too. Making detailed shopping lists helps prevent impulse buying and picking up extras as you are not sure what you are cooking and stops you throwing as much away that wasn't used or needed.

- Write down a weekly menu plan, from packed lunches to snacks and main meals. Obviously if your weekly plans change slightly don't worry just re-jig the menu or make and freeze a dish for another day and carry on!
- When you are planning, try to think about how you may use leftovers or excess ingredients another day. For example, if you are having a roast chicken one day then you could make a delicious stock with the carcass then together with any leftover meat they could both be used in a tasty risotto the next day, along with some added veggies.
- Also if you have the oven on for some jacket potatoes, could you prepare a casserole for the next day at the same time? Where appropriate could you double up on recipes so you can pop half in the freezer for another day?
- Keep your shopping lists from week to week this way you can use them again making adjustments where necessary. If you are shopping online you can often refer to previous shops you have made and quickly add things to your basket from these.

- Try to make the most of offers, freeze extra portions or even shop with a friend and do some swaps on your bargains!
- Make the most of seasonal ingredients – not only are they cheaper when in season they often have a far better flavour. Also look out for locally produced goods to keep down those food miles! Take some time to look around your local farmers markets for really good quality, honest fresh food – you'll be amazed how good it tastes.

Look at the label

You have read all the advice, made your shopping list so don't let panic set in once you start looking at the labels. Labels on foods and drinks give essential information, like the ingredients in the product as well as the nutrients (such as fats, calories, sugars and salt) and how much they contribute to what you're eating each day.

On the back

'Back of pack' labelling is compulsory and gives detailed information about the ingredients, nutritional composition and known allergens. The ingredients are listed in order, starting with the highest-quantity ingredient first, down to the lowest-quantity ingredient last. So if you see sugar appear in the first three ingredients, that food is likely to be high in sugar.

On the front

The colour-coded labelling (like a traffic light) on the front of the pack, while still voluntary, has been around for a while now. It's an easy way to check at a glance how healthy a food or drink is, based on how much fat, saturated fat, sugars and salt it contains. These amounts are colour coded to show whether a particular nutrient is low (green), medium (amber) or high (red). Try to choose foods with more greens and few ambers. Limit foods with many reds; only have these occasionally and in smaller quantities.

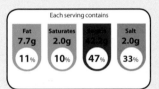 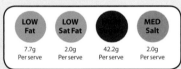

If the traffic lights aren't available, check the 'per 100g' column on the back of pack nutritional label to compare similar products.

Nutritional claims

Nutritional claims, such as fat free or low fat, can be confusing. Here's the difference:

- Fat free: has to have no fat, but check the ingredients list for free (added) sugar, which is often used to replace the fat.
- Sugar free: the product doesn't contain sugar. Check the ingredients list to see what the sugar has been replaced with.
- No added sugar: although no sugar is added, there may be naturally occurring sugar in the food.

- Low fat: the product has 3g or less of fat per 100g.
- Low sugar: has less than 5g of sugar per 100g.
- Reduced fat or sugar: contains 30 per cent less fat or sugar than the standard version of the product. This doesn't necessarily mean it's healthy and in some cases the reduced-fat version of, say, crisps can contain the same amount of calories and fat as the standard version of another brand.

Adapting your own recipes

Being diagnosed with diabetes doesn't mean that you have to learn a whole new way of cooking or banish all your favourite recipes. With a little modification most recipes can be made healthier and more suited to someone with diabetes, and you won't need to cook separate dishes for the rest of the family either. You can modify your usual recipes by:

- Reducing the amount of fat and type of fat you use.
- Cutting down on the salt.
- Cut down on the amount of sugar they contain – try replacing some sugar with dried fruit in baking.
- Increasing the amount of fibre by using more pulses, fruits and vegetables and wholegrain and wholemeal ingredients.

Make your store-cupboard and fridge work for you

Having a well and imaginatively stocked kitchen cupboard and fridge, makes life in the kitchen so much easier. Add a few things each time you do a shop then you should never be stuck for something to cook. Some of the recipes in this book use ingredients you may not have heard of or have to hand. Take a look around the larger supermarkets who have fantastic selections of weird and wonderful ingredients from all around the world. Alternatively, visit specialist shops – it really is worth making the effort as it makes the end dishes superb.

Rice

Different types of rice are suited for different dishes.

- Short-grain rice such as arborio or risotto rice and paella rice. Giving risotto rice a stir during cooking releases some of the starch and creates a fabulous creamy dish. The Japanese use short-grain rice which when cooked becomes sticky and this is great for sushi and other dishes.
- Long-grain rice – the best is probably basmati, giving fluffy individual grains when cooked. Brown basmati is delicious and is higher in fibre.
- Wild rice (which is actually a grain) gives a delicious nutty texture and taste to dishes and is great in salads too.

Pasta

Different shapes are suited to different dishes and sauces.

- The best pasta is made from durum wheat. Buy the shapes you like or those specified in a recipe. I find if you have lots of different types of pasta in the cupboard you seem to end up with lots of bags with not quite enough for a serving and each with slightly different cooking times!

Noodles

- Rice and egg noodles are quick and easy to prepare – an important player in Asian cuisine.
- Udon noodles are a must for Japanese cookery.

Pulses

- Beans and lentils are a great addition to stews and salads. Dried or tinned are great but obviously for convenience tinned are much quicker.
- Lentils don't require pre-soaking so are quick and easy. Puy lentils are wonderful with a deep earthy flavour and nutty texture and are wonderful in salads and with grilled meat or fish.

Oily fish

- Tinned fish in spring water or oil – great for a quick lunch with salad and bread.
- Anchovies can be very salty, but a little can add great depth of flavour to dishes, especially pasta sauces.

Sauces

- Fish sauce (nam pla) – an essential in Thai and Vietnamese cooking. It is very salty so you only need a little.
- Soy sauce and Worcestershire sauce – great for adding flavour. Again, they are quite salty so only use a little or use a lower salt version.

- Ketjap manis – an Indonesian thick, sweet soy sauce. It can be used as a dip, and also as a substitute for dark soy sauce in recipes.

Grains
- Bulgar – a staple of the middle east. Once the grains are soaked and softened they are a wonderful addition to salads and as an accompaniment to main dishes.
- Couscous – an essential in Moroccan and north African cuisine, simple to prepare and a must with tagines to soak up those fragrant juices
- Polenta (cornmeal) – a staple in the Italian kitchen it can either be served served hot – known as wet polenta – or left to cool and set in a dish and then cut into squares or slices which are fried or grilled to give a light crust.

Herbs and spices
Buy in small quantities if you don't use them that often as they don't keep their freshness once opened.

Fab fridge
Light crème fraiche – a great standby for sweet or savoury dishes, also it doesn't split on heating so perfect for sauces.

Parmesan – a little goes a long way as it has such a good strong flavour.

Cottage cheese – virtually fat free, is great mixed with other ingredients like tuna and onion, or a little pesto and grilled bacon for a super healthy lunch on a sandwich or on a jacket potato.

Eggs – always a great standby for omelettes or scrambled eggs – a meal in moments.

And from the freezer …
Keep a few frozen veggies on standby for those days when the fridge is bare or you are feeling lazy. Frozen berries too for super smoothies and instant puddings.

Diets from around the world
Within each country and continent there are a huge range of cultures and traditions when it comes to food and its relationship within society. It is fascinating to see how different countries embrace their recipes passed down from generation to generation, and to see how these recipes are interpreted across the globe. But with time at an all time premium, many traditions are being eroded by the arrival of ready-made foods and takeaways which potentially can be much less healthy for you.

India
Spices in all their glory and variety form an intrinsic part of cooking and life itself. Indians take their food very seriously. Cooking is considered an art and mothers usually begin to teach their daughters and pass down family recipes from an early age. Mealtimes are important occasions for family to get together. Most meals comprise of several dishes ranging from staples like rice and breads to meat and vegetables and rounded off with a dessert. In a lot of Indian homes, foods are made from scratch with fresh ingredients. This is changing in bigger cities where people have increasingly hectic lives and ready made ingredients are more readily used. The different regions of India have varying dishes which use the staples and

produce that their particular climate and terrain determine.

In the north of India where summers are hot and winters cold there is an abundance of fruit and vegetables that are used in a huge array of vegetarian dishes. North Indian curries tend to be quite thick and creamy and are usually served with the preferred breads like naan, parathas and kulchas. Rice is popular in dishes like pilafs and biryanis.

Eastern India is the biggest rice-growing region due to the fact that it has a huge annual rainfall, so most dishes are based around rice, and dishes are kept simple with fish being used on the coast and pork more inland. The people from Eastern India love their sweet foods and desserts!

The folk from Southern India have a love of hot spicy dishes based on rice.

Over to the west a Thaali or large plate of mixed foods is usually served with rices, breads, meat and vegetable dishes and usually something sweet too! Again coastal areas use an abundance of the wonderful fresh fish and seafood on offer where inland the style is a little more frugal.

Indian food at home

Whether you are eating out or you are cooking at home there are a few tips you should bear in mind to keep the fat and calories down. Indian food is renowned for its use of ghee (clarified butter) which is high in fat and saturates so use just a little oil instead. If you are dining out you could ask them to use less or just opt for healthier dishes like tandoori (cooked in a clay oven), tikka or grilled kebab dishes. Choose plain rice as pilau rice is fried in oil. Also ask for your naan plain before it is brushed with ghee.

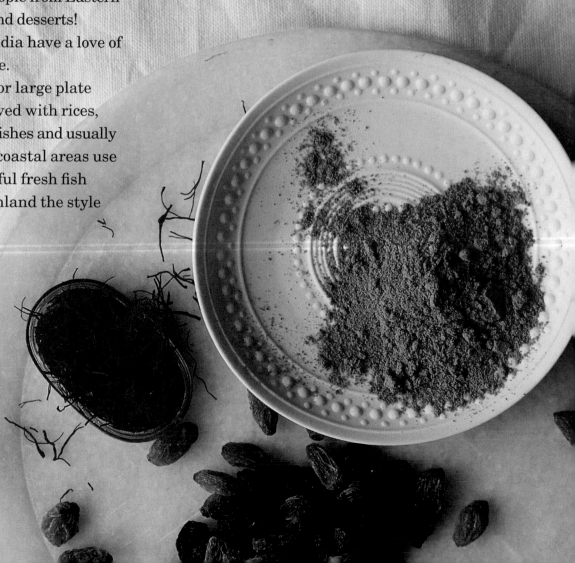

Far Eastern diets

The cooking of Japan, Korea, China and Vietnam are among the most exotic in the world. Looking around our towns and cities we can see a huge number of restaurants offering these foods showing how popular this way of cooking has become.

In China there are many styles of cooking but the majority use a simple base of flavourings like, ginger, garlic and spring onions and soy sauce. Northern China is a great producer of wheat so many meals are based on noodles. To the East rice is more plentiful and more widely used. Onto Southern China where seafood is plentiful and used in many fabulous dishes, including many steamed delicacies.

Think of Japanese food and you probably think of sushi, rice and a filling wrapped in wafer-thin pieces of seaweed – a really healthy dish as it is almost fat free. But there are a myriad of other techniques and traditions using many ingredients unfamiliar to most of us. Soy beans, made into tofu, miso and soy sauce are main players in Japanese cuisine. It is thought that Japanese fondness for soya products explains why they have much lower risk of heart disease and cancer than other countries. Rice and noodles are the main staples. Meals generally consist of a variety of dishes with meat each prepared in a different way from raw, grilled, steamed or deep fried. These dishes are served with rice (or noodles), a light soup and pickles. While rice is the staple food, several kinds of noodles (udon, soba and ramen) are cheap and very popular for light meals.

As an island nation, the Japanese take great pride in their seafood. A wide variety of fish, squid, octopus, eel, and shellfish appear in all kinds of dishes from sushi to tempura.

Tips for healthier Far Eastern foods at home

The Chinese use so many different cooking techniques from baking, stewing and braising to steaming and poaching, some of which are obviously very healthy as they use little or no fat. Stir-frying is what many of us think about when we think of Chinese food and this is a great way to cook healthily. Heat a wok with a little oil until smoking then quickly add your finely prepared ingredients and cook for a few minutes and then flavour. Don't be tempted to add more oil – if it is looking a little dry add a little stock or flavourings instead. If eating out opt for steamed dishes with steamed rice instead of fried ones.

The Americas

America is a true melting pot of food cultures. The traditional good basic native American foods are now heavily influenced by Italian, Mexican and Chinese which have so ingrained in the diet.

Immigrants from Europe stamped their mark on much of North America, each wave of new arrivals making recipes from their native countries, using the ingredients they found available.

Further South, food becomes more soulful – a wonderful blend of native Indian, European, Caribbean and African cultures with such dishes as jambalayas epitomising great American recipes.

Cooking the American way at home

South American foods from countries like Mexico, Peru and Brazil are dominated by spice and, in particular chilli, which seems to appear at the table at every meal in one form or another. The main staples of rice and beans are also a common thread that runs through this vast land.

Think of American food however, and I am sure most of us would conjure up visions of burger and chips. If you are making this at home use these tips to keep things healthy. Grill or barbecue your burger instead of frying, allowing the fat to drip away during cooking. Try not to add cheese and sauces as this can pile on the calories too. Fill the bun with plenty of salad and if you really must have chips go for oven baked ones or make your own thick cut chips, brush with a little oil and bake until crisp.

Beware if you have a large burger and regular fries at 'you know where', – you could tip the balance and be consuming a whopping 700 plus calories and over 40g fat!

Down Under

In the past 30 years or so Australian and New Zealand cooking and cuisine has exploded from good basic and staple foods to the ultra modern style it is today and to what is referred to as 'Pacific Rim'. Influences are gleaned from all over the world, but it is Thailand, Malaysia, Indonesia and Japan where it draws most of its ideas. Adding spice and flavourings to great home-produced seafood and meats and adding twists on recipes from home and southern Europe is its mainstay.

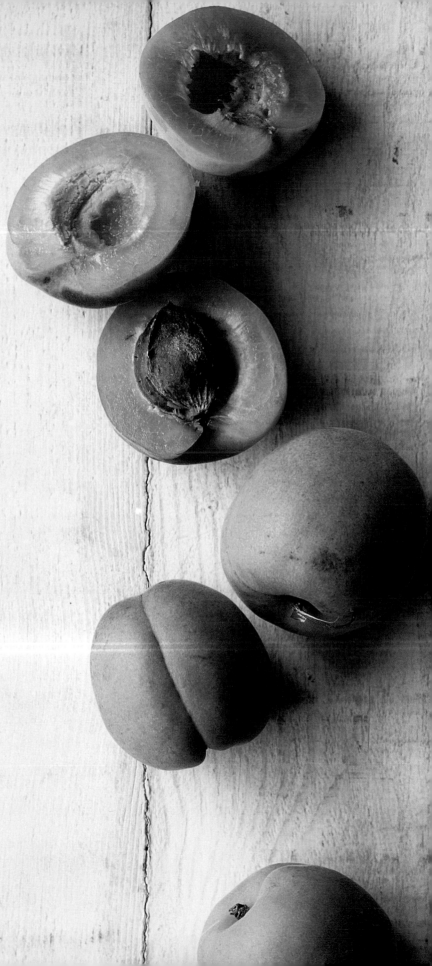

Middle East

Morocco evokes thoughts of spices and plentiful fruits, vegetables, dried fruits and nuts. Fragrant tagines with couscous is the North African staple.

Further on into Egypt there is less use of fruits and vegetables but a wider use of pulses and salads and bread becoming a main staple mainly in the form of pitta. On to Turkey where the fertile land provides an abundance of fresh fruit and vegetables and where meals take the form of meze or mixed plates with lots of different salads purées and breads to whet the appetite.

Magical Mediterranean

So many countries constitute the Mediterranean that there is no single country's diet to follow, it is really just using the common characteristics and putting them into practise.

It has been scientifically proven that the Mediterranean diet offers many healthy benefits, including helping to protect against arthritis, obesity, diabetes, asthma and cardiovascular disease.

The Mediterranean diet prides itself on simplicity and freshness. It is not all about superfoods, it is about combining many wonderful foods for a long-term overall health benefit.

There is an abundance and huge array of pulses to even out blood glucose levels. Fresh fruit and vegetables and salads, which contain many health-giving properties including antioxidants which are found in vitamins A, C and E, lycopene and beta carotene. Antioxidants are chemical compounds that can bind to free oxygen radicals which are produced naturally in the body, and preventing these radicals from damaging healthy cells.

Most dishes use onions and garlic and this may help to thin the blood and in turn reduce blood pressure and fight infections.

Fish and seafood are plentiful and are eaten several times a week. It is the good oils (omega-3) in the oily fish combined with the fact that the diet is low in red meat and dairy products which helps to reduce the incidence of heart disease.

Probably the biggest difference between the Mediterranean diet and that of the rest of the world is the source of fat. Roughly 40 per cent of the daily calorie intake in the Mediterranean comes from fat but it is mainly from plant sources such as avocados and of course olive oil. It is these mono-unsaturated oils that lower bad cholesterol, lower blood pressure, contain antioxidants to help fight cancer and protect against ulcers.

Lets not forget that the people of the Med know how to enjoy a glass of red wine. Raising a glass is not only enjoyable but by stroke of luck also has hidden benefits. Apart from the obvious relaxing and de-stressing qualities we all know the odd drink can give, red wine aids digestion and it contains the antioxidant flavonoid which has an anti-clotting effect and may prevent the oxidation of LDL cholesterol in the blood. One small glass of wine a day can have significant health benefits. But remember drink alcohol in moderation!

Top Mediterranean tips for you at home

- Use tomatoes where you can, in pasta sauces on homemade pizzas, fresh in salads, anyway you can to boost your antioxidant intake.
- Use olive oil in cooking or in dressings.
- Include pasta, wholegrains and pulses where you can on a daily basis – try replacing some red meat in dishes with pulses for less saturated fat and lower GI too!
- Aim for more oily fish in the diet in place of meat.
- Use fresh herbs for flavour instead of salt.

All the information in this book is general. Before undertaking any lifestyle and dietary changes it important that you liaise with your local diabetes team who will give you specific advice tailored to your needs.

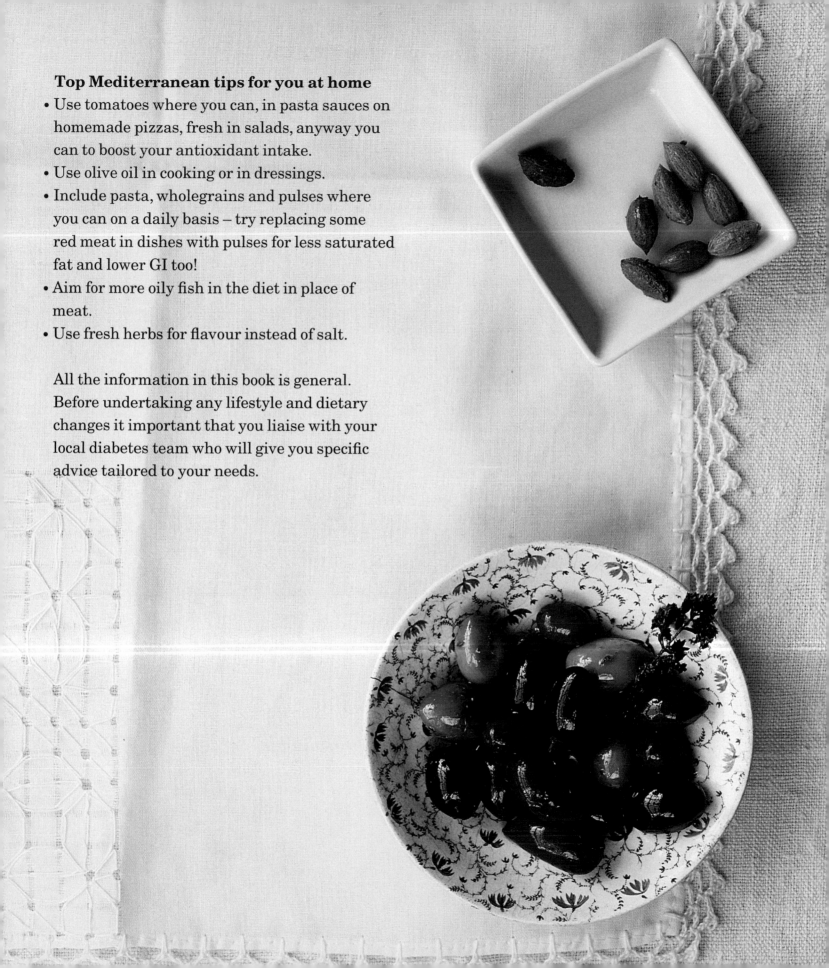

nd Herbs An Omelette with a Touch of India French Toast w
aquet – Catalan Tomato Bread Seeded Fig and Walnut Loa
idge with Oat Bran, Honey and Sunflower Seeds Red and Br
Asparagus and Herbs An Omelette with a Touch of India Fre
mb Tomaquet – Catalan Tomato Bread Seeded Fig and Wal
erry Porridge with Oat Bran, Honey and Sunflower Seeds Re
Asparagus and Herbs An Omelette with a Touch of India Fre
mb Tomaquet – Catalan Tomato Bread Seeded Fig and Wal
erry Porridge with Oat Bran, Honey and Sunflower Seeds Re
Asparagus and Herbs An Omelette with a Touch of India Fre

Breakfasts and breads

mb Tomaquet – Catalan Tomato Bread Seeded Fig and Wal
erry Porridge with Oat Bran, Honey and Sunflower Seeds Re
with Oat Bran, Honey and Sunflower Seeds Red and Brown B
nd Herbs An Omelette with a Touch of India French Toast wi
aquet – Catalan Tomato Bread Seeded Fig and Walnut Loaf
idge with Oat Bran, Honey and Sunflower Seeds Red and Br
Asparagus and Herbs An Omelette with a Touch of India Fre
mb Tomaquet – Catalan Tomato Bread Seeded Fig and Wal
erry Porridge with Oat Bran, Honey and Sunflower Seeds Re
Asparagus and Herbs An Omelette with a Touch of India Fre

Fruity Fresh Soft-Style Muesli

The Swiss tend to soak their muesli the night before and pop it in the fridge, ready for the morning. Are you that organised? If so, this one's for you.

Serves 2
25g rolled oats
25g toasted wheat flakes
25g bran flakes
25g mixed seeds (linseed, sunflower, pumpkin)
25g dried blueberries
1 dessert apple (Cox's Orange Pippin, Braeburn)
25g grated carrot
2 teaspoons cider vinegar 150ml unsweetened apple juice
6 tablespoons low-fat natural yogurt

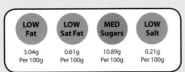

LOW Fat	LOW Sat Fat	MED Sugars	LOW Salt
3.04g Per 100g	0.61g Per 100g	10.89g Per 100g	0.21g Per 100g

1 In a bowl combine the rolled oats, wheat and bran flakes, seeds and dried blueberries.

2 Grate the apple, unpeeled, into the bowl. Mix in the grated carrot and the cider vinegar (this prevents the apple from browning).

3 Beat together the apple juice and yogurt and mix well with the muesli and apple mixture. The muesli is now ready ... for the morning. Cover and refrigerate until then.

Amount per portion (for 2)
Energy 305 kcals, Protein 9.5g, Fat 7.5g, Saturated fat 1.5g, Carbohydrate 53.0g, Total sugars 26.9g, Salt 0.53g, Sodium 209mg

Amount per portion (for 3)
Energy 203 kcals, Protein 6.4g, Fat 5.0g, Saturated fat 1.0g, Carbohydrate 35.3g, Total sugars 17.9g, Salt 0.35g, Sodium 139mg

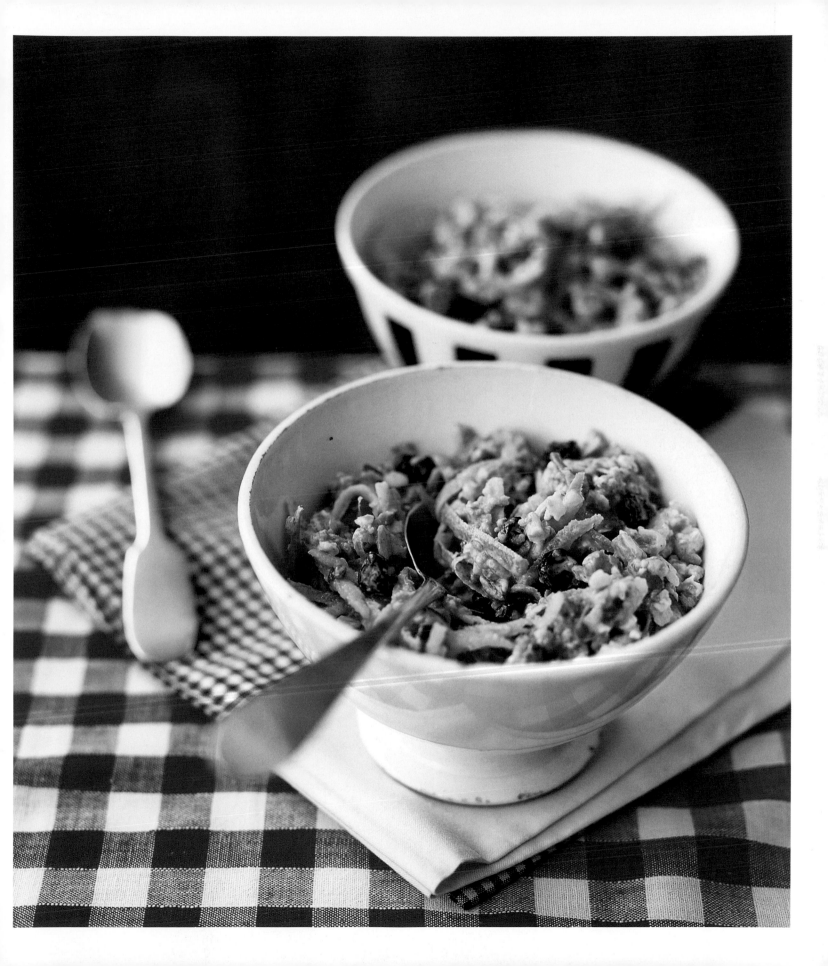

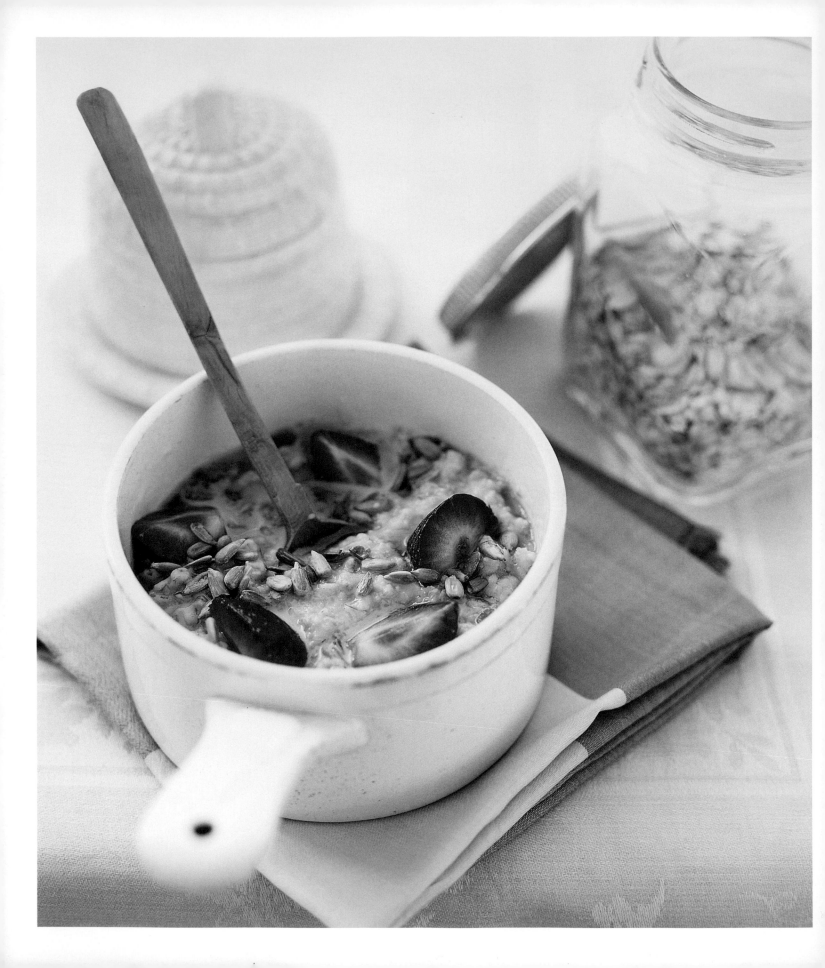

Strawberry Porridge with Oat Bran, Honey and Sunflower Seeds

Porridge is the perfect low GI breakfast food, but let's not get too frugal – add some fruit and seeds for extra pleasure.

Serves 2
100g whole rolled oats
2 tablespoons oat bran
2 tablespoons sunflower seeds, toasted
1 tablespoon honey
100g strawberries, hulled and roughly chopped
3–4 tablespoons semi-skimmed milk

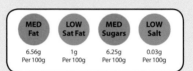

MED Fat	LOW Sat Fat	MED Sugars	LOW Salt
6.56g Per 100g	1g Per 100g	6.25g Per 100g	0.03g Per 100g

1 Put the oats and oat bran in a small saucepan with 500ml of cold water. Bring to a simmer then simmer for 5 minutes, stirring occasionally, until thickened. Add a little more water if you prefer a runnier porridge.

2 Divide the porridge between two individual bowls, sprinkle with the sunflower seeds and drizzle with honey. Top with the strawberries and milk and serve.

Variation You can vary the berries to suit your taste.

Amount per portion
Energy 344 kcals, Protein 14.0g, Fat 10.5g, Saturated fat 1.6g, Carbohydrate 51.5g, Total sugars 10.1g, Salt 0.05g, Sodium 19mg

LEFT Strawberry Porridge with Oat Bran, Honey and Sunflower Seeds

Scrambled Eggs on Grilled Field Mushrooms

Taking breakfast just that little bit further, a lovely weekend dish. Serve with a slice of toast.

Serves 2

2 large field mushrooms,
    85–100g each, wiped clean
spray olive oil
freshly ground white pepper
½ teaspoon chopped fresh thyme leaves
4 eggs, lightly beaten
½ teaspoon chopped fresh tarragon
1 teaspoon chopped fresh parsley
1 teaspoon chopped fresh chives
15g monounsaturated spread

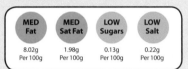

MED Fat	MED Sat Fat	LOW Sugars	LOW Salt
8.02g Per 100g	1.98g Per 100g	0.13g Per 100g	0.22g Per 100g

1 Preheat the grill to high. Spray the mushrooms on both sides with a little oil, season generously with pepper and sprinkle with thyme. Put the mushrooms in the grill pan and add 1 tablespoon of water. Cook under the grill for about 10 minutes until tender, turning once.

2 Meanwhile, combine the eggs with the tarragon, parsley and chives and season with pepper. Some 3 minutes before the mushrooms are ready, gently heat a non-stick saucepan or frying pan and melt the monounsaturated spread. Add the eggs, stir for 30 seconds then draw the sides of the egg mixture to the centre, creating lumpy curds. Cook until done to your liking.

3 Set the mushrooms on to two plates, then spoon the scrambled eggs over the top and serve immediately.

Tips If you have any leftover tarragon, immerse it in a bottle of white wine vinegar or cider vinegar for a delicious splash over grilled fish and chicken, or a soup.

Some people prefer scrambled eggs French style, very smooth with no lumps – very much like baby food – but if you're one of those people, use a whisk instead of a spoon when cooking.

Amount per portion
Energy 235 kcals, Protein 17.0g, Fat 19.0g, Saturated fat 4.7g, Carbohydrate 1.0g, Total sugars 0.3g, Salt 0.53g, Sodium 209mg

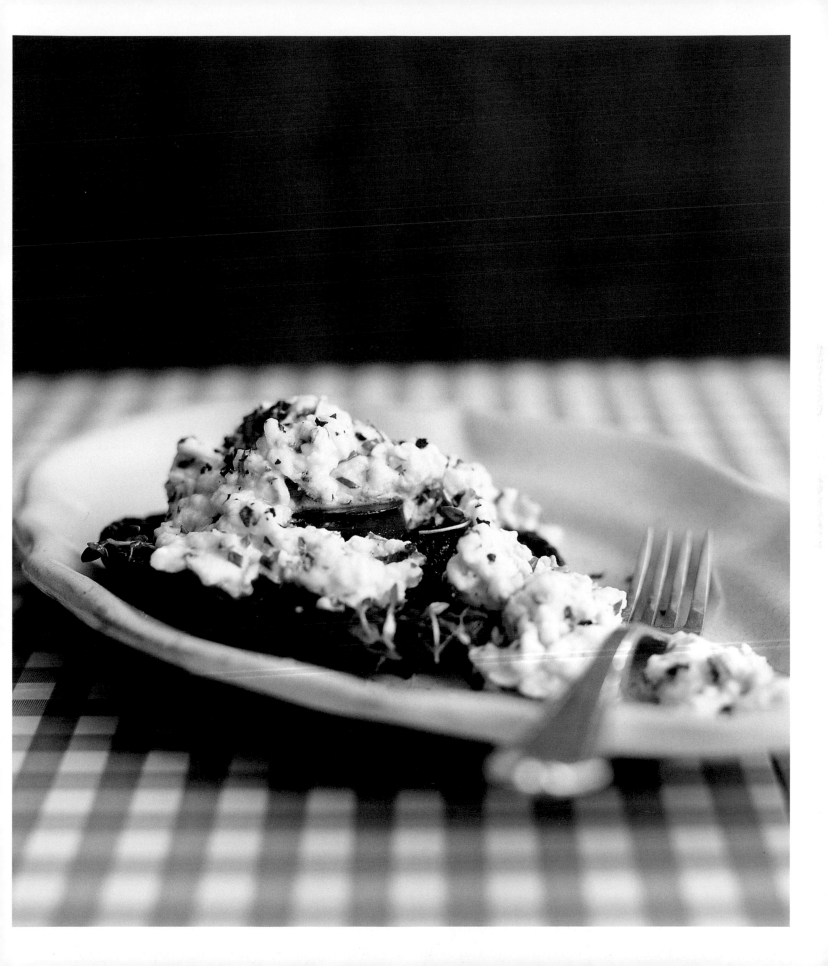

Egg White Omelette with Asparagus and Herbs

Egg-white omelettes are very popular in the USA.

Serves 2

4 egg whites (keep the yolks for
 another use)
1 tablespoon finely chopped fresh mixed
 herbs (chives, tarragon, chervil)
15g monounsaturated spread
8 asparagus spears, cooked, cut into
 2.5cm pieces and kept warm
2 slices wholegrain bread, toasted
cherry tomatoes, halved, to serve
salt and freshly ground black pepper

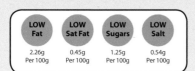

LOW Fat	LOW Sat Fat	LOW Sugars	LOW Salt
2.26g Per 100g	0.45g Per 100g	1.25g Per 100g	0.54g Per 100g

1 Whisk the egg whites with a fork and add the herbs, a pinch of salt and some pepper.

2 Melt half the monounsaturated spread in a small non-stick omelette pan over a medium heat. Pour half the egg white into the pan and with a fork quickly pull the edges to the centre, so the omelette cooks evenly. When the omelette is cooked but still soft, place half the warm asparagus in the centre and leave on the heat for a second longer. Then fold the omelette in half, giving the pan a light tap to loosen the omelette.

3 Slide the omelette out on to a slice of warm toast and serve with halved cherry tomatoes. Melt the remaining spread and cook the remaining egg white in the same way.

Amount per portion

Energy 196 kcals, Protein 14.0g, Fat 6.0g, Saturated fat 1.2g, Carbohydrate 22.0g, Total sugars 3.3g, Salt 1.42g, Sodium 559mg

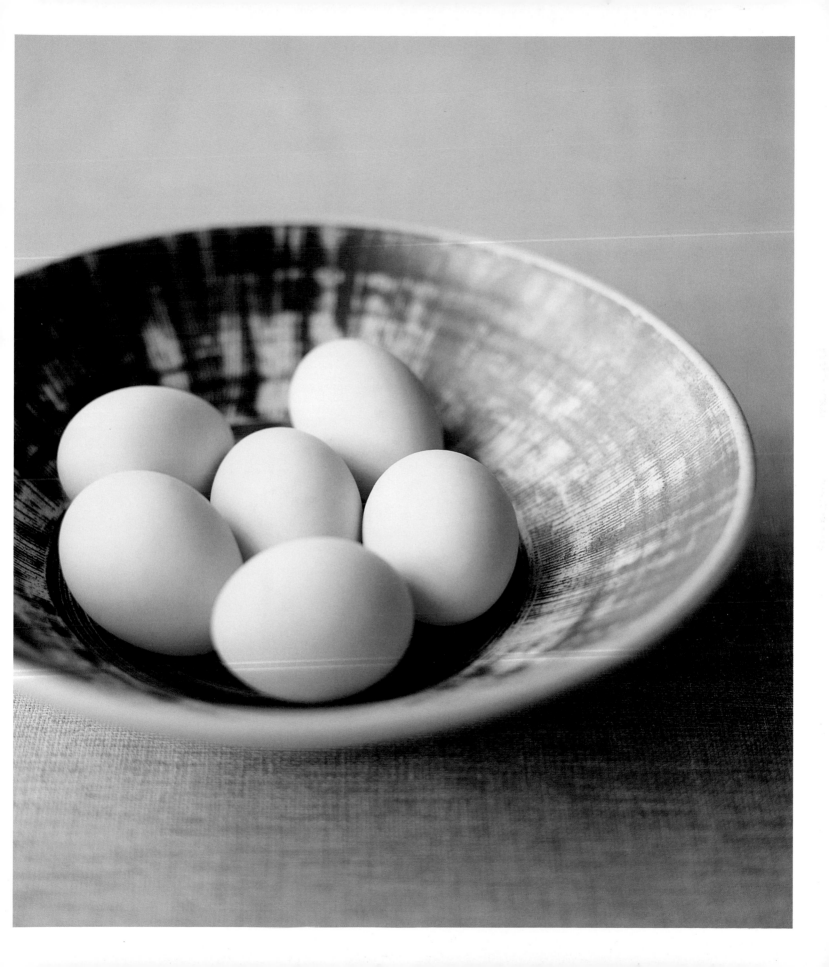

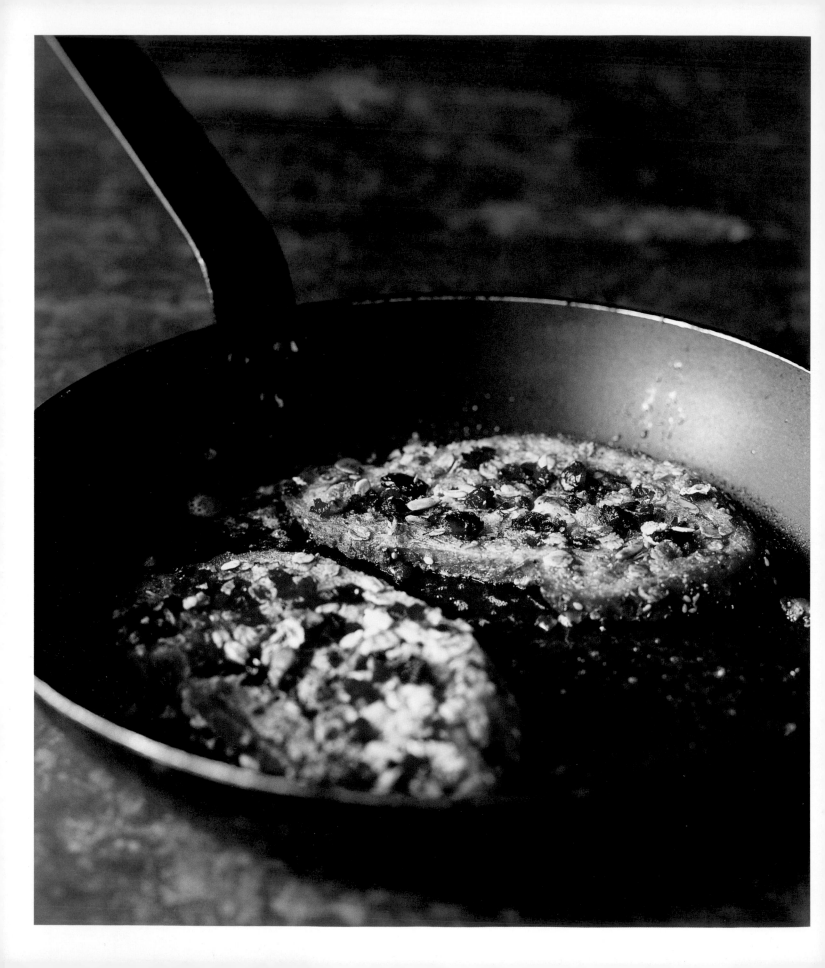

French Toast with a Crunch

Everyone loves eggy bread or French toast, and by using a multigrain bread and muesli you can make it extra healthy as you are lowering the GI.

Serves 4
1 egg white, lightly beaten
75ml skimmed milk
juice and grated zest of 1 lime
1 teaspoon sugar or low-calorie
    granulated sweetener
50g unsweetened muesli
25g dried cranberries,
    finely chopped
4 slices multigrain bread,
    each slice halved
1 tablespoon olive oil

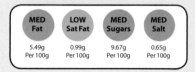

Note: this traffic light analysis is using sweetener instead of sugar

1 In a bowl whisk together the egg white, milk, lime juice and zest and sweetener. Place the muesli and cranberries on a flat plate and stir to mix well. Dip each piece of bread into the liquid and then into the muesli.

2 Heat half the oil in a large frying pan over a medium to low heat. Place half the bread in the pan and gently cook for 3 minutes each side. Heat the remaining oil and cook the remaining bread in the same way.

Variations Have some fun and instead of cranberries use any other dried berries, such as blueberries or raspberries, or bing cherries. You can also substitute orange for the lime.

Amount per portion
Energy 197 kcals, Protein 7.0g, Fat 5.0g, Saturated fat 0.9g, Carbohydrate 33.0g, Total sugars 8.8g, Salt 0.59g, Sodium 235mg

Spiced Tomatoes on Toast

These spices give fresh tomatoes that extra little kick of flavour, because, let's be honest, unless you grow your own, they can be very bland.

Serves 2
spray olive oil
¼ teaspoon ground coriander
¼ teaspoon fennel seeds
2 spring onions, sliced
¼ teaspoon ground cumin
2 garlic cloves, sliced
½ teaspoon chilli powder
4 medium tomatoes, each cut into
    3 thick slices
2 slices seeded bread, toasted
chopped fresh coriander leaves,
    to garnish

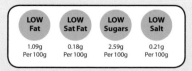

1 Spray a frying pan with oil and place on a medium heat. Add the ground coriander, fennel seeds, spring onions, ground cumin and garlic, and stir-fry until the spices start releasing their fragrant bouquet. Add the chilli powder and the tomatoes, and cook for 3 minutes or until the tomatoes start to soften.

2 With a slotted spoon, arrange the tomato slices on top of the toast, retaining the tomato juices. Garnish the tomatoes with chopped coriander leaves and drizzle with the tomato juices.

Amount per portion
Energy 136 kcals, Protein 5.2g, Fat 2.4g, Saturated fat 0.4g, Carbohydrate 24.9g, Total sugars 5.7g, Salt 0.47g, Sodium 185mg

LEFT French Toast
with a Crunch

A Textured Kedgeree

This colonial dish, invented in India to be eaten by the Brits, makes a great weekend brunch. Here I've made a few add-ons to improve the GI rating and by chance, they also heighten the flavour.

Serves 4

1 teaspoon sunflower oil
1 onion, finely diced
1 red chilli, deseeded and diced
2 teaspoons hot curry paste
275g quick-cook brown rice
2 tomatoes, deseeded and diced
275g hot-smoked salmon, flaked
1 teaspoon ground turmeric
1 tablespoon chopped pistachio nuts
1 tablespoon chopped fresh coriander
1 teaspoon chopped fresh mint
2 teaspoons chilli seeds (spiced seeds)
3 tablespoons 0 per cent fat Greek yogurt
salt and freshly ground black pepper

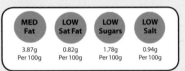

MED Fat	LOW Sat Fat	LOW Sugars	LOW Salt
3.87g Per 100g	0.82g Per 100g	1.78g Per 100g	0.94g Per 100g

1 Heat the oil in a frying pan and over a gentle heat cook the onion, chilli and curry paste for approximately 8 minutes.

2 Meanwhile, in a microwave cook the rice according to the instructions on the packet.

3 Add the cooked rice to the spiced onions in the frying pan. Increase the heat and stir in the tomatoes, salmon, turmeric and pistachios – use a gentle action so as not to pulp the salmon.

4 Add in the remaining ingredients and mix. Season to taste and serve warm.

Amount per portion

Energy 407 kcals, Protein 23.9g, Fat 10.4g, Saturated fat 2.2g, Carbohydrate 58.2g, Total sugars 4.8g, Salt 2.52g, Sodium 994mg

Pa Amb Tomaquet – Catalan Tomato Bread

Tomato bread, served all over Spain, makes a great breakfast or mid-morning snack. This recipe uses seeded bread, to improve the GI rating, but you could go for a rustic country bread instead if you feel it would give a more authentic result.

Serves 2
2 slices seeded bread
1 garlic clove
2 large tomatoes, halved
2 teaspoons extra virgin olive oil
salt and freshly ground pepper

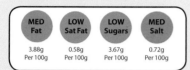

MED Fat	LOW Sat Fat	LOW Sugars	MED Salt
3.88g Per 100g	0.58g Per 100g	3.67g Per 100g	0.72g Per 100g

1 Toast the bread, then rub the garlic all over – the toast's rough surface will act as a grater. Then rub the cut sides of the tomatoes over the toast until you are left with the skin, which you discard. Season to taste then drizzle modestly with the olive oil.

Variations If you fancy a treat, a little scattering of crispy bacon would be nice, or if you're on your best behaviour scatter with a few of your favourite seeds – sunflower, pumpkin, that sort of thing.

Amount per portion
Energy 153 kcals, Protein 4.3g, Fat 5.4g, Saturated fat 0.8g, Carbohydrate 23.2g, Total sugars 5.1g, Salt 1.06g, Sodium 417mg

Seeded Fig and Walnut Loaf

It's a cliché, but you can't beat the smell of freshly baked bread, and you certainly can't beat that touchy-feely experience of hand-crafting loaves. This recipe makes a lovely, dense, crunchy loaf – great for a treat.

Serves 8
170g unbleached white bread flour, plus extra for dusting
60g wholemeal flour
12g fast-acting dried yeast
½ teaspoon salt
1 teaspoon caster sugar
135ml lukewarm water
30g chopped dried figs
30g mixed seeds (sunflower, linseed)
30g chopped walnuts

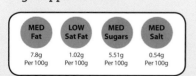

MED Fat	LOW Sat Fat	MED Sugars	MED Salt
7.8g Per 100g	1.02g Per 100g	5.51g Per 100g	0.54g Per 100g

1 Put both flours, the yeast, salt and sugar in the bowl of your mixer or food processor with the dough hook attached. With the machine switched on, slowly add the water and when a dough forms, fold in the fruit, seeds and nuts.
2 Turn out on to a lightly floured work surface, then start kneading and continue for 10 minutes (give yourself a short break from time to time). Shape into a loaf, place on a baking tray, and leave in a warm spot till doubled in size. Meanwhile, preheat the oven to 190°C/375°F/gas mark 5.
3 When the dough has risen, dust the surface of the loaf with a light snowfall of white flour and bake for 35–40 minutes depending on the shape of the loaf; when cooked, the loaf will sound hollow when tapped on the base. Transfer to a rack and leave to cool.

Amount per portion
Energy kcals 154, Protein 5.5g, Fat 4.6g, Saturated fat 0.6g, Carbohydrate 24.3g, Total sugars 3.3g, Salt 0.32g, Sodium 128mg

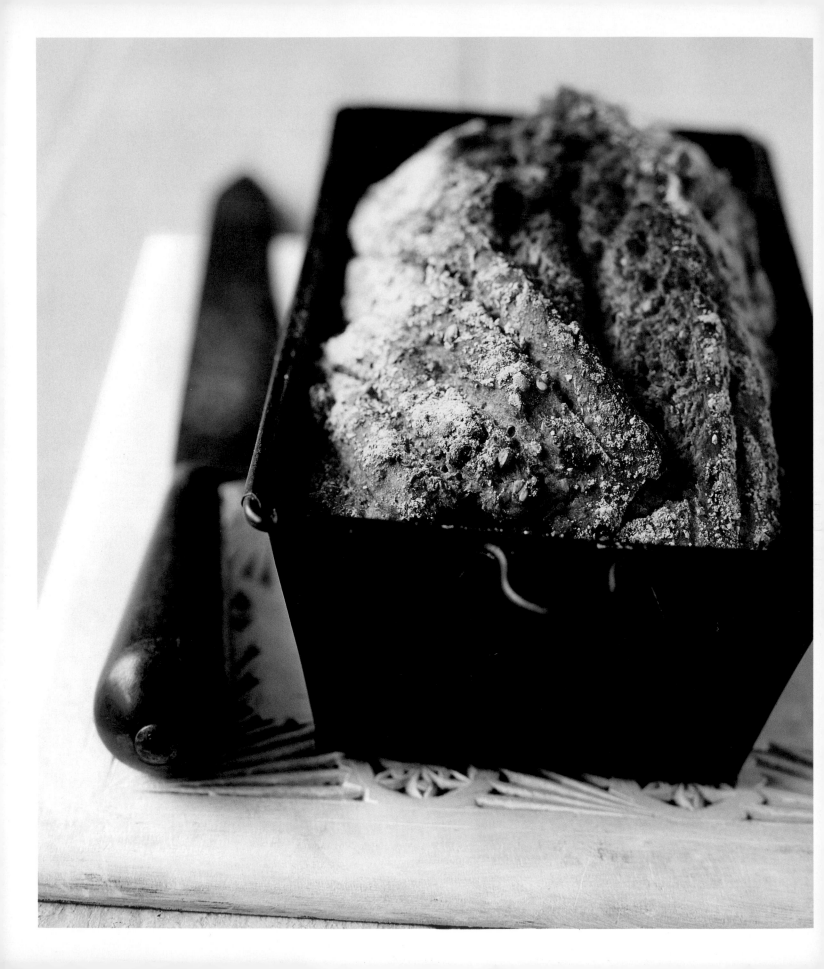

Bake Your Own Seeded Bread

This delicious nutty seeded bread is fantastic – it doesn't need proving so is quick to make, there is no heavy kneading, and it contains loads of slow-release nuts and seeds for lower GI.

Makes 1 small loaf (serves 4)
500g spelt flour
15g fast-acting dried yeast
¼ teaspoon salt
25g chopped walnuts
25g sesame seeds
25g hemp seeds
25g linseed
25g pumpkin seeds
15g dried seaweed, chopped (optional)
500ml warm water

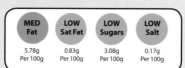

MED Fat	LOW Sat Fat	LOW Sugars	LOW Salt
5.78g Per 100g	0.83g Per 100g	3.08g Per 100g	0.17g Per 100g

1 Preheat the oven to 200°C/400°F/gas mark 6 and lightly grease a 900g loaf tin. Combine all the dry ingredients in a large bowl, then gradually add the water, drawing in the sides of the flour mixture until the dough comes together.

2 Pop the dough into the prepared tin (no, you don't need to let it rise first, that all happens in the oven). Slash the surface and pop in the oven, and bake for 1 hour. The bread will rise nicely and come away from the sides of the tin. The base of the loaf will sound hollow when cooked.

3 Remove the loaf from the tin and set on a rack to cool. Alternatively, if you prefer crisp sides, take the loaf out of its tin and return it to the oven for 6–8 minutes.

Variations Many types of seed are available, you don't have to follow this formula; have a play – you could even add a little dried fruit.

Amount per portion
Energy 573,kcals, Protein 24.2g, Fat 16.7g, Saturated fat 2.4g, Carbohydrate 86.9g, Total sugars 8.9g, Salt 0.49g, Sodium 194mg

Snacks, starters and soups

Spinach and Red Pepper Omelette Roll

This Korean roll is so versatile – it makes a great snack or supper dish, and is also good for breakfast, though it would probably be best to make it ahead of time as it requires some preparation.

Serves 4

225g frozen spinach, defrosted
3 roast peppers from a jar, drained
   and chopped
1 tablespoon sesame oil
1 tablespoon sesame seeds
2 garlic cloves, crushed to a paste
2 mild green chillies, deseeded
   and finely chopped
½ teaspoon chilli powder
2 spring onions, finely chopped
3 tablespoons reduced-salt soy sauce
6 eggs, beaten
1 tablespoon dry sherry
spray oil, for frying
salt and freshly ground black pepper

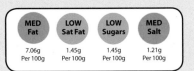

MED Fat	LOW Sat Fat	LOW Sugars	MED Salt
7.06g Per 100g	1.45g Per 100g	1.45g Per 100g	1.21g Per 100g

1 Squeeze excess liquid from the spinach, then chop it. In a bowl, mix it with the roast peppers, sesame oil and seeds, garlic, chilli and chilli powder, spring onions and half the soy sauce. Set aside. Mix together the eggs, remaining soy sauce and sherry, and season to taste with salt and pepper.

2 Heat a non-stick frying pan and spray with a light coating of oil. Spoon or pour in a quarter of the egg mix, immediately tipping the pan so the egg covers the whole of the pan in a thin layer. Cook gently for 1½ minutes until cooked all the way through, then tip it on to a clean work surface or plate. Cook the remaining egg mix in the same manner, in three batches.

3 Spread a quarter of the spinach mixture carefully over one of the 'omelettes' and roll it up into a tight cylinder, then cut it into 2cm lengths. Repeat the process with the other rolls.

Tip The rolls can be eaten either at room temperature or hot – warm them up in the microwave, or wrap them in foil and pop into the oven. For breakfast, serve it on seeded toast, and for a more substantial meal accompany it with new potatoes and a salad.

Amount per portion
Energy 241 kcals, Protein 15.0g, Fat 18.0g, Saturated fat 3.7g, Carbohydrate 5.0g, Total sugars 3.7g, Salt 3.08g, Sodium 1211mg

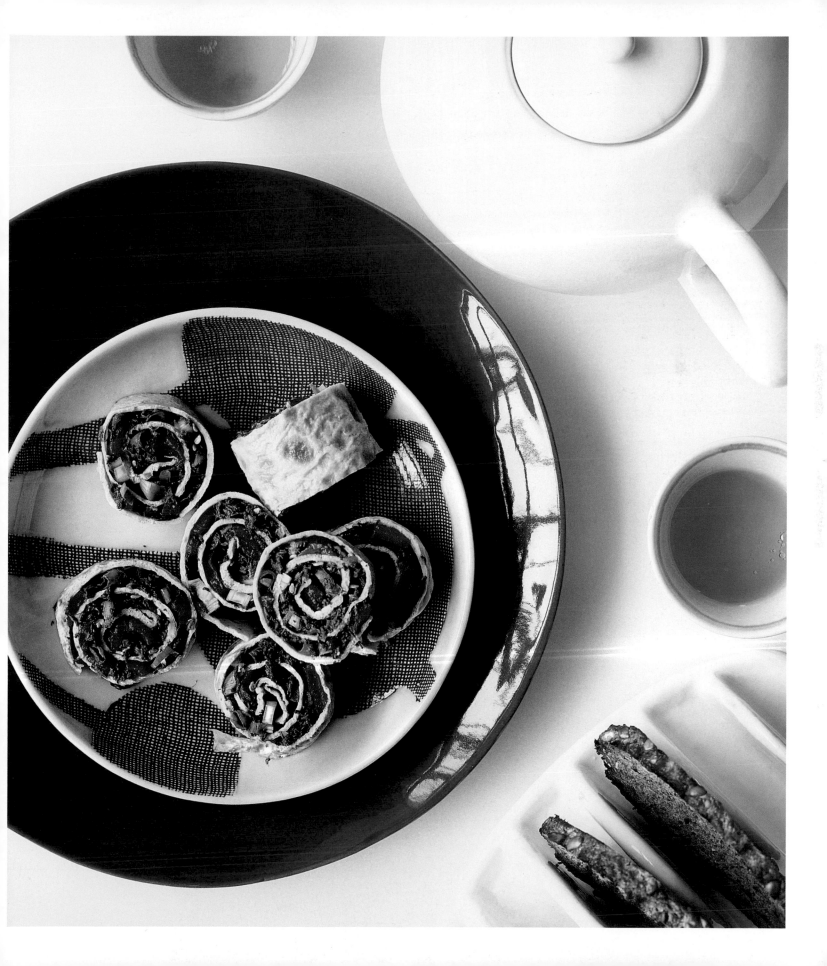

Asparagus with Egg and Cauliflower Sauce

Australians have fab produce and some particularly inventive chefs, such as Bill Granger and Donna Hay. This recipe would be delicious served with toasted wholemeal pitta bread.

Serves 4

110g cauliflower, broken into tiny florets
16 asparagus spears, trimmed
3 eggs
2 anchovy fillets
½ teaspoon chopped fresh rosemary
60ml aged sherry vinegar
60ml extra virgin olive oil
1 teaspoon snipped fresh chives

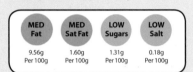

MED Fat	MED Sat Fat	LOW Sugars	LOW Salt
9.56g Per 100g	1.60g Per 100g	1.31g Per 100g	0.18g Per 100g

1 In a large pan of boiling water, cook the cauliflower florets for 3 minutes. Remove the cauliflower with a slotted spoon, cover to keep warm and set aside. Plunge the asparagus into the pan and cook for a few minutes (5–6 minutes for thick spears), then drain and set aside.

2 Bring a smaller pan of water to the boil and cook the eggs for precisely 4 minutes (set the timer). While the eggs are cooking, chop the anchovy together with the rosemary into a cohesive paste, then place in a warm bowl and beat in the vinegar and the olive oil. Set aside.

3 Once the eggs have cooked, and working quickly, lift them out and hold each with a cloth. Break them in half with the back of a spoon or knife, and scoop the contents into the anchovy dressing. Mash together, leaving some texture to the egg white, then fold in the cauliflower.

4 Divide the asparagus between four warmed plates, add the chives to the egg and cauliflower sauce and spoon over the top of the asparagus.

Amount per portion
Energy 229 kcals, Protein 10.1g, Fat 19.7g, Saturated fat 3.3g, Carbohydrate 3.0g, Total sugars 2.7g, Salt 0.38g, Sodium 148mg

Boiled Eggs with Asparagus Soldiers

Boiled eggs are a great fast food, packed with nutrients – a real superfood. Egg and toast soldiers are a firm British favourite, but here they are wonderfully partnered with crunchy new-season asparagus instead. Serve with a slice or two of toast as well if you need extra carbohydrate.

Serves 4
24 thick asparagus spears, trimmed
8 large eggs
50g Dukkah (see page 257)

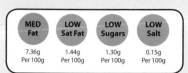

MED Fat	LOW Sat Fat	LOW Sugars	LOW Salt
7.36g Per 100g	1.44g Per 100g	1.30g Per 100g	0.15g Per 100g

1 Bring one large and one medium pan of water to the boil and lightly salt the large pan. Set your timer for 4 minutes 30 seconds, then put the eggs gently into the non-salted water and the asparagus into the salted water. Start the timer.

2 When ready, drain the asparagus and pop the eggs into eggcups, allowing 2 eggs per person. Immediately cut the tops off the shells, revealing runny eggs. Place 6 asparagus beside each pair of eggs, and serve with a little pot of dukkah. Then get the gang to dip the asparagus into the egg yolk then roll it in the dukkah – delish.

Tip It's important not to overcook the asparagus, so that it remains green and crunchy; floppy asparagus makes for a messy, dribbly experience.

Amount per portion
Energy 298 kcals, Protein 22.3g, Fat 20.9g, Saturated fat 4.1g, Carbohydrate 5.5g, Total sugars 3.7g, Salt 0.44g, Sodium 175mg

Spicy Mushrooms on Toast with Asian Salad

Mushrooms on toast are always popular, but sometimes they cry out for a little extra. Here it is.

Serves 2
1 teaspoon sesame oil
1 teaspoon sunflower oil
1 onion, finely diced
1 teaspoon grated fresh ginger
1 garlic clove, finely chopped
1 fresh chilli, deseeded and finely chopped
275g button mushrooms, quartered
150ml vegetable stock
2 tablespoons ketjap manis
    (Indonesian sweet soy sauce)
salt and freshly ground black pepper
2 slices granary bread

For the salad
juice of 1 lime
1 teaspoon sugar
1 teaspoon fish sauce (nam pla)
8 cherry tomatoes, halved
2 spring onions, sliced
1 tablespoon chopped fresh coriander
1 tablespoon chopped fresh mint

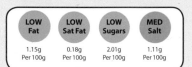

1 Heat the oil over a moderate heat, add the onion, ginger, garlic and chilli and cook until the onion is soft. Increase the heat, add the mushrooms and cook for 5 minutes. Add the stock and ketjap manis and cook for a further 5 minutes. Season to taste.
2 Meanwhile, make the salad. Mix together the lime juice, sweetener and fish sauce, then toss with the rest of the salad ingredients. Toast the bread.
3 With a slotted spoon, lift the mushrooms and place them on the toast. Boil the juices remaining in the pan until no more than 4 tablespoons remain. Pour these juices over the mushrooms and serve with the salad and a slice of lime.

Tip When preparing mushrooms, treat them gently as they are fragile; and unless they are old, they rarely need peeling.

Amount per portion
Energy 184 kcals, Protein 9.0g, Fat 5.0g, Saturated fat 0.8g, Carbohydrate 27.0g, Total sugars 8.7g, Salt 2.43g, Sodium 959mg

Tuna Carpaccio with Cucumber and Yogurt

This is such a lovely healthy starter or light lunch dish but make sure you use sustainable yellow fin tuna, never blue fin.

Serves 4
325g good-quality tuna loin
3 tablespoons 0 per cent fat natural
    Greek yogurt
1 garlic clove, crushed to a paste
    with a little salt
2 teaspoons chopped fresh mint
grated zest and juice of 2 lemons
2 tablespoons extra virgin olive oil
1 European (a small ridge type) cucumber
    or ½ English, cut into 1cm dice
salt and freshly ground black pepper
seeded bread, to serve

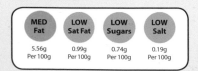

1 Freeze the tuna for 1 hour – this makes it easier to slice it really thinly. While it is in the freezer, mix together the yogurt, garlic and mint. Season with a little salt and black pepper and loosen with a little of the lemon juice.
2 With a sharp knife, cut the fish into very thin slices. Arrange the slices onto individual cold plates, and drizzle each plate with olive oil and the remaining lemon juice. Scatter over the diced cucumber and lemon zest, then dot over the minted yogurt in small puddles. Serve with a seeded bread.

Amount per portion
Energy 173 kcals, Protein 21.0g, Fat 9.0g, Saturated fat 1.6g, Carbohydrate 2.0g, Total sugars 1.2g, Salt 0.75g, Sodium 293mg

RIGHT Spicy Mushrooms on Toast with Asian Salad

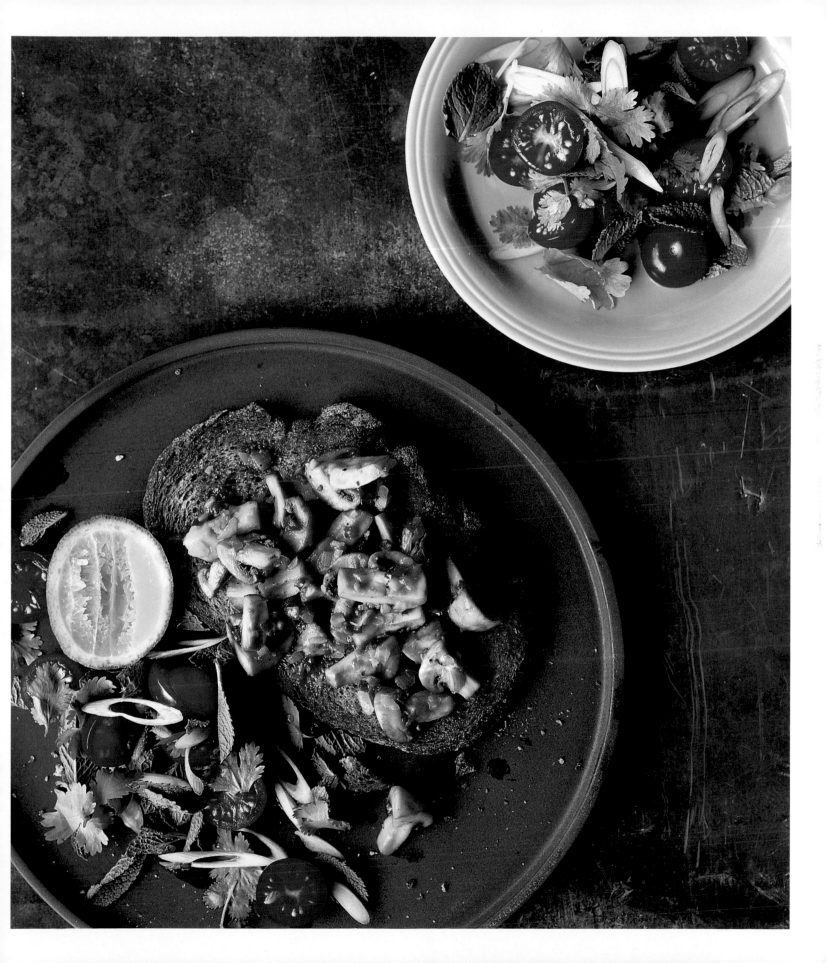

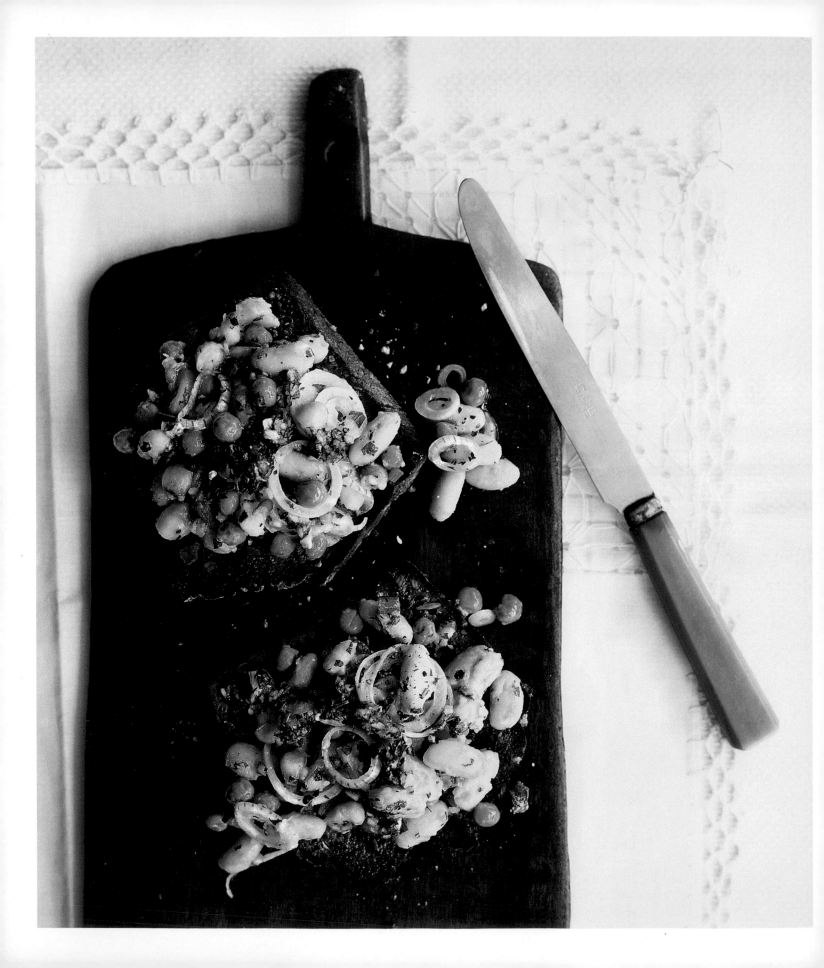

White Bean and Rosemary Bruschetta

There are plenty of times when you need a good comforting carbohydrate meal, and this Italian one ticks all the boxes. Personally, I can't usually be bothered to soak dried beans and then cook them, especially when there are so many different varieties of tinned beans and pulses available and they're all perfectly cooked and ready to use.

Serves 4
4 garlic cloves
½ tablespoon fresh rosemary leaves
1 tablespoon fresh parsley leaves
1 tablespoon extra virgin olive oil
1 x 400g tin cannellini beans, drained
2 spring onions, chopped
3 tablespoons frozen petit pois, defrosted
4 thick slices seeded bread
freshly ground black pepper

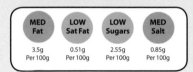

MED Fat	LOW Sat Fat	LOW Sugars	MED Salt
3.5g Per 100g	0.51g Per 100g	2.55g Per 100g	0.85g Per 100g

1 With a mortar and pestle or in a mini food processor, crush or blitz together 3 garlic cloves, the rosemary and the parsley with the olive oil and a splash of water.

2 Take half the garlic-rosemary paste and cook in a non-stick frying pan for 3 minutes over a gentle heat. Add the beans and toss to coat thoroughly, then cook until heated through. With a fork or a potato masher, roughly crush the beans, leaving some whole. Fold in the spring onions and peas.

3 Toast or grill the bread, then rub each slice with the remaining garlic clove. Spread with the bean mash, then top each slice with a little of the remaining garlic-rosemary paste.

Amount per portion
Energy 219 kcals, Protein 9.8g, Fat 4.8g, Saturated fat 0.7g, Carbohydrate 36.3g, Total sugars 3.5g, Salt 1.16g, Sodium 457mg

Moutabel with Chickpeas and Hazelnuts

Moutabel is a bit like that other Middle Eastern aubergine purée, baba ganoush – very moreish, and even more so with my addition of chickpeas and hazelnuts. Serve with vegetable crudités or warm wholemeal pitta bread to scoop up this delicious dip.

Serves 4–6
2 large aubergines
2 garlic cloves
4 tablespoons tahini (sesame paste)
juice of 1 lemon
2 tablespoons 0 per cent fat natural
    Greek yogurt
1 tablespoon extra virgin olive oil
1 x 400g tin chickpeas, drained
50g chopped hazelnuts
freshly ground black pepper

To garnish
2 tablespoons pomegranate seeds
½ teaspoon sweet paprika
chopped fresh parsley

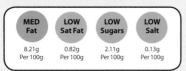

MED Fat	LOW Sat Fat	LOW Sugars	LOW Salt
8.21g Per 100g	0.82g Per 100g	2.11g Per 100g	0.13g Per 100g

1 Preheat the oven to 230°C/450°F/gas mark 8. Set the aubergines on a baking tray and cook for 25 minutes, turning every 5 minutes, until the skin is charred. Transfer the aubergines to a bowl and cover with clingfilm and set aside to cool. When cool enough to handle, peel off the skin under running water.

2 In a food-processor blend together the aubergine flesh and garlic until smooth, then add the tahini, lemon juice, yogurt and olive oil. Pulse briefly to combine. Spoon into a bowl then fold in the chickpeas and hazelnuts, and season with pepper. Serve scattered with pomegranate seeds, paprika and parsley.

Tip For the best flavour, it's important that the aubergines are well charred.

Amount per portion
Energy 317 kcals, Protein 12.0g, Fat 23.0g, Saturated fat 2.3g, Carbohydrate 16.7g, Total sugars 5.9g, Salt 0.37g, Sodium 146mg

Tzatziki

This yogurt and cucumber mixture is a staple of Greek mezes. The various brands available in the shops are usually very high in fat, so why buy it when it is so easy to make?

Serves 4 as part of a meze
1 cucumber, peeled, deseeded and
    grated or diced
1 teaspoon salt
1 tablespoon extra virgin olive oil
2–3 garlic cloves, crushed with a little salt
2 teaspoons white wine vinegar
¼ teaspoon freshly ground black pepper
225g 0 per cent fat natural Greek yogurt
12 mint leaves, chopped
pitta bread, to serve

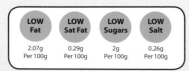

LOW Fat	LOW Sat Fat	LOW Sugars	LOW Salt
2.07g Per 100g	0.29g Per 100g	2g Per 100g	0.26g Per 100g

1 Put the cucumber into a colander, sprinkle the salt over and mix well, then set aside for 30 minutes to drain some of the cucumbers' natural liquid. Rinse and pat dry.

2 Meanwhile, combine the oil with the garlic, vinegar and pepper. Whisk in the yogurt and fold in the cucumber and chopped mint. Taste and adjust the seasoning if liked, and serve with pitta bread.

Tip The easiest way of deseeding a cucumber is to cut it in half lengthways and run a teaspoon down the centre of each half.

Amount per portion
Energy 66 kcals, Protein 6.4g, Fat 2.9g, Saturated fat 0.4g, Carbohydrate 3.9g, Total sugars 2.8g, Salt 0.36g, Sodium 141mg

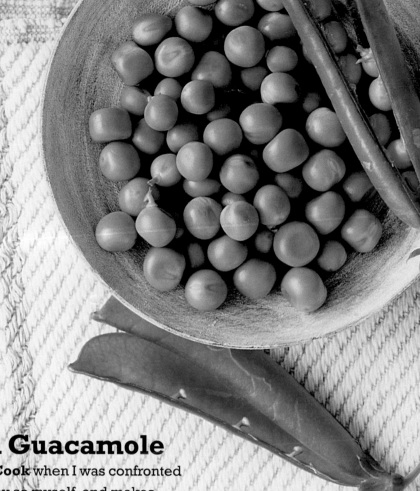

Sweet Pea and White Bean Guacamole

I produced this US-inspired dish on **Ready Steady Cook** when I was confronted with a bag of frozen peas. It's rather good, even if I say so myself, and makes a great dip or accompaniment to a bowl of chilli con carne.

Serves 4
1 tablespoon extra virgin olive oil
2 tablespoons lime juice
2 tablespoons fresh coriander leaves
2 hot red chillies, deseeded and diced
500g cooked frozen peas, drained
½ teaspoon ground cumin
½ teaspoon ground coriander
1 teaspoon salt
½ teaspoon freshly ground black pepper
2 plum tomatoes, deseeded and diced
½ red onion, peeled and finely diced
1 x 400g tin cannellini beans or other white beans, drained and rinsed

1 In a food processor blend together the oil, lime juice, coriander leaves and chillies until reasonably smooth. Add the peas, spices, salt and pepper and blend until smooth (a few lumps may remain).
2 Tip the mixture into a bowl and fold in the tomatoes, onion and beans. Adjust the seasoning to taste.

Variation Fold in 4 tablespoons of 0 per cent fat yogurt along with the beans at the end.

Amount per portion
Energy 196 kcals, Protein 13.2g, Fat 4.9g, Saturated fat 0.4g, Carbohydrate 26.6g, Total sugars 7.2g, Salt 2.21g, Sodium 871mg

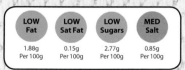

LOW Fat	LOW Sat Fat	LOW Sugars	MED Salt
1.88g Per 100g	0.15g Per 100g	2.77g Per 100g	0.85g Per 100g

Hot Stuffed Vine Leaves

I know these won't be everyone's cup of tea, but there is a certain satisfaction in making your own dolmades and you can make them to your own personal specification.

Serves 4
120g long-grain brown rice
225g lean minced beef or lamb
1 x 200g tin chopped tomatoes
1 small onion, finely chopped
1 teaspoon dried oregano
3 tablespoons finely chopped fresh parsley
3 tablespoons finely chopped celery
1 tablespoon tomato purée
12 preserved vine leaves, drained
2 tomatoes, sliced
2 garlic cloves, sliced
juice of 1 lemon, or more to taste
salt and freshly ground black pepper

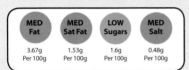

MED Fat	MED Sat Fat	LOW Sugars	MED Salt
3.67g Per 100g	1.53g Per 100g	1.6g Per 100g	0.48g Per 100g

1 Preheat the oven to 180°C/350°F/gas mark 4. Mix together the rice, meat, chopped tomatoes, onion, oregano, parsley, celery, and some salt and pepper. Fold in the tomato purée.

2 Place a vine leaf on a plate, vein-side up. Put a heaped teaspoon of the rice and meat filling in the centre, near the stem edge. Fold the stem end up over the filling, then fold both sides towards the middle and roll up like a small cigar. Don't roll too tightly, as the rice will need room to expand. Repeat the process with the remaining filling and leaves.

3 Line the bottom of an ovenproof dish with a layer of tomato slices (or leftover vine leaves) to prevent the stuffed leaves from sticking to the pan and burning. Pack the stuffed leaves in layers over that, pushing slices of garlic here and there between them. Sprinkle with lemon juice and pour over about 300ml water. Cover with oiled aluminium foil.

4 Cook in the preheated oven for 45 minutes or until tender, adding extra water if necessary. Serve as part of a meze selection.

Tip Vine leaves are usually sold vacuum-packed, but if you can't find them try cabbage leaves or spring greens.

Amount per portion
Energy 264 kcals, Protein 15.1g, Fat 10.3g, Saturated fat 4.3g, Carbohydrate 29.7g, Total sugars 4.5g, Salt 1.36g, Sodium 536mg

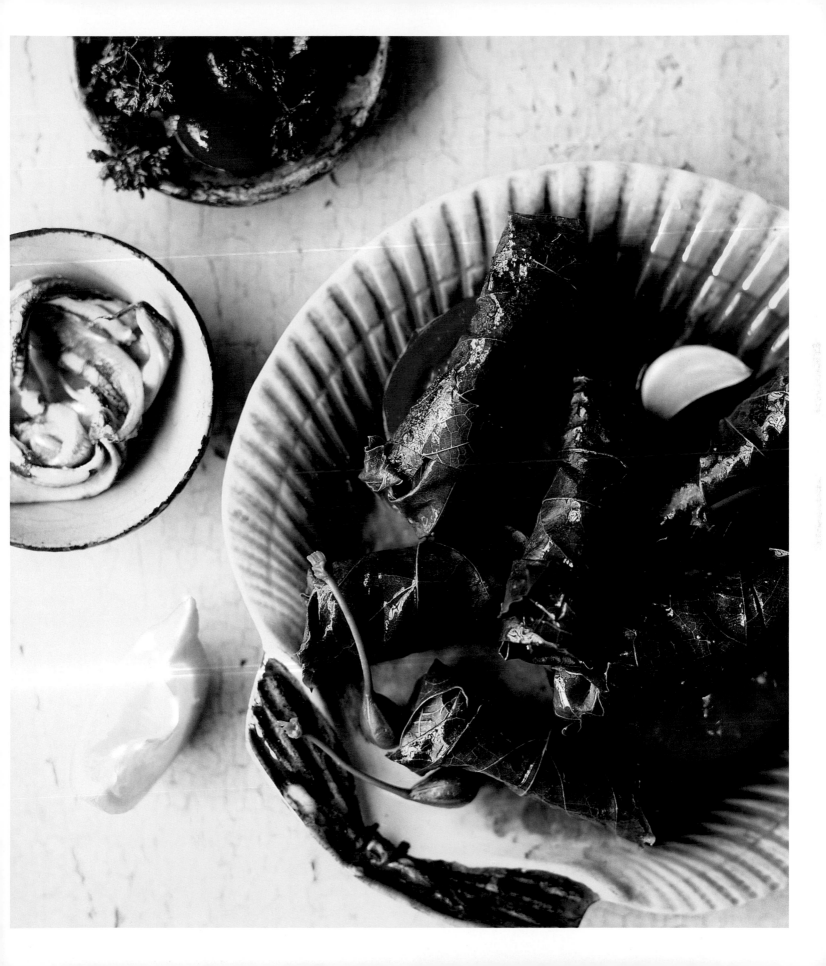

Little Ham Pots

Classic flavours, lovely finish. This twist on a great British favourite makes for a perfect light meal with some toasted seeded bread, or a very acceptable starter for a dinner. With the exception of the ham and yogurt, you can leave out any of the other ingredients without it being a problem.

Serves 4

115g extra fine French beans, cut into
 1cm pieces
115g frozen petit pois, defrosted
225g thickly cut cooked ham, cut in strips
4 cornichons (baby gherkins), quartered
8 baby white pickled onions
1 shallot, diced
1 teaspoon non-pareille capers
 (baby capers), drained and rinsed
1 tablespoon chopped fresh parsley
120g 0 per cent fat natural Greek yogurt
2 teaspoons Dijon mustard
1 egg, hard-boiled and chopped
freshly ground black pepper
leaf salad and seeded toast, to serve

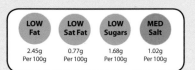

LOW Fat	LOW Sat Fat	LOW Sugars	MED Salt
2.45g Per 100g	0.77g Per 100g	1.68g Per 100g	1.02g Per 100g

1 In a pan of lightly salted boiling water cook the beans for 3 minutes, then add the peas and cook for a further 1 minute. Drain and refresh under cold running water.

2 In a bowl mix together the ham, beans and peas, cornichons, pickled onions, shallot, capers and parsley, and season with pepper. In another bowl combine the yogurt with the mustard, stir in the chopped egg and the ham mixture, and adjust the seasoning to taste. Spoon the mixture into four ramekins and serve with a leaf salad and seeded toast.

Amount per portion
Energy 148 kcals, Protein 19.5g, Fat 5.1g, Saturated fat 1.6g, Carbohydrate 6.4g, Total sugars 3.5g, Salt 2.13g, Sodium 838mg

Potted Orange Duck with Hazelnuts

Potting is a great British tradition, a classic way of preserving foods. The 'authentic' method uses too much fat for a healthy diet, so I've worked out a leaner version, best saved for special occasions.

Serves 8

the raw meat from 6 duck legs, skin
   and fat removed
175ml orange liqueur (Cointreau,
   Grand Marnier)
grated zest of 2 oranges
115g chopped toasted hazelnuts
1 teaspoon green peppercorns in brine
225g duck or chicken livers, trimmed
2 egg yolks
2 tablespoons chopped fresh parsley
2 teaspoons chopped fresh mint
sunflower oil, for greasing
freshly ground black pepper
seeded bread, pickles and green salad,
   to serve

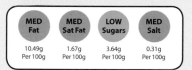

MED Fat	MED Sat Fat	LOW Sugars	MED Salt
10.49g Per 100g	1.67g Per 100g	3.64g Per 100g	0.31g Per 100g

1 In a food processor, dice half the duck meat with a pulse action. Transfer to a bowl and mix with half the liqueur, all the orange zest, the hazelnuts and peppercorns. In the food processor, mince the remaining meat together with the duck livers and egg yolks. Transfer to a clean bowl, add the parsley and mint, plenty of pepper and the remaining liqueur, and mulch with your hands to combine all. Cover both bowls and leave to marinate for 2 hours.

2 Preheat the oven to 180°C/350°F/gas mark 4. Lightly oil a 750ml terrine mould or terracotta bowl. Place half the minced mixture in the bottom of the terrine mould, then tip in all the diced duck, then layer on the remaining mince. Cover with foil, put the dish in a deep roasting tin, and pour in hot water around the dish to come halfway up its side. Pop the dish in the preheated oven and cook for 1 hour 15 minutes.

3 Remove the dish from the oven, cover with a plate or similar that fits inside the mould and rests on the potted duck, and weigh the plate down with a couple of full tins. Allow to cool, then refrigerate until ready to serve. Serve with crunchy pickles and a green salad.

Tip When the potted duck is ready it should have shrunk from the sides of the mould.

Amount per portion
Energy 316 kcals, Protein 22.5g, Fat 17.0g, Saturated fat 2.7g, Carbohydrate 6.3g, Total sugars 5.9g, Sodium 124mg

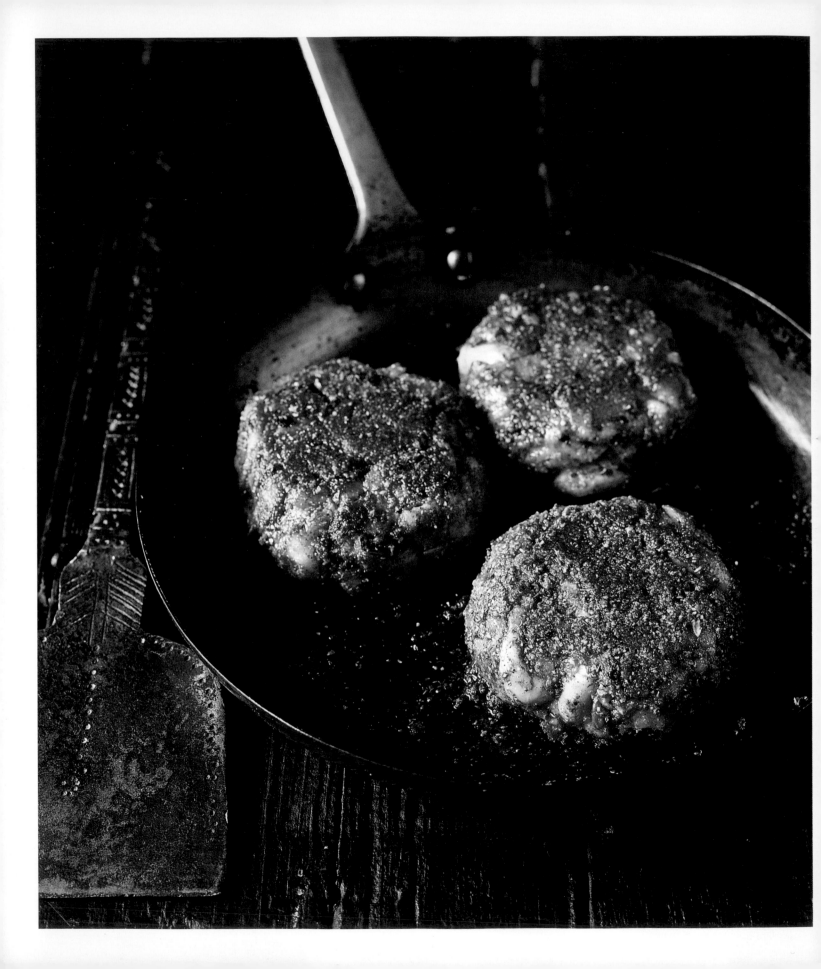

Potato, Garlic and Prawn Fritters

There's no deep-frying for these fritters – this Indian-influenced version is delicious oven-baked or lightly fried and served with a salad.

Serves 4
550g new potatoes, quartered
1 tablespoon sunflower oil

For the dukkah spice mix
2 tablespoons sunflower seeds
2 spring onions, finely sliced
½ teaspoon ground turmeric
2 garlic cloves, finely chopped
1 teaspoon black mustard seeds
2 tablespoons chopped fresh coriander
1 teaspoon chopped fresh mint
¼ teaspoon asafoetida powder (optional)
1 teaspoon curry leaves, broken
    or finely chopped
100g cooked, North Atlantic prawns,
    shell-off
1 egg yolk
2 tablespoons Dukkah (see page 257)
crunchy salad, to serve

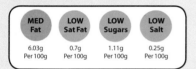

MED Fat	LOW Sat Fat	LOW Sugars	LOW Salt
6.03g Per 100g	0.7g Per 100g	1.11g Per 100g	0.25g Per 100g

1 Cook the new potatoes in boiling salted water until tender, about 20 minutes. Drain then mash half the potatoes with a fork or masher, and lightly crush the remainder. Tip them into the same bowl and keep warm.

2 Meanwhile, make the spice mix. Heat the oil in a saucepan over a low heat, then add the sunflower seeds, spring onions, turmeric, garlic and mustard seeds. Cook very gently for 4 minutes, stirring often. Add the coriander, mint, asafoetida and curry leaves and mix well. Add the spice mix to the potatoes while both are still warm, then leave to cool.

3 Fold the prawns into the potatoes, then mix in the egg yolk to help bind the mix. Shape into 4 cakes, squeezing them firmly. Refrigerate them for an hour or so to firm up.

4 If baking the fritters, preheat the oven to 180°C/350°F/gas mark 4. Dip the cakes top and bottom in the Dukkah, pushing the seeds in well. Bake for 20 minutes, turning once. Serve with a salad with loads of crunch from cucumber, carrot and radish.

Amount per portion
Energy 248 kcals, Protein 12g, Fat 12g, Saturated fat 1.4g, Carbohydrate 25g, Total sugars 2.2g, Salt 0.5g, Sodium 197mg

Smoked Haddock, White Bean and Honey

Think of smoked haddock in the same way as you would smoked salmon. It's good value, and because it has a 'cooked' texture it is extremely easy to use and makes for a lovely starter or supper ingredient, as in this easy-peasy Spanish recipe.

Serves 4

375g undyed smoked haddock, skinned
    and cut into small dice
1 x 200g tin white beans, drained and rinsed
3 tomatoes, deseeded and diced
1 small red onion, thinly sliced
1 tablespoon extra virgin olive oil
1 teaspoon sherry vinegar or balsamic
    vinegar
2 teaspoons medium sherry
1 teaspoon runny honey
8 gem lettuce leaves
salt and freshly ground black pepper
crusty seeded bread, to serve

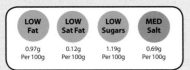

1 Mix together all the ingredients except the lettuce leaves, and season to taste. Spoon the mixture into the lettuce leaves, and serve with crusty seeded bread.

Amount per portion
Energy 159 kcals, Protein 21.0g, Fat 3.9g, Saturated fat 0.5g, Carbohydrate 10.1g, Total sugars 4.8g, Salt 2.77g, Sodium 1093mg

Aubergine and Red Pepper Salsa

This makes a refreshing salad when tossed with a few jumbo prawns
and some leaves, but it also forms a great partnership with plain grilled
fish. Serve with crusty bread for extra carbohydrate.

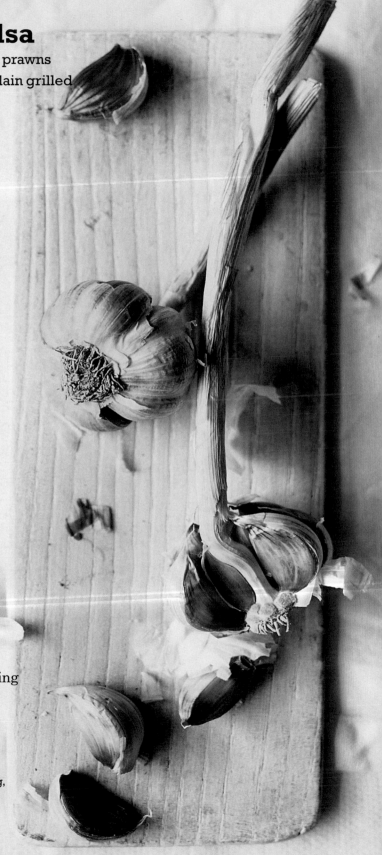

Serves 4
1 large aubergine
20ml sunflower oil
90ml reduced-salt soy sauce
90ml rice vinegar
2 red peppers, roasted, peeled, deseeded and
   cut into 2.5cm dice
2 tablespoons fish sauce (nam pla)
1 tablespoon soft dark brown sugar
1 teaspoon hot chilli sauce
4 spring onions, finely sliced
1 tablespoon grated fresh ginger
2 tablespoons chopped fresh coriander leaves
1 tablespoon chopped fresh mint
2 tablespoons chopped fresh flat-leaf parsley
3 garlic cloves, finely chopped
1 teaspoon finely grated lemon zest

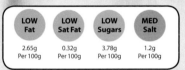

LOW Fat	LOW Sat Fat	LOW Sugars	MED Salt
2.65g Per 100g	0.32g Per 100g	3.78g Per 100g	1.2g Per 100g

1 Cut the aubergine into 5mm slices. Mix together the oil,
soy sauce and vinegar. Marinate the aubergine in this mix
for 1 hour, turning and basting regularly. Drain well over
a bowl to catch any marinade.

2 Cook the aubergine slices – ideally over a barbecue, but
failing that over a high heat on a griddle pan or frying pan
for 4–5 minutes each side. The aubergine slices should be
very dark and thoroughly cooked. Leave to cool.

3 Cut the aubergine slices to match the red pepper dice.
Mix together all the remaining ingredients and any remaining
marinade, then mix in the aubergine and red pepper.
Refrigerate until just before you wish to use, then bring
up to room temperature.

Amount per portion
Energy 115 kcals, Protein 3.2g, Fat 6.6g, Saturated fat 0.8g, Carbohydrate 11.4g,
Total sugars 9.4g, Salt 3.75g, Sodium 1480mg

Caribbean Salmon Tartare

In the past I would have used tuna or swordfish for this but as they seem to be threatened with extinction, it's best to use a sustainable fish.

Serves 4 as a starter, or 8 for meze
325g raw salmon fillet, finely diced
4 spring onions, finely chopped
2 tablespoons lime juice
1 teaspoon finely diced fresh red chilli
2 tablespoons avocado or rapeseed oil
1 teaspoon runny honey
2 tablespoons finely chopped fresh
    coriander leaf
1 teaspoon grated ginger
1 mango, cut into small dice
¼ pineapple, peeled and finely diced
fresh coriander leaves, to garnish
lime wedges, to serve

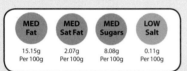

MED Fat	MED Sat Fat	MED Sugars	LOW Salt
15.15g Per 100g	2.07g Per 100g	8.08g Per 100g	0.11g Per 100g

1 About 1 hour 30 minutes before serving, combine all the ingredients except the coriander leaves and lime wedges.
2 Place an oiled ring mould on to an individual plate and push a quarter of the mixture into the mould or an eighth if serving as meze, then remove the mould. Repeat with the remaining tartare mixture. Serve garnished with coriander leaves and lime wedges and bread on the side.

Tip Rubbing your hands with oil will protect them from the heat of the chillies.

Amount per portion
Energy 484 kcals, Protein 36.5g, Fat 30.6g, Saturated fat 4.1g, Carbohydrate 16.6g, Total sugars 16.1g, Fibre (Englyst) 2.5g, Salt 0.21g, Sodium 84mg

Salmon Tartare

Based on that French classic, steak tartare – lovely as a starter or light lunch served with toasted seeded bread for an added crunch.

Serves 4
325g very fresh salmon, skinned
    and finely diced
1 teaspoon English mustard
2 teaspoons capers, rinsed and
    finely chopped
2 spring onions, finely chopped
1 sweet gherkin, finely diced
1 teaspoon Worcestershire sauce
½ teaspoon Tabasco sauce
juice of 1 lemon
1 tablespoon good-quality olive oil
2 teaspoons chopped fresh parsley
freshly ground black pepper
seeded bread, to serve

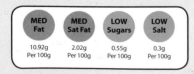

MED Fat	MED Sat Fat	LOW Sugars	LOW Salt
10.92g Per 100g	2.02g Per 100g	0.55g Per 100g	0.3g Per 100g

1 Combine all the ingredients, mixing well to combine the flavours, and season to taste. Line 4 moulds with clingfilm and fill with the mixture, then refrigerate for 20 minutes to set the shape. Turn out on to chilled plates and serve with seeded bread or toast.

Variations To take the powerful ingredients you need a strongly flavoured fish with an oily base, so very fresh tuna or mackerel also work well.

Amount per portion
Energy 178 kcals, Protein 16.8g, Fat 11.9g, Saturated fat 2.2g, Carbohydrate 0.9g, Total sugars 0.6g, Fibre (Englyst) 0.2g, Salt 0.33g, Sodium 131mg

RIGHT Caribbean
Salmon Tartare

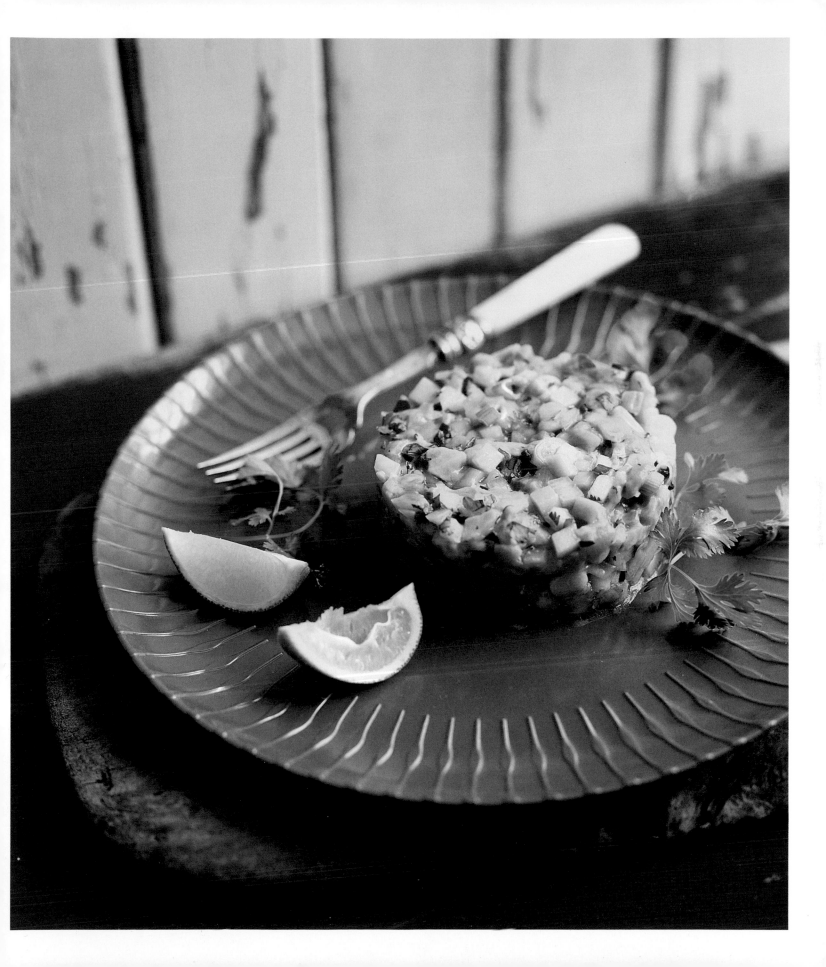

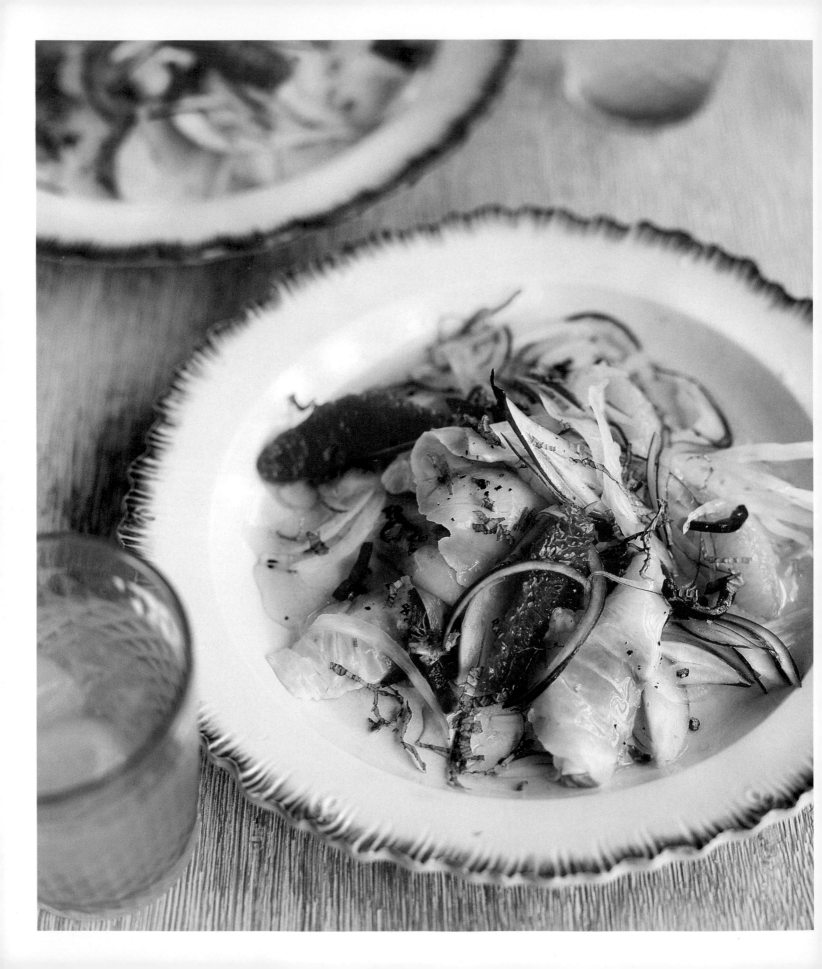

Sea Bass, Fennel and Citrus Ceviche

Raw fish must be über fresh, then it is delicious. With this recipe and its marinade there is a cooked effect, so you don't even have to tell your friends it's raw. Serve with bread if you need extra carbohydrate.

Serves 4

2 sea bass fillets, about 325g in total, skinned and pin-boned
juice of 2 limes
2 mild fresh red chillies, deseeded and cut into thin strips
1 garlic clove, crushed to a paste with a little salt
1 red or pink grapefruit
1 navel orange
½ red onion, very thinly sliced
1 fennel bulb, very thinly sliced
1 tablespoon shredded fresh mint leaves, to garnish
2 teaspoons extra virgin olive oil
salt and freshly ground black pepper

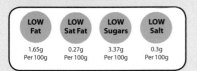

LOW Fat	LOW Sat Fat	LOW Sugars	LOW Salt
1.65g Per 100g	0.27g Per 100g	3.37g Per 100g	0.3g Per 100g

1 Slice the bass fillets into 1cm-wide strips. Place them in a bowl and sprinkle over about ½ teaspoon salt, then set aside for 20 minutes during which time the fish will 'tighten' and start to 'cook'. Rinse and dry them well with kitchen paper, return them to a clean bowl and add the lime juice, chillies and garlic. Toss to coat all the fish pieces and leave for 15 minutes to 'cook' by marinating in the acid lime juice.

2 Meanwhile, peel the grapefruit and orange. Hold the fruit over a bowl to catch the juice and with a small sharp knife cut down both sides of each segment, as close to the membrane as you can, then ease the flesh out into the bowl. Squeeze the membranes over the bowl to release any remaining juice. Mix in the onion and fennel.

3 Just before serving, add the citrus fruit mix to the fish and its juices, and season with pepper. Arrange between 4 cold plates, scatter with mint and drizzle with olive oil.

Variations Use any really fresh fish, such as salmon or mackerel. A few sprouting seeds scattered over the top of the ceviche makes for good GI.

Amount per portion
Energy 143 kcals, Protein 17.3g, Fat 4.3g, Saturated fat 0.7g, Carbohydrate 9.4g, Total sugars 8.8g, Salt 0.79g, Sodium 310mg

Soft Boiled Eggs with Mustard Beans

This variation on a great British tradition is so simple but so delicious, especially if you grow your own beans in the garden. Just remember not to overcook the eggs, as you want semi-runny yolks to bring a gooey sunshine to the plate.

Serves 4

4 large eggs
225g extra fine French beans
   or thinly sliced runner beans
2 shallots, thinly sliced
4 radishes, thinly sliced
25g toasted chopped hazelnuts

For the dressing

2 tablespoons extra virgin olive oil
2 tablespoons 0 per cent fat natural
   Greek yogurt
1 tablespoon Dijon mustard
1 tablespoon cider vinegar
salt and freshly ground black pepper

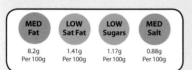

MED Fat	LOW Sat Fat	LOW Sugars	MED Salt
8.2g Per 100g	1.41g Per 100g	1.17g Per 100g	0.88g Per 100g

1 In a pan of boiling water, cook the eggs for 5 minutes 30 seconds. Drain, refresh under cold running water, and peel when cool enough to handle.

2 In a pan of boiling salted water, cook the beans for 4 minutes, then drain but do not refresh. While the beans are still hot, toss in the shallots, radishes and hazelnuts.

3 Make the dressing by whisking together all the ingredients; add a little water if necessary to thin down. Stir the dressing into the beans and arrange on to individual plates. Cut the eggs in half and place on top of the beans. This is excellent served as a bruschetta on seeded toast.

Tip If you're a fan of the runner bean, as I am, buy yourself a beaner, the perfect little gadget for topping, tailing, stringing and slicing in a couple of moves.

Amount per portion

Energy 206 kcals, Protein 10.6g, Fat 16.8g, Saturated fat 2.9g, Carbohydrate 3.3g, Total sugars 2.4g, Salt 1.14g, Sodium 448mg

Curried Pickled Eggs

I'm a bit of a pickled egg fan, but usually ones you can buy are submerged in a boring vinegar solution, so this recipe will produce a snack egg that says, 'Hello', and 'Wow!'

Serves 12
600ml cider vinegar
2 dried chillies
6 green cardamom pods
2 tablespoons coriander seeds
½ teaspoon celery seeds
½ teaspoon yellow mustard seeds
1 teaspoon curry paste or powder
2 cloves
1 teaspoon ground turmeric
6 garlic cloves, lightly crushed
½ teaspoon sugar
1 red onion, sliced into rings
12 eggs, hard-boiled and peeled
salt

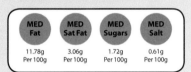

MED Fat	MED Sat Fat	MED Sugars	MED Salt
11.78g Per 100g	3.06g Per 100g	1.72g Per 100g	0.61g Per 100g

1 In a non-reactive saucepan combine all the ingredients except the onion and eggs, and add about ¼ teaspoon salt. Bring to the boil and simmer for 10 minutes. Set aside to cool.

2 Meanwhile, layer the onion rings and eggs in a large clean preserving jar. Strain the vinegar on to the eggs to cover completely, topping up if necessary with extra vinegar. Seal tightly and allow the flavours to develop for at least 1 week before eating. Refrigerate after opening. Chop up and add to a mixed leaf salad.

Variation Quail's eggs make a nice cocktail nibble (they are hard-boiled in 5 minutes). Allow four quail's eggs for every hen's egg.

Amount per portion
Energy 106 kcals, Protein 8.23g, Fat 7.1g, Saturated fat 1.83g, Carbohydrate 2.53g, Total sugars 1.03g, Salt 0.36g, Sodium 143mg

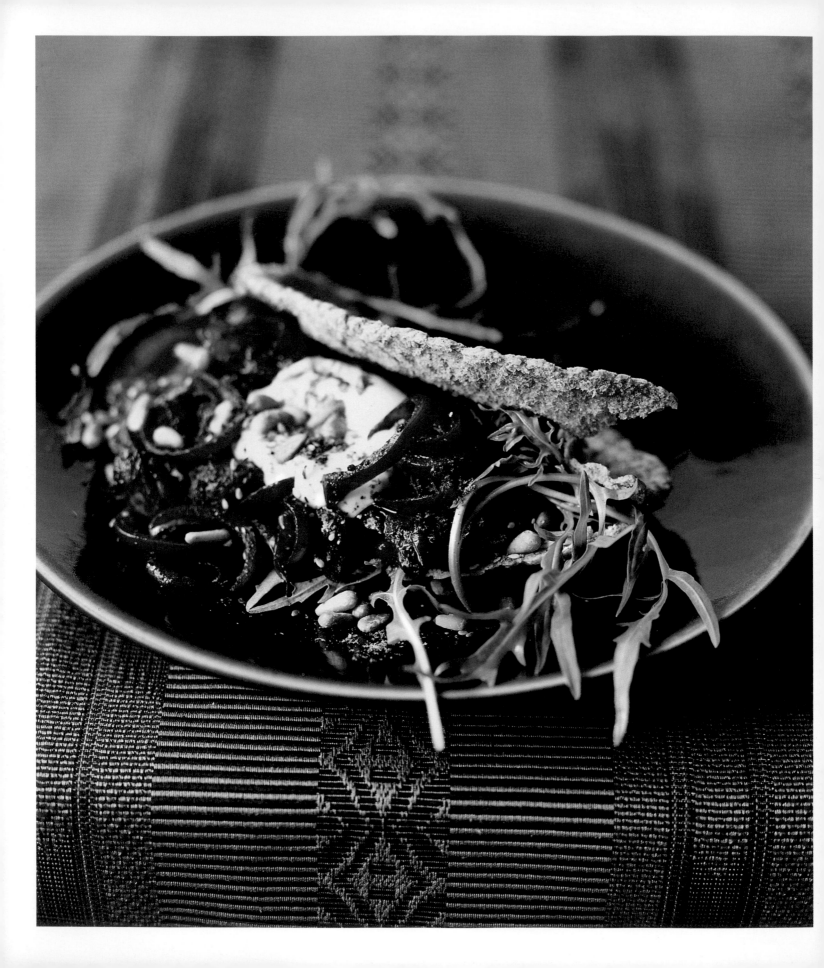

The Ultimate Chicken Sandwich

This is a fab sandwich, but to make it you'll have to stock your store cupboard with a couple of Middle Eastern products. Sumac and za'atar are well worth having and can be found in Middle Eastern food shops or via the internet.

Serves 4
2 chicken breasts, thinly sliced
2 small red onions, thinly sliced
½ tablespoon harissa chilli paste
3 garlic cloves, crushed to a paste
    with a little sea salt
1 teaspoon allspice
½ teaspoon ground cinnamon
1 tablespoon sumac
2 tablespoons extra virgin olive oil
grated zest and juice of ½ lemon
1 tablespoon za'atar
salt and freshly ground black pepper

To serve
4 wholemeal pitta breads
a handful of rocket leaves
2 tomatoes, thinly sliced
2 tablespoons 0 per cent fat natural
    Greek yogurt
25g toasted pine nuts

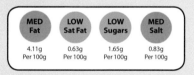

1 In a large bowl, mix together the chicken slices, onions, harissa, garlic, spices, oil, lemon juice and zest, and add salt and pepper to taste. Leave to marinate for a couple of hours or overnight if possible.

2 Heat a large frying pan and cook the chicken and its marinade over a medium heat for 8–10 minutes, stirring regularly, until caramelised with lovely brown onions. Sprinkle with za'atar.

3 Just before the chicken is ready, toast or warm the pitta breads, and cut a pocket along the side of each. Place a little rocket in each, along with a few slices of tomato. Spoon in the chicken mix and top with a bit of yogurt and a few pine nuts. Serve immediately.

Amount per portion
Energy 352 kcals, Protein 26g, Fat 13g, Saturated fat 2g, Carbohydrate 35g, Total sugars 5.2g, Salt 2.63g, Sodium 1034mg

Chicken, Bacon and Avocado Sandwich

Avocado is a misunderstood fruit – certainly it is not low in calories but it has good monounsaturated fat and its superfood benefits (it's rich in antioxidants and high in potassium) must surely outweigh its downside. In any case, for this classic American sandwich I'm only giving a quarter avocado per person, so no need to worry.

Serves 4

1 ripe avocado
200g tinned chickpeas, drained and rinsed
½ teaspoon ground cumin
juice of 1 lime
2 tomatoes, deseeded and diced
1 red chilli, deseeded and finely chopped
1 teaspoon chopped fresh coriander, plus
    4 sprigs to garnish
4 rashers back bacon, rinds removed
1 cooked chicken breast, sliced into
    8 pieces
4 slices country-style seeded bread
salt and freshly ground black pepper

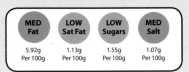

MED Fat	LOW Sat Fat	LOW Sugars	MED Salt
5.92g Per 100g	1.13g Per 100g	1.55g Per 100g	1.07g Per 100g

1 Mash the avocado, leaving a little texture. Fold in the chickpeas, cumin, lime juice, tomatoes, chilli and coriander and season to taste. Cover tightly with clingfilm and leave for the flavours develop.

2 Grill the bacon until crisp, and cut each rasher into 4. Spoon the avocado mixture on to the bread slices, scatter bacon and 2 pieces of chicken on each. Garnish each with a sprig of coriander.

Amount per portion
Energy 307 kcals, Protein 21.5g, Fat 12.6g, Saturated fat 2.4g, Carbohydrate 28.6g, Total sugars 3.3g, Salt 2.27g, Sodium 896mg

Fried Chicken Livers with Herbs and Chilli

India meets Italy – big flavours, lovely starter.

Serves 4

200g chicken livers, cleaned and cut in half
1 teaspoon grated ginger
2 teaspoons finely chopped garlic
¼ teaspoon ground turmeric
¼ teaspoon ground cumin
¼ teaspoon ground coriander
1 tablespoon lemon juice
1 tablespoon sunflower oil
1 small red onion, sliced
2 handfuls of baby spinach
2 tablespoons chopped fresh coriander
2 teaspoons chopped fresh mint
1 tablespoon pine nuts
2 green chillies, deseeded and sliced
4 thick slices seeded country loaf, toasted
salt

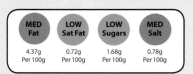

1 In a bowl, mix together the chicken livers, ginger, garlic, turmeric, cumin, coriander and lemon juice. Leave to marinate for 10 minutes.
2 Heat the oil in a frying pan, then add the livers and fry them for 3 minutes each side, turning once only. Remove them from the pan and keep warm. Add the onion to the pan and cook for 3 minutes, then add the spinach, coriander and mint and cook until wilted.
3 Add the livers, pine nuts and chillies, adjust the seasoning to taste and toss to combine. Spoon on to the toasted bread and serve immediately.

Amount per portion
Energy 220 kcals, Protein 14.5g, Fat 7.3g, Saturated fat 1.2g, Carbohydrate 25.9g, Total sugars 2.8g, Salt 1.30g, Sodium 514mg

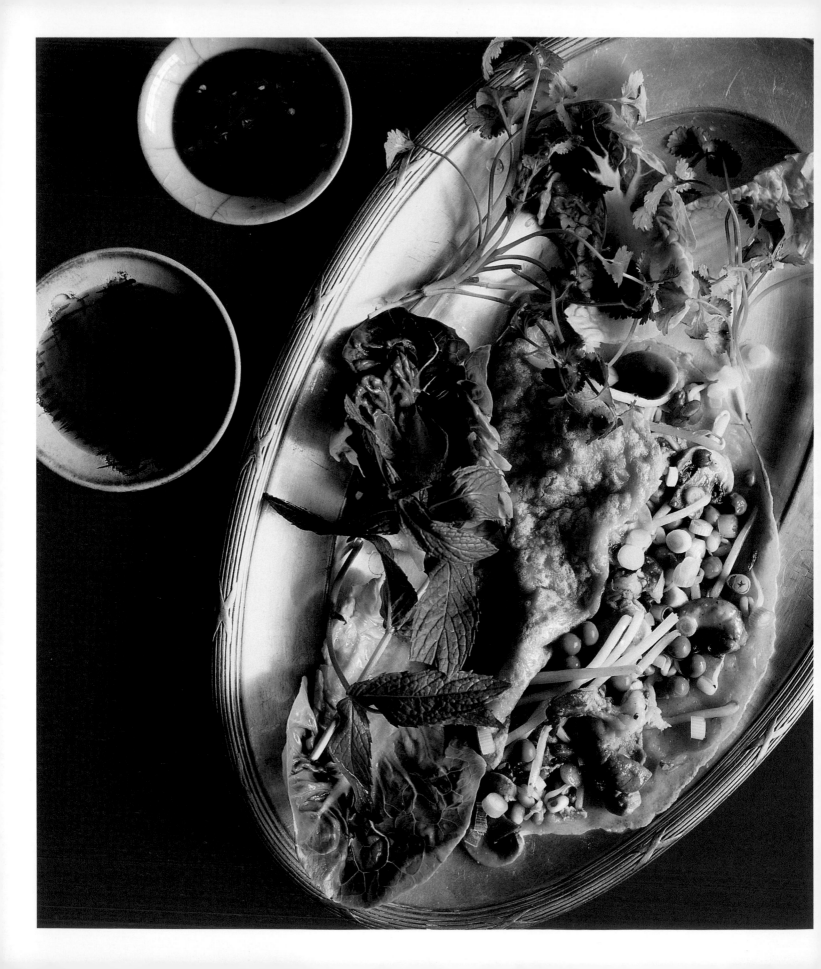

Asian Surf and Turf Crêpes

Pancakes are always a useful package for all sorts of fillings. Oriental flavours make this a very moreish dish.

Serves 8 as a starter or 4 as a main

For the batter
85g cornflour
300g rice flour
180ml low-fat coconut milk
180ml semi-skimmed milk

For the filling
175g pork fillet, thinly cut
16 raw tiger prawns, shell-off,
    deveined and split in half lengthways
2 tablespoons fish sauce (nam pla)
1 teaspoon crushed garlic
2 shallots, finely chopped
4 spring onions, finely sliced
115g sprouting seeds (mung beans)
1 tablespoon caster sugar or granulated
    low-calorie sweetener
1 teaspoon freshly ground black pepper
2 tablespoons sunflower oil
50g beansprouts
50g frozen peas, defrosted
85g button mushrooms, sliced

To serve
Baby gem lettuce leaves
fresh mint leaves
fresh coriander leaves

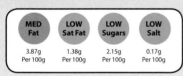

MED Fat	LOW Sat Fat	LOW Sugars	LOW Salt
3.87g Per 100g	1.38g Per 100g	2.15g Per 100g	0.17g Per 100g

1 To make the batter, put all the batter ingredients in a food processor and add 300ml water. Whizz until smooth, then pass through a fine sieve into a jug and set aside.

2 Put the pork and prawns together in a large bowl. Add the fish sauce, garlic, shallots, spring onions, mung beans, sweetener and pepper and mix well. Set aside to marinate for at least 30 minutes.

3 Heat half the oil in a frying pan. Add the pork and prawn mix and stir-fry over a fierce heat for 2 minutes. Transfer the pork and prawn to a flat dish and divide into 8 portions.

4 Heat some oil in a small frying pan. Give the batter a whisk, then pour a small amount into the pan and swirl to cover the base. Immediately add one-eighth of the pork and prawn and a scattering of the vegetables. Reduce the heat to low, cover with a lid and cook for 5 minutes. Fold the crepe in half and then in half again, slide it onto a plate and keep warm. Repeat the process to make 8 stuffed crêpes.

5 To eat, rip off a piece of crêpe, pop in a piece of lettuce then top with mint and coriander.

Amount per portion
Energy 292 kcals, Protein 13.7g, Fat 7g, Saturated fat 2.5g, Carbohydrate 42.5g, Total sugars 3.9g, Salt 0.3g, Sodium 359mg

A Sort of Tom Yam

I say sort of, because to make this classic Asian soup more GI-friendly I've added a few extra ingredients – but it's just as delicious as the original.

Serves 4
4 boneless skinless chicken thighs,
    each cut into 6 pieces
1.5 litres chicken stock
2 stalks of lemongrass, heavily bruised
    with the back of a knife
2cm piece of galangal (optional), bruised
2cm piece of fresh ginger, peeled
    and bruised
1 large onion, roughly chopped
1 sweet potato, cut into 1cm dice
1 carrot, cut into thin rounds
100g cauliflower, broken into small florets
1 x 400g tin white cannellini beans,
    drained and rinsed
6 baby sweetcorn, halved
2 bird's eye chillies, deseeded
    and finely chopped
4 kaffir lime leaves
3 tablespoons fresh coriander leaves
2 spring onions, sliced
1 tablespoon fish sauce (nam pla)
2 tablespoons lime juice

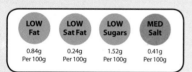

LOW Fat	LOW Sat Fat	LOW Sugars	MED Salt
0.84g Per 100g	0.24g Per 100g	1.52g Per 100g	0.41g Per 100g

1 Wash the chicken pieces then put them in a large saucepan with the stock, lemongrass, galangal if using, ginger, onion, sweet potato and carrot. Bring to the boil then reduce the heat and simmer for 15 minutes.
2 Add the cauliflower, beans, sweetcorn, chillies and kaffir lime leaves, and cook for a further 8 minutes. Remove the lemongrass, galangal and ginger and discard.
3 Add the coriander, spring onions, fish sauce and lime juice, and serve immediately.

Amount per portion
Energy 358 kcals, Protein 48.8g, Fat 5.6g, Saturated fat 1.6g, Carbohydrate 30.3g, Total sugars 10.1g, Salt 2.75g, Sodium 1086mg

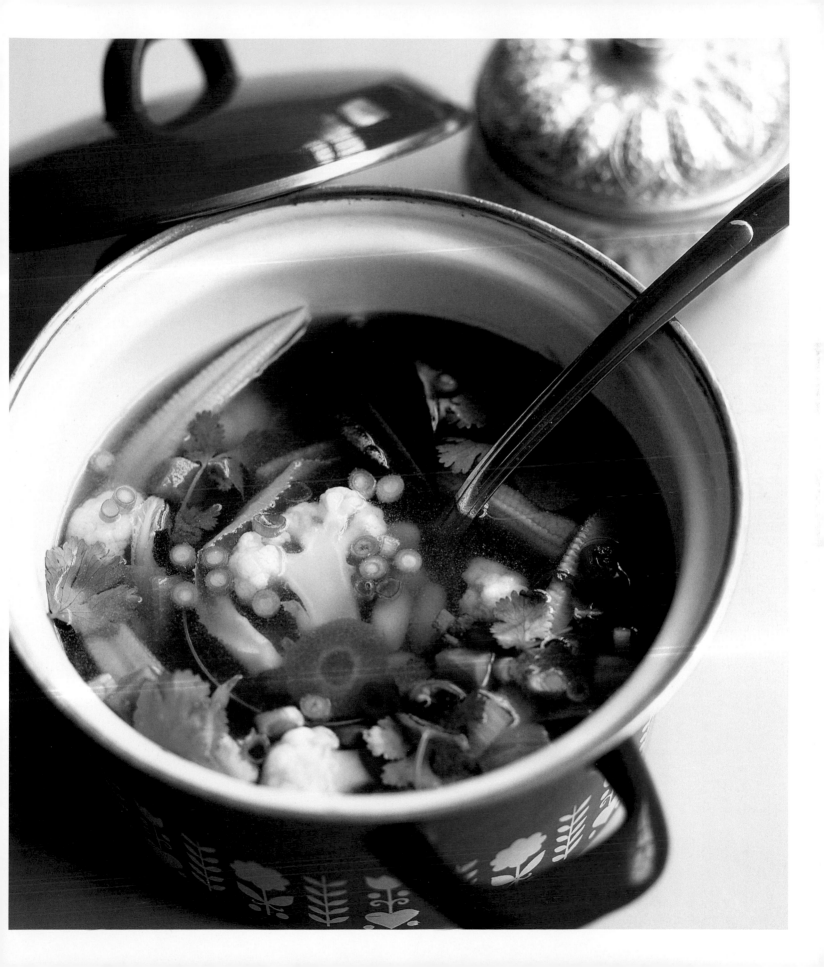

Spiced Tomato and Coconut Soup

An unusual and delicious soup with a strong Indian background. The coconut makes it quite high in fat but it is quick and easy to make so maybe keep it for special occasions.

Serves 4
115g desiccated coconut
300ml warm water
1 tablespoon sunflower oil
1 large onion, finely chopped
1 small carrot, cut into 1cm dice
2 garlic cloves, finely chopped
1 teaspoon brown mustard seeds
1 teaspoon cumin seeds
¼ teaspoon asafoetida powder (optional)
8 curry leaves, crumbled
2 x 400g tins chopped tomatoes
1 x 400g tin white haricot beans, drained
1 teaspoon chilli powder
1 teaspoon ground turmeric
1 teaspoon garam masala
1 teaspoon caster sugar
salt and freshly ground black pepper

1 Soak the desiccated coconut in the warm water for 20 minutes.

2 Meanwhile heat the oil in a saucepan, add the onion, carrot, garlic, mustard seeds, cumin, asafoetida and curry leaves and cook gently for 8 minutes to soften the onions. Add the tomatoes, beans, chilli powder and turmeric and simmer for 15 minutes.

3 Put the coconut and its soaking water into a blender and blend to a smoothish paste. Mix with the tomato and bean mixture, along with the garam masala and sugar, and heat gently but do not allow to boil. Season to taste and serve with crusty seeded bread.

Amount per portion
Energy 320 kcals, Protein 9.2g, Fat 22.1g, Saturated fat 15.8g, Carbohydrate 22.6g, Total sugars 11.4g, Salt 1.01g, Sodium 401mg

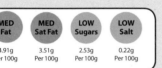

MED Fat	MED Sat Fat	LOW Sugars	LOW Salt
4.91g Per 100g	3.51g Per 100g	2.53g Per 100g	0.22g Per 100g

Chilled Cucumber and Honeydew Soup with Mint

In the UK it is a rare occasion when we fancy a chilled soup, and then it's usually a Spanish tomato gazpacho or French potato and leek vichyssoise. I was offered this in Brunei, it's lovely and really refreshing for a hot summer's day.

Serves 4
1 honeydew melon, peeled and deseeded
1 cucumber
200g 0 per cent fat natural Greek yogurt
12 mint leaves, plus extra shredded leaves
    for garnish
grated zest and juice of 2 limes
½ teaspoon salt
¼ teaspoon ground pepper
½ teaspoon caster sugar
1 tablespoon toasted sunflower seeds
1 mild red chilli, deseeded and finely diced
2 teaspoons mint sauce

1 Cut three quarters of the melon and cucumber into large chunks, and the remainder into small dice.

2 In a food processor, blend together the large chunks, the yogurt, whole mint leaves, lime zest and juice, salt and pepper and sugar. When the mixture is smooth, stir in the small dice of melon and cucumber and the sunflower seeds. Spoon into individual chilled bowls and garnish with shreds of mint leaves, chilli and a drizzle of mint sauce.

Amount per portion
Energy 106 kcals, Protein 7.4g, Fat 1.8g, Saturated fat 0.2g, Carbohydrate 16.0g, Total sugars 14.7g, Salt 0.89g, Sodium 352mg

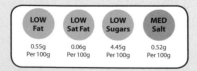

LOW Fat	LOW Sat Fat	LOW Sugars	MED Salt
0.55g Per 100g	0.06g Per 100g	4.45g Per 100g	0.52g Per 100g

Roast Butternut Squash Soup with Crushed Chickpeas

A fabulous Australian recipe. Butternut squash is one of my favourite vegetables.

Serves 4

2 onions, each cut into 6 wedges
8 garlic cloves
1 butternut squash, unpeeled, cut in half
    lengthways, deseeded, each half cut
    into 4 wedges
2 teaspoons chopped fresh thyme
spray olive oil
1.5 litres vegetable stock
1 x 400g tin chickpeas, drained and rinsed
1 tablespoon extra virgin olive oil
115g petit pois, defrosted
1 fresh red chilli, deseeded and chopped
1 tablespoon chopped fresh parsley
salt and freshly ground black pepper

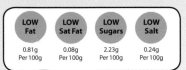

LOW Fat	LOW Sat Fat	LOW Sugars	LOW Salt
0.81g Per 100g	0.08g Per 100g	2.23g Per 100g	0.24g Per 100g

1 Preheat the oven to 200°C/400°F/gas mark 6. Put the onions into a bowl, add 6 of the garlic cloves, all the squash and thyme, and grind over some black pepper. Spray with oil and toss to coat everything with oil. Tip into a roasting tin, pop in the oven and roast for about 35 minutes, tossing regularly – keep an eye on the garlic, you don't want it burning.

2 Remove from the oven. When cool enough to handle, scrape the butternut flesh from the skin and pop it into a food processor, along with the roast onion and garlic and any juices from the tray, and blitz until semi-smooth (it's nice to retain a little texture). Tip this combo into a pan along with the stock and bring to the boil, then check the seasoning and adjust to taste.

3 Meanwhile, in a bowl mash half the chickpeas with a fork and mix with the remaining whole chickpeas. Chop the remaining garlic. Heat the olive oil in a frying pan and cook the garlic along with the mixed chickpeas, the peas, chilli and parsley, for 3 minutes at most.

4 Season to taste and pour the soup into warmed bowls, then spoon the chickpea mix on to the surface.

Variations Where do you stop? I could suggest using coriander instead of parsley, or adding some cumin seeds to the roasting process, or a teaspoon of harissa to the chickpeas – all would go together incredibly well.

Amount per portion
Energy 248 kcals, Protein 10.8g, Fat 6.3g, Saturated fat 0.6g, Carbohydrate 39.6g, Total sugars 17.3g, Salt 1.89g, Sodium 746mg

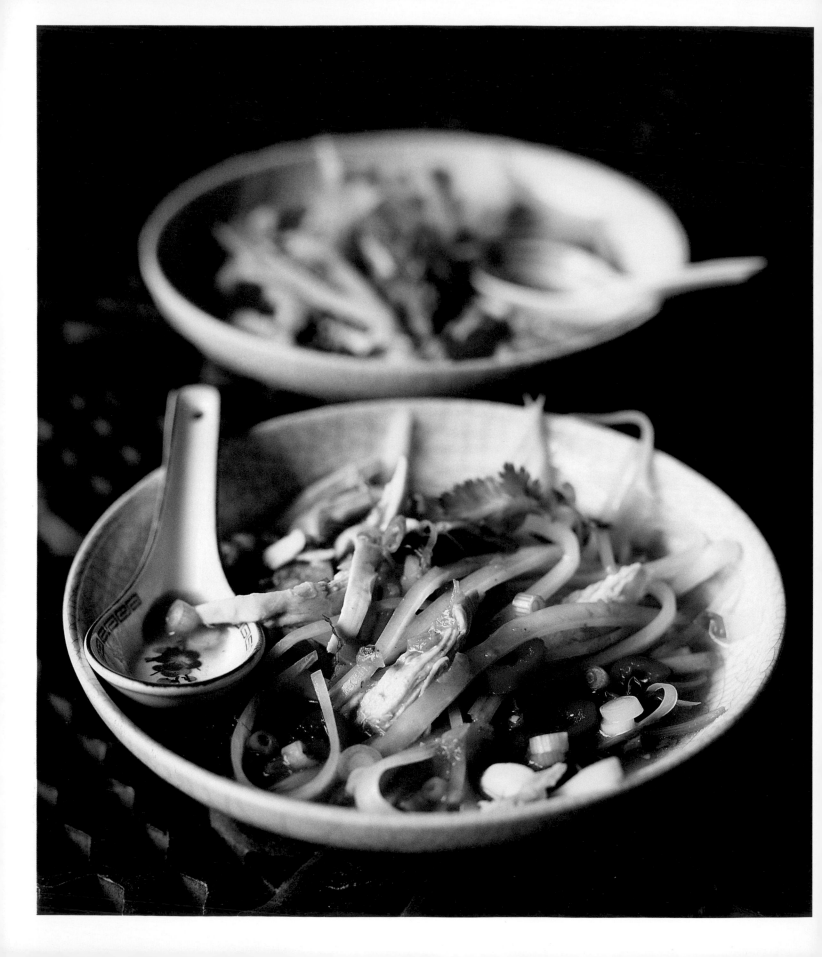

Quick Sweet-and-Sour Chicken Soup

Whenever I was unwell, my Mum would give me a bowl of chicken soup, I think it's a Jewish tradition. This soup has all the benefits, but loads more flavour.

Serves 4

3 shallots, chopped
1 teaspoon crushed black peppercorns
5 garlic cloves, finely chopped
1 tablespoon shrimp paste (balchan)
1 tablespoon sunflower oil
1.2 litres chicken stock
1 tablespoon chopped fresh ginger
1 hot fresh chilli, deseeded and finely sliced
125ml tamarind juice (use 1 part tamarind
   paste to 3 parts water)
1 unripe papaya, cut into matchsticks
450g cooked chicken, thinly shredded
a handful of baby spinach leaves
1 tablespoon runny honey
juice of 1 lime
1 tablespoon fish sauce (nam pla)
4 spring onions, finely chopped

To garnish

1 tablespoon fresh coriander leaves
2 teaspoons shredded fresh mint leaves

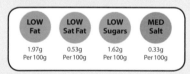

LOW Fat	LOW Sat Fat	LOW Sugars	MED Salt
1.97g Per 100g	0.53g Per 100g	1.62g Per 100g	0.33g Per 100g

1 In a mini food processor blend together the shallots, peppercorns, garlic and shrimp paste.

2 Heat the oil in a large pan over a medium heat, then fry the shallot paste for 1 minute. Add the chicken stock and bring to the boil. Add the ginger, chilli and tamarind juice and cook for 3 minutes.

3 Fold in the papaya, chicken, spinach, honey, lime juice, fish sauce and spring onions. Heat for 2 minutes to warm through. Garnish with coriander and mint leaves.

Tip Shrimp paste (balchan) and fish sauce (nam pla) are readily available in Asian food stores.

Amount per portion
Energy 339 kcals, Protein 42.4g, Fat 11.9g, Saturated fat 3.2g, Carbohydrate 16.8g, Total sugars 9.8g, Salt 1.97g, Sodium 778mg

Fava Bean and Pasta Soup

Tins of beans are always a useful store-cupboard ingredient and an excellent way of saving time rather than having to soak beans overnight.

Serves 4
1 tablespoon olive oil
2 onions, finely chopped
1 fennel bulb, finely diced
1 teaspoon fennel seeds
2.3 litres vegetable stock
2 x 400g tins fava, broad or flageolet beans, drained and rinsed
225g small macaroni or ditalini
4 tomatoes, deseeded and diced
1 tablespoon chopped fresh fennel fronds or dill fronds
salt and freshly ground black pepper
crusty seeded bread, to serve

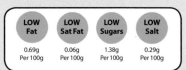

1 Heat the oil in a large saucepan then over a low heat cook the onions and fennel until softened, about 10–12 minutes. Add the fennel seeds and stock, bring to the boil and simmer for 20 minutes.
2 Add half the beans, return to the boil then remove from the heat. Leave to cool slightly, then purée in a liquidiser or blender.
3 Return the smooth soup to the saucepan, then add the pasta and cook for 10–12 minutes, stirring regularly, until the pasta is cooked but retains some firmness. Add the remaining beans, along with the tomatoes and fennel fronds, bring back to temperature and season to taste. Serve with hot crusty seeded bread.

Amount per portion
Energy 418 kcals, Protein 19.8g, Fat 6.5g, Saturated fat 0.6g, Carbohydrate 74.8g, Total sugars 13.0g, Salt 2.73g, Sodium 1077mg

Chickpea and Cabbage Soup

A wonderful warming French soup for cold winter days.

Serves 4
1 tablespoon extra virgin olive oil,
1 onion, finely chopped
3 garlic cloves, finely chopped
2 bay leaves
1 teaspoon fresh thyme leaves
1 chilli, deseeded and finely diced
4 tablespoons roughly chopped fresh flat-leaf parsley
1 tablespoon chopped fresh marjoram
1 x 400g tin chopped tomatoes
1 x 400g tin chickpeas and their liquor
1 litre vegetable stock
450g greens (Savoy, cavolo nero, spring greens), shredded
grated Parmesan cheese, to serve
salt and freshly ground black pepper

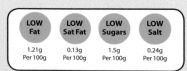

1 In a large saucepan heat the oil over a medium heat, then add the onion, garlic, bay leaves, thyme and chilli and cook for about 10 minutes or until the onions have softened without colouring.
2 Add the parsley, marjoram and tomatoes and cook for a further 3 minutes. Add the chickpeas, their liquor and the stock and cook for a further 30 minutes at a steady simmer.
3 Add the shredded greens and cook for a further 10 minutes. Adjust the seasoning to taste. To serve, pour into individual bowls, sprinkle with grated Parmesan and drizzle with olive oil.

Amount per portion
Energy 200 kcals, Protein 9.5g, Fat 8.6g, Saturated fat 0.9g, Carbohydrate 22.6g, Total sugars 10.6g, Salt 1.71g, Sodium 674mg

Pappa al Pomodoro
with Borlotti Beans

The Italians eat a lot of bread, and they like it fresh. Being a thrifty nation they created this soup to use up leftovers, and very good it is too. I of course have gone a step further by adding beans for a better GI rating.

Serves 4

1 tablespoon olive oil
3 garlic cloves, finely chopped
2 shallots, finely diced
500g ripe tomatoes, deseeded
    and roughly chopped
500ml vegetable stock
500ml tomato passata
¼ teaspoon salt
1 teaspoon freshly ground black pepper
1 teaspoon caster sugar
400g day-old seeded bread, crusts removed
    and discarded, cut into 1cm cubes
leaves from 1 small bunch of basil, ripped
1 x 400g tin borlotti beans, drained
    and rinsed
1 tablespoon freshly grated Parmesan cheese

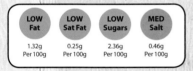

LOW Fat	LOW Sat Fat	LOW Sugars	MED Salt
1.32g Per 100g	0.25g Per 100g	2.36g Per 100g	0.46g Per 100g

1 Heat the oil in a large saucepan and over a medium heat cook the garlic and shallots for 4 minutes. Add the tomatoes and cook for a further 5 minutes. Add the stock, passata, salt and pepper and bring to the boil. Reduce the heat, add the sugar, bread and basil, cover and simmer for 30 minutes, stirring from time to time. Fold in the borlotti beans and warm through.
2 Adjust the seasoning to taste, spoon into individual bowls and sprinkle with a little Parmesan.

Amount per portion
Energy 402 kcals, Protein 16.3g, Fat 7.5g, Saturated fat 1.4g, Carbohydrate 72.0g, Total sugars 13.4g, Salt 2.62g, Sodium 1035mg

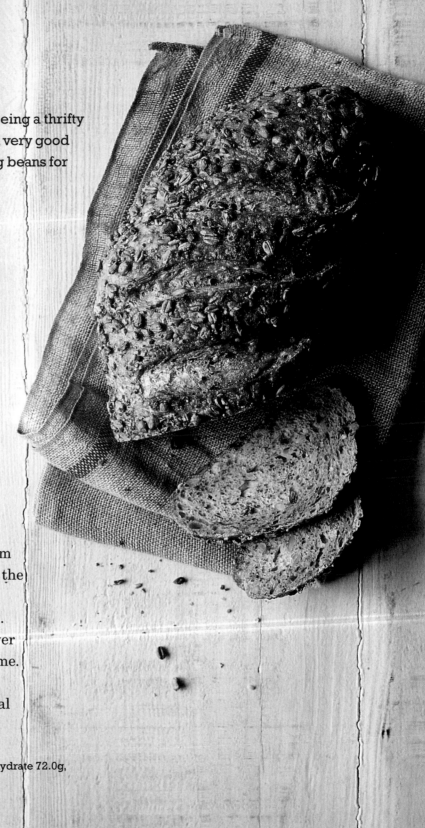

Pistou

A French version of the classic Italian minestrone, finished off with a small dollop of pistou sauce – similar to pesto but without the pine nuts. The good low-GI beans and chunky vegetables make this a great main-course soup.

Serves 4

2 tablespoons olive oil
1 large onion, roughly chopped
2 leeks, roughly chopped
4 new potatoes, roughly diced
2 carrots, sliced
1 celery stalk, thinly sliced
1.3 litres vegetable stock
3 bay leaves
1 x 400g tin chopped tomatoes
2 teaspoons tomato purée
2 courgettes, thickly sliced
85g extra fine French beans, cut into
    1cm pieces
50g frozen petit pois
1 x 400g tin cannellini beans, rinsed
1 x 400g tin flageolet beans, rinsed
salt and freshly ground black pepper

For the pistou sauce

4 garlic cloves
40g grated Parmesan cheese
14 fresh basil leaves

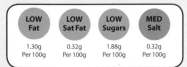

1 Heat half the oil in a large saucepan, then add the onion and leeks and cook over a medium heat for 8 minutes, stirring occasionally. Add the potatoes, carrots, celery, stock, bay leaves, tomatoes and tomato purée and stir. Bring to the boil and simmer for 20 minutes.

2 Add the courgettes, French beans, petit pois and tinned cannellini and flageolet beans, return to the boil and cook for a further 5 minutes. Season to taste.

3 Meanwhile, make the pistou. With a mortar and pestle or in a mini food processor blend the garlic, Parmesan and basil together with the remaining oil and a little water if necessary to make a smooth paste. Serve a small dollop on top of each bowl of soup.

Amount per portion
Energy 354 kcals, Protein 20.5g, Fat 11.5g, Saturated fat 2.8g, Carbohydrate 45.1g, Total sugars 16.6g, Salt 2.79g, Sodium 1099mg

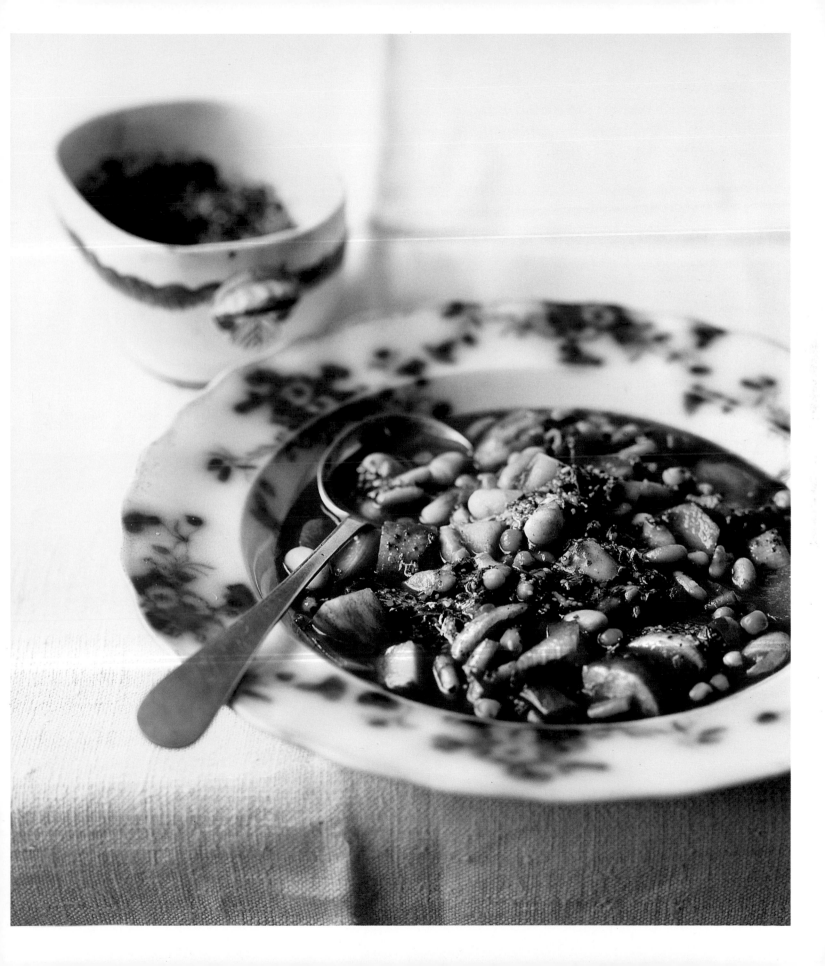

Harira

Harira is a chunky North African lamb and chickpea soup that is substantial enough to work as a good lunch when served with some crusty seeded bread. It's got loads of lovely flavours, a few of which I've added to the traditional recipe.

Serves 4

2 tablespoons olive oil
2 onions, chopped
2 garlic cloves, crushed to a paste with
    a little salt
200g lamb neck fillet, cut into 1½ cm cubes
2 tablespoons tomato purée
1 tablespoon harissa chilli paste
2 small sweet potatoes, cut into 1cm dice
1 x 400g tin chopped tomatoes
1 teaspoon ground ginger
a pinch of saffron
1 x 400g tin chickpeas, drained
1 litre lamb stock
85g fresh spinach, tough stems removed
2 tablespoons chopped fresh coriander
juice of 1 lemon
salt and freshly ground black pepper

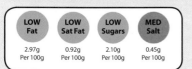

1 In a large saucepan heat the olive oil over a medium heat, then add the onions and garlic and fry gently until the onion has softened without colouring. Increase the heat and fry the lamb, stirring regularly, until brown all over, about 3 minutes.
2 Stir in the tomato purée and harissa, then add the sweet potatoes, tomatoes, ginger, saffron, chickpeas and lamb stock. Bring to the boil, reduce the heat and simmer gently for 1 hour.
3 Add the spinach, coriander and lemon juice, and cook until the spinach has wilted. Adjust the seasoning to taste and serve.

Amount per portion
Energy 391 kcals, Protein 21.2g, Fat 17.8g, Saturated fat 5.5g, Carbohydrate 39.0g, Total sugars 12.6g, Salt 2.71g, Sodium 1067mg

Avgolemono Soup

This is one of the first soups Jacinta, my wife, cooked for me – a legacy from her Greek ex-boyfriend. Simple and delicious.

Serves 4
1.5 litres good-quality chicken stock
115g quick cook long-grain brown rice
4 large eggs, beaten
juice of 2 large lemons
3 tablespoons chopped fresh parsley
salt and freshly ground pepper

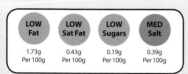

1 Bring the stock to the boil. Pour in the rice and cook over a medium heat for 15 minutes or until the rice is tender and cooked. Do not drain.

2 Combine the eggs with the lemon juice. When the rice is cooked, allow the stock to cool slightly then add a little to the egg mixture and whisk well. Pour the mix into the stock, stir, place over a low heat and stir continuously until the liquid has thickened and coats the back of a spoon. Do not allow to boil. Fold in the chopped parsley, season to taste and serve.

Tip Wash the rice under the cold running water before cooking to remove some of the starch. If using traditional brown rice, you will need to cook it for about 25 minutes.

Amount per portion
Energy 246 kcals, Protein 20.9g, Fat 8.0g, Saturated fat 2.0g, Carbohydrate 24.4g, Total sugars 0.9g, Salt 1.8g, Sodium 707mg

Fassoulada

Chock-full of vegetables and beans, this Greek soup is a wonderful main-course soup for a really cold day – and as a bonus, you just throw everything in together.

Serves 4
1 large onion, roughly chopped
2 carrots, sliced
2 leeks, sliced
2 celery stalks, sliced
4 garlic cloves, sliced
1 x 400g tin chopped tomatoes
2 tablespoons tomato purée
2 bay leaves
1 dried chilli, chopped
1 x 400g tin white butter beans, drained
1 litre vegetable stock
salt and freshly ground black pepper

To serve
4 slices seeded bread
2 tablespoons extra virgin olive oil

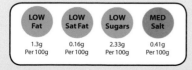

1 Put all the soup ingredients together in a large saucepan and stir, bring to the boil and simmer for 1 hour 15 minutes–1 hour 30 minutes. Season to taste.

2 Just before the soup is ready, toast the bread, drizzle each slice with a little olive oil and place in the bottom of individual warmed soup bowls. Pour on the soup and enjoy.

Amount per portion
Energy 286 kcals, Protein 11g, Fat 8g, Saturated fat 1g, Carbohydrate 44g, Total sugars 14.4g, Salt 2.56g, Sodium 1008mg

e Tuna Salade Niçoise Oinamul – Korean Cucumber Salad

nsalada Mista A Crunchy Pear and Walnut Salad A Lemong

h Cold Chicken and Two Cucumber Salad with Yogurt Dres

ad Spicy Lentil and Salmon Salad Posh Fried Rice Saffron P

Onions Charred Cauliflower, Tartare Flavours Spiced Chic

pice and Rice Dhal with Added Spice Green Vegetables w

es and Asian Influence Californian Cobb Salad Borlotti and

n and Prawn Salad Thai Papaya Salad Rare Tuna Salade Niç

Crunch An Eastern Salad Spanish Ensalada Mista A Crunc

nzanella Nutty, fruity Tabbouleh Cold Chicken and Two Cuc

nge, Cumin and Carrot Salad Spicy Lentil and Salmon Sala

Roasted Carrots and Baby Onions Charred Cauliflower, Ta

Curried Beans Fattoush Spice and Rice Dhal with Added S

ews Butterbeans with Chillies and Asian Influence Californ

Shoot, Mushroom and Prawn Salad Thai Papaya Salad Rare

almon, Beans and Crunch An Eastern Salad Spanish Ensala

se Dipping Sauce Panzanella Nutty, fruity Tabbouleh Cold C

essing Greek Salad Orange, Cumin and Carrot Salad Spicy

e Beans and Pine Nuts Roasted Carrots and Baby Onions C

s, Goat's Cheese & Mint Nutty Curried Beans Fattoush Spic

kpea and Potato Salad A Salad of Salmon, Beans and Crunc
Chicken and Peanut Salad Vietnamese Dipping Sauce Pan
Tomato Salad with Sumac and Garlic Dressing Greek Sala
laff Smashed Roast Butternut Salad with White Beans and P
s Griddled Courgettes with Chickpeas, Goat's Cheese & M
mond and Orange Stir-Fried Greens with Mustard Seeds a
tage Cheese Salad French Potato Salad Seafood and Lime S
Oinamul – Korean Cucumber Salad Chickpea and Potato S
ear and Walnut Salad A Lemongrass, Chicken and Peanut S
er Salad with Yogurt Dressing Tomato Salad with Sumac an

Salads and sides

sh Fried Rice Saffron Pea Pilaff Smashed Roast Butternut Sal
Flavours Spiced Chickpeas Griddled Courgettes with Chi
Green Vegetables with Almond and Orange Stir-Fried Gre
obb Salad Borlotti and Cottage Cheese Salad French Potat
a Salade Niçoise Oinamul – Korean Cucumber Salad Chick
ista A Crunchy Pear and Walnut Salad A Lemongrass, Chic
ken and Two Cucumber Salad with Yogurt Dressing Tomato
il and Salmon Salad Posh Fried Rice Saffron Pea Pilaff Smas
d Cauliflower, Tartare Flavours Spiced Chickpeas Griddle
d Rice Dhal with Added Spice Green Vegetables with Almo

Californian Cobb Salad

Americans love their salads, and this one is a classic, often served in neat lines of different ingredients, but, to be honest, if you want to toss it all together, please feel free to do so.

Serves 8

1 iceberg lettuce
1 romaine or cos lettuce
1 bunch of watercress
1 small head of chicory, leaves separated
8 medium tomatoes, peeled, deseeded and diced
2 cooked chicken breasts, diced
100g crisp cooked bacon, crumbled
1 avocado, diced
3 eggs, hard-boiled and chopped
2 tablespoons chopped fresh chives
50g Roquefort blue cheese, crumbled into pieces
toast or cornbread, to serve

For the dressing

1 tablespoon red wine vinegar
1 teaspoon sugar or granulated low-calorie sweetener
1 teaspoon lemon juice
½ teaspoon ground black pepper
1 teaspoon Worcestershire sauce
1 teaspoon English mustard
3 garlic cloves, chopped
3 tablespoons olive oil

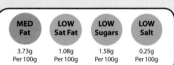

MED Fat	LOW Sat Fat	LOW Sugars	LOW Salt
3.73g Per 100g	1.08g Per 100g	1.58g Per 100g	0.25g Per 100g

1 First make the dressing by putting all the dressing ingredients in a clean jam jar, sealing and shaking to emulsify. Chill until required and shake before serving.

2 Shred the lettuces and in a salad bowl combine them with the watercress and chicory. Scatter the tomatoes over the top, together with the chicken and bacon, then decorate with pieces of avocado and sprinkle over the chopped eggs, chives and Roquefort. Just before serving pour over some dressing and mix thoroughly. Delicious served with toast or cornbread.

Tip Depending on the degree of oiliness desired, you can add a little water to the dressing.

Amount per portion
Energy 242 kcals, Protein 17.8g, Fat 14.9g, Saturated fat 4.3g, Carbohydrate 6.3g, Total sugars 6.1g, Salt 1g, Sodium 402mg

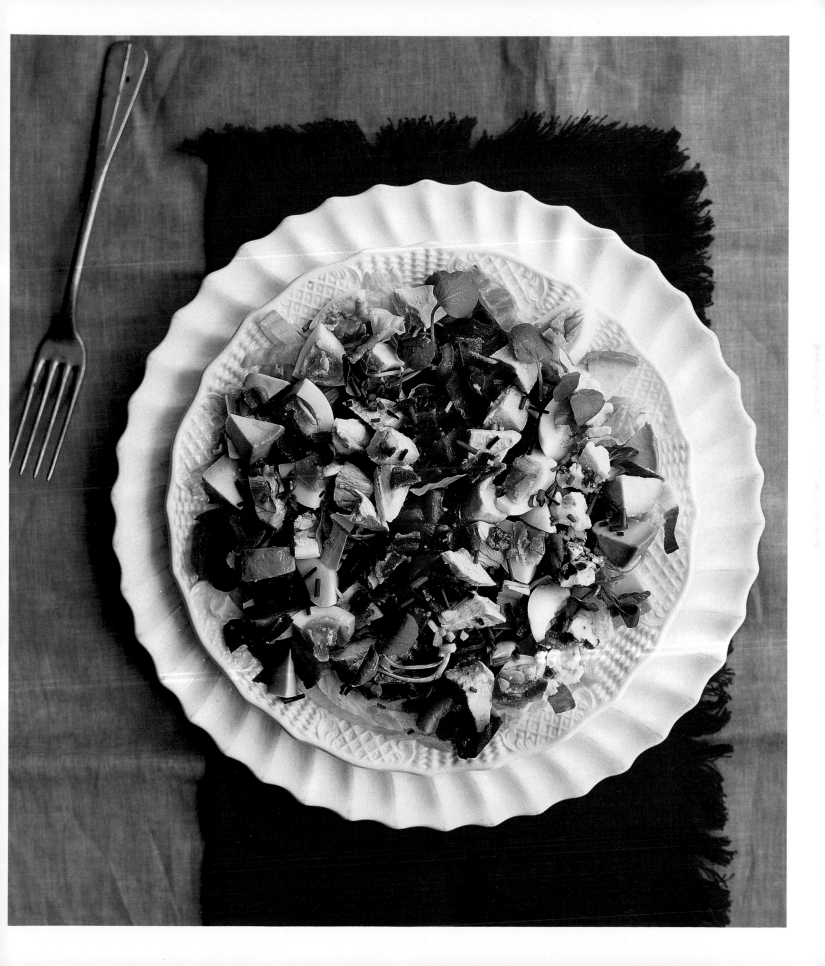

Borlotti and Cottage Cheese Salad

In this simple Italian salad, it's important that the beans be warm when you add the other ingredients.

Serves 4

1 x 400g tin borlotti beans, drained
    and rinsed
2 tablespoons extra virgin olive oil
1 tablespoon fresh lemon juice
1 teaspoon dried oregano
¼ teaspoon crushed chilli flakes
110g cottage cheese
3 tablespoons roughly chopped fresh
    flat-leaf parsley, to garnish
salt and freshly ground black pepper

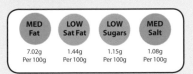

1 Put the beans in a saucepan, add cold water to cover and heat until warmed through but do not allow to boil.

2 Drain the hot beans well and transfer to a large mixing bowl. Stir in the remaining ingredients except the parsley, being careful to retain some consistency to the cottage cheese.

3 Just before serving adjust the seasoning to taste. Garnish with parsley and serve immediately.

Amount per portion
Energy 140 kcals, Protein 7.9g, Fat 7.3g, Saturated fat 1.5g, Carbohydrate 11.3g, Total sugars 1.2g, Salt 1.12g, Sodium 444mg

French Potato Salad

Most people associate potato salad with mayonnaise, but actually a vinaigrette-style dressing is excellent.

Serves 4

16 waxy new potatoes (Charlotte,
    Ratte, Pink Fir)
2 slices rustic seeded bread, cut into
    1cm pieces
1 garlic clove, crushed to a paste
    with a little salt
80ml dry white wine
40ml extra virgin olive oil
2 teaspoons Dijon mustard
1 tablespoon white wine vinegar
2 shallots, finely chopped
5 cornichons (baby gherkins), finely sliced
1 tablespoon non-pareille capers
    (baby capers)
2 tablespoons chopped fresh parsley
salt and freshly ground black pepper

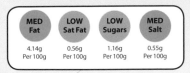

1 Preheat oven to 180°C/350°F/gas mark 4. Cook the potatoes in boiling salted water until tender, about 20 minutes. Drain and when cool enough to handle, cut into 1cm slices.

2 Meanwhile, place the bread pieces on a baking tray and toast in the preheated oven until they have turned into crispy croûtons, about 12 minutes.

3 While they are toasting, whisk together the garlic, white wine, olive oil, mustard and vinegar. Season to taste then fold in the shallots, cornichons, capers and parsley. Pour this flavoured vinaigrette over the warm potatoes. Just before serving, fold in the croûtons.

Tip Non-pareille is a type of small caper generally considered to be of the finest quality.

Amount per portion
Energy 240 kcals, Protein 4.4g, Fat 10.3g, Saturated fat 1.4g, Carbohydrate 31.0g, Total sugars 2.9g, Salt 1.36g, Sodium 536mg

Seafood and Lime Salad

This Middle Eastern-style salad is just right for a summer lunch or supper, with loads of citrus and fennel flavours, and can be eaten warm or cold. You can vary the choice of seafood, but the balance in this recipe works well for me.

Serves 4
500g mussels in their shells, cleaned
    and any open mussels discarded
100ml dry white wine
2 shallots, finely diced
3 garlic cloves, crushed to a paste
    with a little salt
1 fennel bulb, outside leaves removed,
    the rest very thinly sliced
1 small red onion, thinly sliced
¼ savoy cabbage, finely shredded
1 carrot, grated
8 new potatoes, cooked and quartered
1 tablespoon chopped fresh dill
1 tablespoon snipped fresh chives
2 tablespoons extra virgin olive oil
12 raw tiger prawns, shell-off and deveined
225g cleaned squid tubes, opened up
    and cut into 2cm squares
1 tablespoon sumac
grated zest and juice of 2 limes
1 mild red chilli, deseeded and thinly sliced
salt and freshly ground black pepper

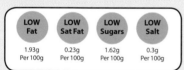

LOW Fat	LOW Sat Fat	LOW Sugars	LOW Salt
1.93g Per 100g	0.23g Per 100g	1.62g Per 100g	0.3g Per 100g

1 Pop the mussels into a large saucepan and add the wine, shallots and a third of the garlic. Cover tightly and cook over a high heat, shaking the pan occasionally, for 4–5 minutes. With a slotted spoon lift the mussels to a bowl, discarding any that have not opened. Return the cooking liquor to the heat and boil until only 2–3 tablespoons remain, then strain into a bowl and retain. When the mussels have cooled enough to handle, scoop the flesh into a bowl and discard the shells.

2 Mix together the fennel, onion, cabbage, carrot, cooked potatoes and herbs.

3 Heat the oil in a frying pan then, in batches, cook the prawns and squid over a high heat for about 1 minute each side. Add them to the vegetables, then fry the mussel flesh briefly (45 seconds) and add them to the salad.

4 Into the oily fish pan pour the mussel juices to combine with the oil, season to taste and heat for 1 minute, then pour this hot liquid over the salad. Add the sumac, lime zest and juice and the chilli, and toss well. Serve immediately, or leave to cool and refrigerate for up to 24 hours.

Amount per portion
Energy 249 kcals, Protein 22.8g, Fat 8.3g, Saturated fat 1.0g, Carbohydrate 20.1g, Total sugars 7.0g, Salt 1.29g, Sodium 512mg

Pea Shoot, Mushroom and Prawn Salad

Fresh, delicious pea shoots, harvested from the growing tips of pea plants, are all the rage at the moment and they're becoming commercially more widely available in Britain. Of course, you could always get gardening and grow your own …

Serves 4
115g pea shoots
50g button mushrooms, quartered
115g cooked North Atlantic prawns, shell-off

For the dressing
2 teaspoons English mustard powder
1 teaspoon sugar or granulated low-calorie
  sweetener
1 tablespoon cider vinegar or white wine
  vinegar
1 tablespoon chopped fresh mint
1 teaspoon snipped fresh chives
freshly ground black pepper

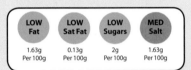

LOW Fat	LOW Sat Fat	LOW Sugars	MED Salt
1.63g Per 100g	0.13g Per 100g	2g Per 100g	1.63g Per 100g

1 In a large bowl, mix together the pea shoots, mushrooms and prawns. Mix together all the dressing ingredients, and thin with a little water if needed. Stir the dressing into the salad.

Tip If you have time, leave the dressing to rest for 30 minutes for the flavours to develop before you mix it into the salad. Delicious served with bread to mop up the juices.

Amount per portion (sugar)
Energy 55 kcals, Protein 9.1g, Fat 1.3g, Saturated fat 0.1g, Carbohydrate 1.9g, Total sugars 1.6g, Salt 0.66g, Sodium 259mg

Amount per portion (low-calorie sweetener)
Energy 52 kcals, Protein 9.1g, Fat 1.3g, Saturated fat 0.1g, Carbohydrate 1.0g, Total sugars 0.6g, Salt 0.66g, Sodium 259mg

Thai Papaya Salad

A refreshing oriental salad, to which you can add prawns and crabmeat for a more substantial offering.

Serves 4
2 hard green papayas, peeled, deseeded
  and grated
2 garlic cloves, finely chopped
2 small red chillies, deseeded and
  finely sliced
4 tomatoes, deseeded and diced
50g peanuts, chopped
4 tablespoons chopped fresh mint
2 tablespoons chopped fresh coriander
grated zest and juice of 2 limes
1½ tablespoons runny honey
1 tablespoon dried shrimp powder
crusty bread, to serve

LOW Fat	LOW Sat Fat	LOW Sugars	LOW Salt
2.55g Per 100g	0.45g Per 100g	3.32g Per 100g	0.15g Per 100g

1 Mix together all the ingredients and allow the flavours to develop for 15 minutes before serving. Serve with crusty bread.

Tip Shrimp powder is ground dried shrimps and is often used as a flavouring in oriental soups, salads and stir-fries.

Amount per portion
Energy 146 kcals, Protein 7.0g, Fat 6.3g, Saturated fat 1.1g, Carbohydrate 16.4g, Total sugars 8.2g, Salt 0.37g, Sodium 149mg

RIGHT Pea Shoot, Mushroom and Prawn Salad

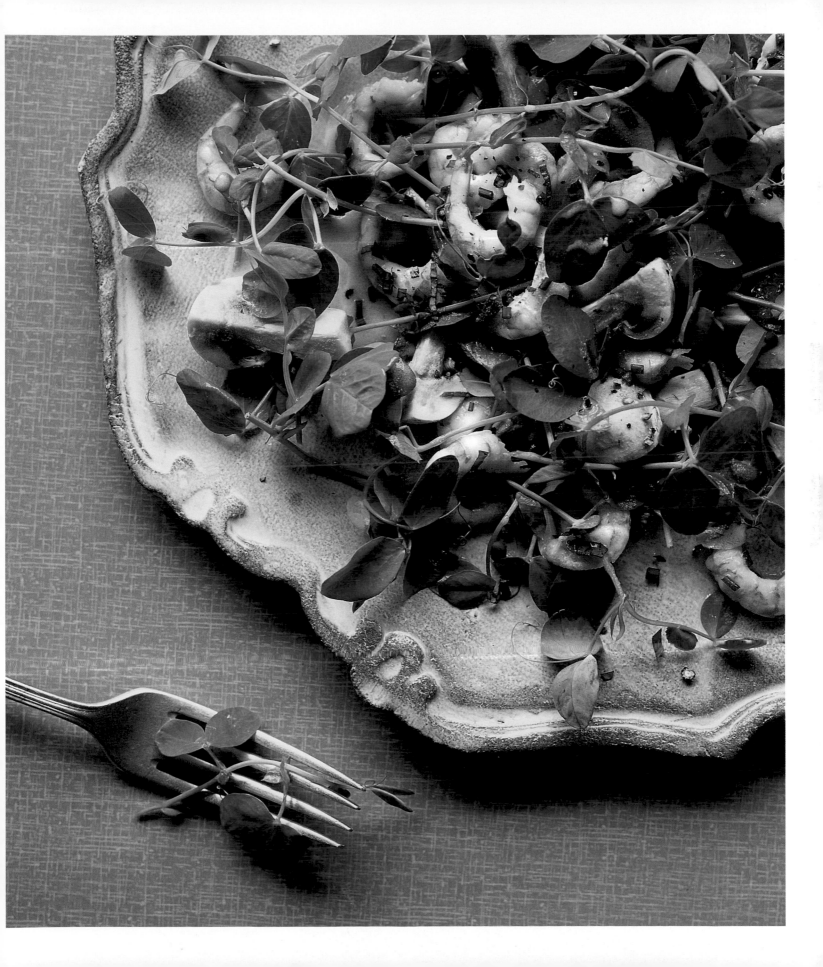

Rare Tuna Salade Niçoise

When in the south of France, I love the Niçoise salad served in the beach shacks on the coast.
They, of course, use tinned tuna, but this version uses fresh.

Serves 4
4 x 115g fresh tuna steaks, each approx
   2.5cm thick
16 new salad potatoes
2 eggs, at room temperature
85g extra fine French beans, trimmed
2 little gem lettuce hearts, quartered
   lengthways and separated into leaves
2 plum tomatoes, roughly chopped
½ red onion, finely sliced
2 anchovy fillets, cut lengthways into
   thin strips
12 stoned black olives in brine, drained
8 fresh basil leaves, torn

For the marinade
2 tablespoons extra virgin olive oil
1 tablespoon aged red wine vinegar
1 tablespoon chopped fresh flat-leaf parsley
1 tablespoon snipped fresh chives
1 garlic clove, finely chopped
salt and freshly ground black pepper

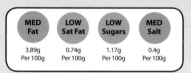

MED Fat	LOW Sat Fat	LOW Sugars	MED Salt
3.89g Per 100g	0.74g Per 100g	1.17g Per 100g	0.4g Per 100g

1 First make the marinade. In a bowl, whisk together the olive oil, vinegar, parsley, chives, garlic and 1 teaspoon each of salt and pepper. Lay the tuna in a shallow non-metallic dish and pour over half the marinade. Cover with clingfilm and refrigerate for 1 hour to allow the flavours to penetrate the tuna, turning the fish over occasionally. Set the remaining marinade aside.

2 Bring a pan of salted water to the boil, add the potatoes, cover and simmer for 10–12 minutes or until just tender. Drain then cut into quarters lengthways.

3 Put the eggs in a small pan and just cover with boiling water, then cook for 8 minutes. Drain and rinse under cold running water, then remove the shells and cut each egg into quarters lengthways – the yolks should still be slightly soft.

4 Plunge the beans into a pan of boiling salted water and blanch for 3 minutes or so, then drain and refresh under cold running water.

5 Heat a griddle pan to very hot. Remove the tuna from the marinade, shaking off any excess. Cook the tuna steaks for about 2 minutes each side, depending on how rare you like your fish.

6 Arrange the lettuce leaves on to individual plates or one large platter and add the potatoes, French beans, tomatoes, onion and anchovies. Place the tuna steaks on top and drizzle over the remaining marinade. Scatter over the eggs, olives and torn basil leaves to serve.

Tip Tuna becomes exceedingly dry when overcooked, so watch it!

Amount per portion
Energy 353 kcals, Protein 34.6g, Fat 15.3g, Saturated fat 2.9g, Carbohydrate 20.6g, Total sugars 4.6g, Salt 1.56g, Sodium 614mg

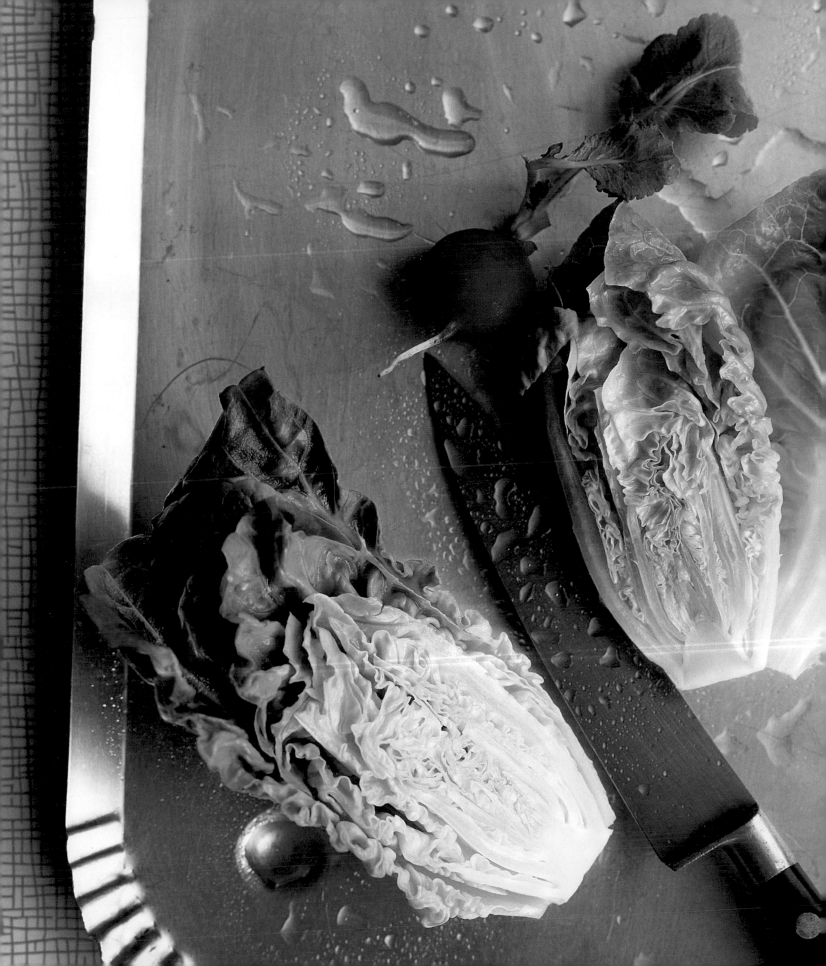

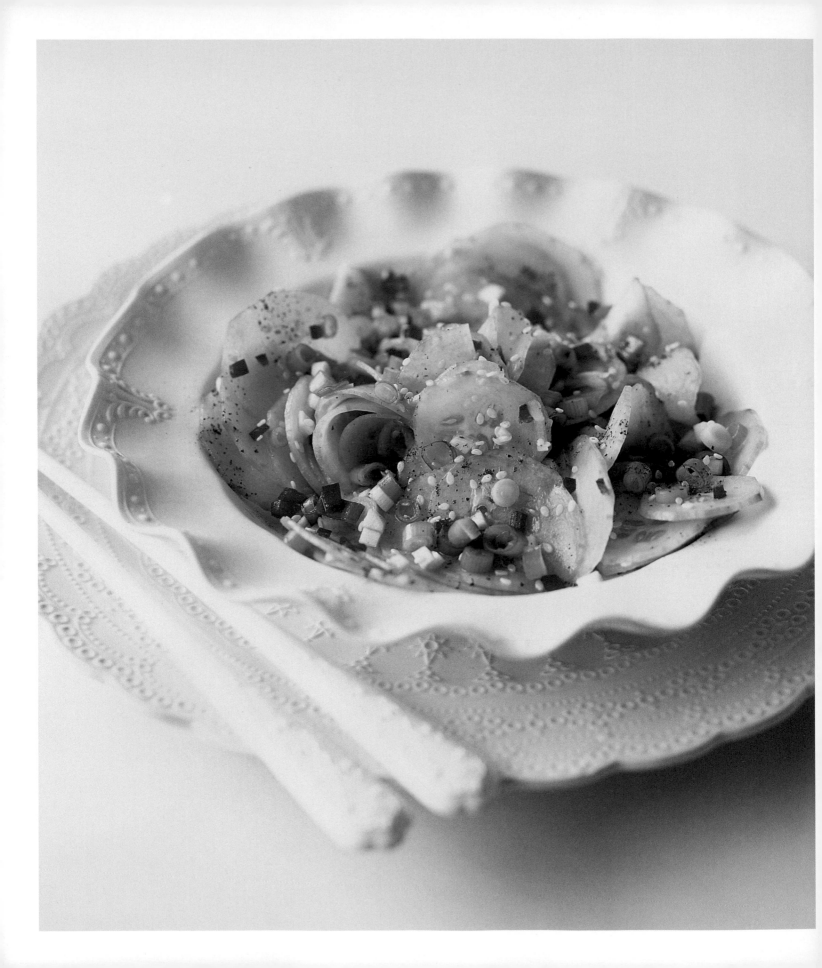

Oinamul – Korean Cucumber Salad

A very refreshing salad that is a good accompaniment to grilled or stewed meats.

Serves 4
1 cucumber, peeled and thinly sliced
1 teaspoon salt
3 spring onions, chopped
1 fresh red chilli, deseeded and
    finely chopped
1 tablespoon sesame oil
3 garlic cloves, finely chopped
1 teaspoon sesame seeds
¼ teaspoon chilli powder
1 teaspoon roasted unsalted
    peanuts, chopped
seeded bread, to serve

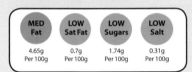

MED Fat	LOW Sat Fat	LOW Sugars	LOW Salt
4.65g Per 100g	0.7g Per 100g	1.74g Per 100g	0.31g Per 100g

1 Put the cucumber into a colander, sprinkle the salt over and mix well, then set aside for 30 minutes to drain some of the cucumbers' natural liquid. Rinse them in fresh water and squeeze them well to remove as much liquid as possible.

2 Mix together all the remaining ingredients then add the cucumber and mix well. This will keep, covered and in the fridge, for 3–4 days. Serve with seeded bread.

Tip You could omit the salting stage but you would then need to eat the salad within an hour or so, otherwise the flavour will become diluted with the cucumber juices.

Amount per portion
Energy 51 kcals, Protein 1.5g, Fat 4.0g, Saturated fat 0.6g, Carbohydrate 2.3g, Total sugars 1.5g, Salt 0.27g, Sodium 104mg

Chickpea and Potato Salad

A beneficial Indian-influenced salad that has great slow-release qualities; it's excellent as a light lunch, with some crusty seeded bread and a bowl of soup. You'll probably find it difficult to source one of the ingredients, anardana – dried pomegranate seeds – so omit it if you haven't got an Asian or Middle Eastern shop nearby.

Serves 4
8 new potatoes, cubed
1 red onion, finely sliced
½ red pepper, cut into 1cm dice
175g watermelon, cut into 2cm dice
1 x 400g tin chickpeas, drained
grated zest and juice of 1 lemon
2 teaspoons chopped fresh mint
1 teaspoon caster sugar
2 tablespoons fresh pomegranate seeds
1 teaspoon anardana (dried pomegranate
    seeds), coarsely ground
salt and freshly ground black pepper

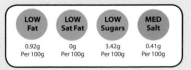

LOW Fat	LOW Sat Fat	LOW Sugars	MED Salt
0.92g Per 100g	0g Per 100g	3.42g Per 100g	0.41g Per 100g

1 Cook the potatoes in boiling salted water until tender, about 10 minutes, and drain them. While the potatoes are still warm, mix them together with the remaining ingredients and season to taste.

Amount per portion
Energy 147 kcals, Protein 6.2g, Fat 2.2g, Saturated fat 0.0g, Carbohydrate 27.3g, Total sugars 8.2g, Salt 0.98g, Sodium 387mg

LEFT Oinamul – Korean
Cucumber Salad

A Salad of Salmon, Beans and Crunch

Choose wild salmon if you can afford it, otherwise look for a farmed salmon with a good pedigree. This salad has some lovely elements, and enough going on for you to not say, 'oh, no, not salmon again!'

Serves 4

1 x 450g salmon fillet
1 carrot, sliced
1 onion, halved
2 bay leaves
12 black peppercorns
3 slices seeded bread, crusts removed, ripped into small pieces
200g extra fine French beans, topped, tailed and cut in 1cm pieces
200g podded broad beans, raw
200g drained and rinsed tinned white beans
1 tablespoon extra virgin olive oil
juice of ½ lemon
2 tablespoons low-fat mayonnaise
1 teaspoon each snipped fresh chives, chopped fresh parsley and chopped fresh tarragon
salt and freshly ground black pepper

To serve

salad leaves
lemon wedges

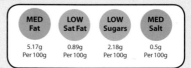

MED Fat	LOW Sat Fat	LOW Sugars	MED Salt
5.17g Per 100g	0.89g Per 100g	2.18g Per 100g	0.5g Per 100g

1 Preheat the oven to 180°C/350°F/gas mark 4. Put the salmon fillet in a saucepan along with the carrot, onion, bay leaves and peppercorns. Cover with water, bring to the boil and immediately switch off the heat. Leave in the water to cool.

2 Put the bread pieces into a food processor and pulse until you have rustic crumbs. Tip them onto a baking tray and bake for 15 minutes until crisp and golden. Set aside.

3 Fill a saucepan three-quarters full with water, season with salt and bring to the boil. Add the French beans and cook for 2 minutes, then add the broad beans and cook for a further 2 minutes. Add the white canned beans and warm through, then drain and stir in the oil and lemon juice and season to taste.

4 Flake the salmon onto individual plates. Mix together the mayonnaise and herbs and place a dollop on top of the salmon. Scatter with the beans and serve with dressed salad leaves and lemon wedges, topped with crispy crumbs.

Amount per portion
Energy 417 kcals, Protein 33g, Fat 18g, Saturated fat 3.1g, Carbohydrate 33g, Total sugars 7.6g, Salt 1.75g, Sodium 688mg

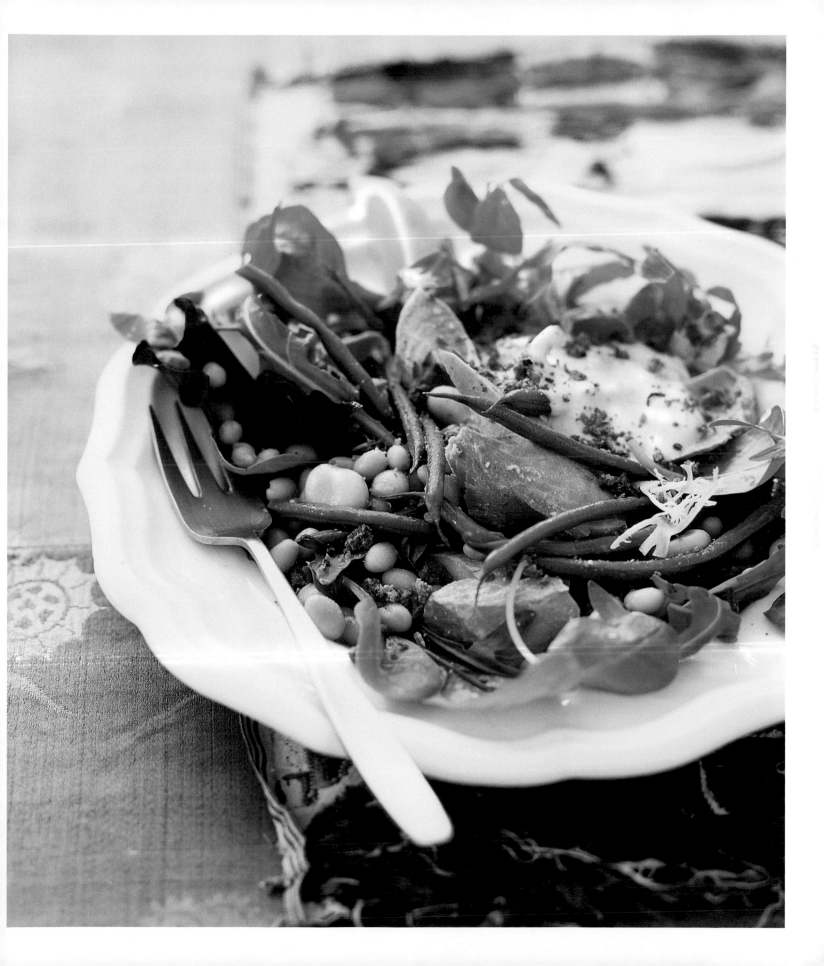

An Eastern Salad

This is the sort of dish I'll have for lunch on a day off – it's easy to prepare, you can use most salad ingredients or vegetables, and when you've finished eating you'll feel satisfied and a little bit virtuous.

Serves 4

For the dressing
85g unsalted roasted peanuts
90ml lime juice
30ml fish sauce (nam pla)
2 teaspoons caster sugar
4 garlic cloves
3 tablespoons roughly chopped
   fresh coriander
2 hot Thai chillies, deseeded

For the salad
1 head of baby gem lettuce, leaves
   separated
2 tomatoes, roughly diced
1 carrot, thinly sliced
½ cucumber, peeled, seeded and cut
   into 1cm half-moons
85g small broccoli florets
2 shallots, thinly sliced
½ red pepper, deseeded and cut into
   small dice
115g tofu, cubed
115g edamame beans, blanched briefly
   in boiling water
½ bunch of coriander leaves
10 fresh basil leaves, shredded
8 fresh mint leaves, shredded
2 hard-boiled eggs, cut into wedges

1 To make the dressing, in a blender or food processor blend together half the peanuts with all the remaining ingredients.
2 Mix together all the salad ingredients except the eggs, and toss with the dressing. Arrange on to individual plates and garnish with the eggs and the remaining peanuts.

Amount per portion
Energy 295 kcals, Protein 18.8g, Fat 17.3g, Saturated fat 3.5g, Carbohydrate 16.9g, Total sugars 10.4g, Salt 1.62g, Sodium 640mg

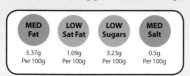

MED Fat	LOW Sat Fat	LOW Sugars	MED Salt
5.37g Per 100g	1.09g Per 100g	3.23g Per 100g	0.5g Per 100g

Spanish Ensalada Mista

Having a house in Spain inevitably means trying out various Spanish dishes, some good, some not so good. Before I tried this salad, I wasn't a fan of tinned asparagus, but it sort of grows on you.

Serves 4

1 head of romaine lettuce
2 tomatoes, each cut into 6 pieces
1 small cucumber, peeled, seeded
    and sliced
½ yellow or red onion, thinly sliced
1 red or yellow pepper, sliced into strips
1 x 280g jar grilled artichoke hearts,
    drained
1 carrot, grated
1 x 185g tin tuna steak in spring water,
    drained
2 eggs, hard-boiled and cut into quarters
1 x 425g tin white asparagus, drained
50g anchovy-stuffed green olives
2 tablespoons extra virgin olive oil
1 tablespoon sherry vinegar
freshly ground black pepper
crusty bread, to serve

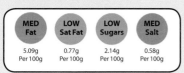

MED Fat	LOW Sat Fat	LOW Sugars	MED Salt
5.09g Per 100g	0.77g Per 100g	2.14g Per 100g	0.58g Per 100g

1 Break up the lettuce into small pieces, and on a large platter make a bed of lettuce. Top with the tomatoes, cucumber, onions, red or yellow pepper, artichoke hearts and carrot. Break the tuna up into small chunks with a fork then spread it out around the bed of lettuce. Place the egg quarters, asparagus and olives all over the salad.

2 Dress with oil and vinegar, and sprinkle with pepper to taste. Serve with some bread.

Tip Every family in Spain has their own version of Ensalada Mista, so it is slightly different in every household – therefore, don't worry if you are missing one of the ingredients.

Amount per portion

Energy 287 kcals, Protein 16.0g, Fat 20.4g, Saturated fat 3.1g, Carbohydrate 10.7g, Total sugars 8.6g, Salt 2.33g, Sodium 917mg

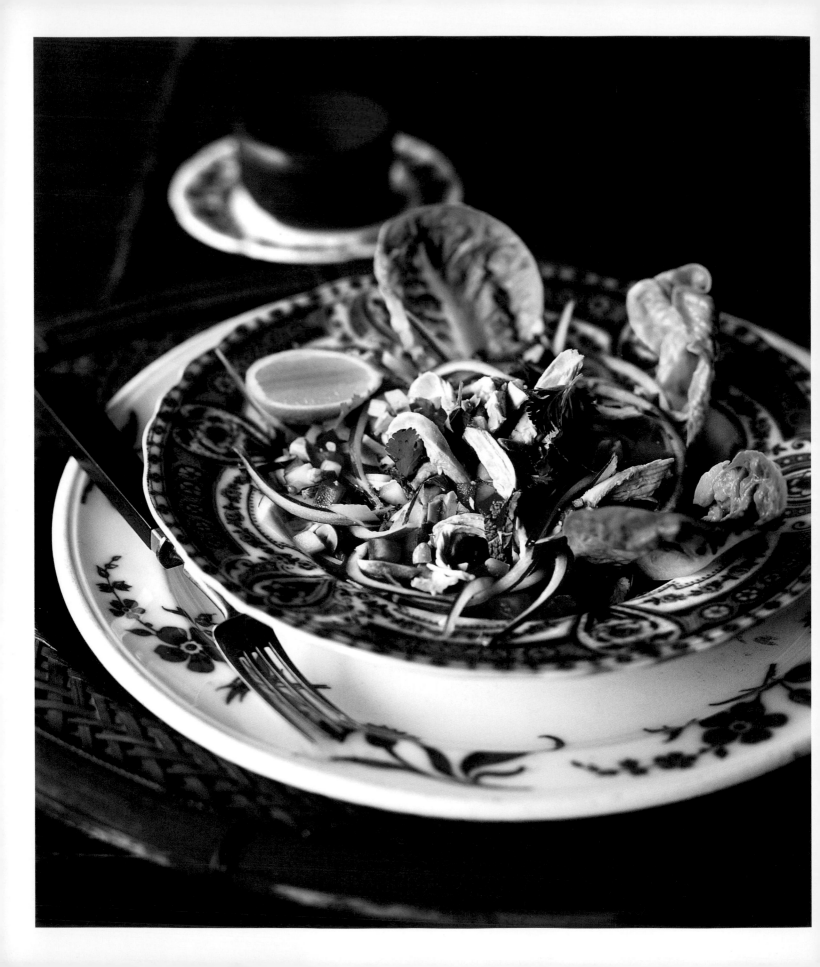

Lemongrass, Chicken and Peanut Salad

I love most Asian salads and now that so many Asian ingredients are readily available in the UK they're easy to put together. This one from Brunei is pretty fiery, but chillies are good for you!

Serves 4

500g cooked chicken breast, shredded
1 red onion, chopped
½ cucumber, deseeded and diced
1 bird's eye chilli, deseeded and finely
    diced
1 each red and green mild chilli, cut in
    thin shreds
1 small bunch of fresh coriander, chopped
12 fresh mint leaves, shredded
2 gem lettuces, leaves separated
3 tomatoes, deseeded and diced
1 tablespoon roasted peanuts, chopped
lime wedges, to serve

For the peanut dressing

2 tablespoons lime juice
1 tablespoon fish sauce (nam pla)
2 teaspoons caster sugar
1 tablespoon crunchy peanut butter

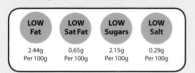

LOW Fat	LOW Sat Fat	LOW Sugars	LOW Salt
2.44g Per 100g	0.65g Per 100g	2.15g Per 100g	0.29g Per 100g

1 In a bowl mix together the chicken, onion, cucumber, chillies, coriander and mint.

2 Make the dressing: In a separate bowl, whisk together the lime juice, fish sauce, sugar and peanut butter, thinning it down with a little water if too thick.

Mix the dressing into the salad.

3 Scatter gem lettuce leaves on to individual plates. Spoon the salad over the lettuce leaves and garnish with diced tomato and chopped peanuts, and serve with lime wedges.

Amount per portion
Energy 272 kcals, Protein 41.4g, Fat 8.3g, Saturated fat 2.2g, Carbohydrate 8.6g, Total sugars 7.3g, Salt 0.98g, Sodium 388mg

Panzanella

This delicious Tuscan salad traditionally makes use of up to 3-day old bread – soaked in water and squeezed dry before being added to the salad – but I prefer to use fresher bread, rubbed with garlic and grilled for an added crunch.

Serves 4

2 tablespoons extra virgin olive oil
3 x 1cm-thick slices ciabatta
3 garlic cloves, 2 of them finely chopped
2 anchovy fillets
1 tablespoon non-pareille capers (baby capers), drained
2 tablespoons aged red wine vinegar
2 tablespoons chopped fresh flat-leaf parsley
4 plum tomatoes, deseeded and cubed
1 small red onion, finely sliced
½ cucumber, cut lengthways, deseeded and cut into 1cm chunks
2 celery stalks, finely sliced
12 fresh basil leaves, ripped
50g stoned black olives, chopped
salt and freshly ground black pepper

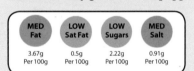

1 Dribble some of the oil on both sides of the ciabatta bread, then grill both sides on a barbecue or under a grill. Rub both sides with the unchopped garlic clove, then rip the bread into 1cm cubes. Set aside.

2 In a mini food processor or with a mortar and pestle, blend together the chopped garlic, anchovies and capers with about half a teaspoon of sea salt. Add the remaining olive oil, vinegar and the parsley and pulse the food processor until the ingredients are combined into a dressing.

3 In a bowl, mix together the bread and all the remaining ingredients, and toss with the anchovy dressing. Season to taste with black pepper.

Amount per portion
Energy 137 kcals, Protein 3.7g, Fat 8.1g, Saturated fat 1.1g, Carbohydrate 13.2g, Total sugars 4.9g, Salt 2.02g, Sodium 799mg

Nutty, Fruity Tabbouleh

So often you see this Middle Eastern salad as a big bowl of white grains with a few flecks of green, when traditionally it's all green with a few flecks of white. This version has a few nice additions too.

Serves 4

75g quick-cook cracked or bulgar wheat
juice of 2 lemons
1 tablespoon extra virgin olive oil
50g fresh flat-leaf parsley, chopped
15g fresh mint, chopped
1 bunch of spring onions, finely sliced
25g pistachio nuts, chopped
25g brazil nuts, chopped
25g sultanas
50g dried apricots, chopped
3 plum tomatoes, deseeded and diced
salt and freshly ground black pepper

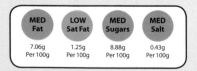

1 Soak the cracked wheat in cold water for 20 minutes, then drain and squeeze dry. Put the wheat in a large glass bowl, season with salt and pepper, and stir in the lemon juice and olive oil. Leave to rest for 30 minutes.

2 Mix in the parsley, mint, spring onions, nuts and fruit. Adjust the seasoning to taste and top with the plum tomatoes.

Amount per portion
Energy 236 kcals, Protein 6.3g, Fat 11.3g, Saturated fat 2.0g, Carbohydrate 29.1g, Total sugars 14.2g, Salt 0.68g, Sodium 268mg

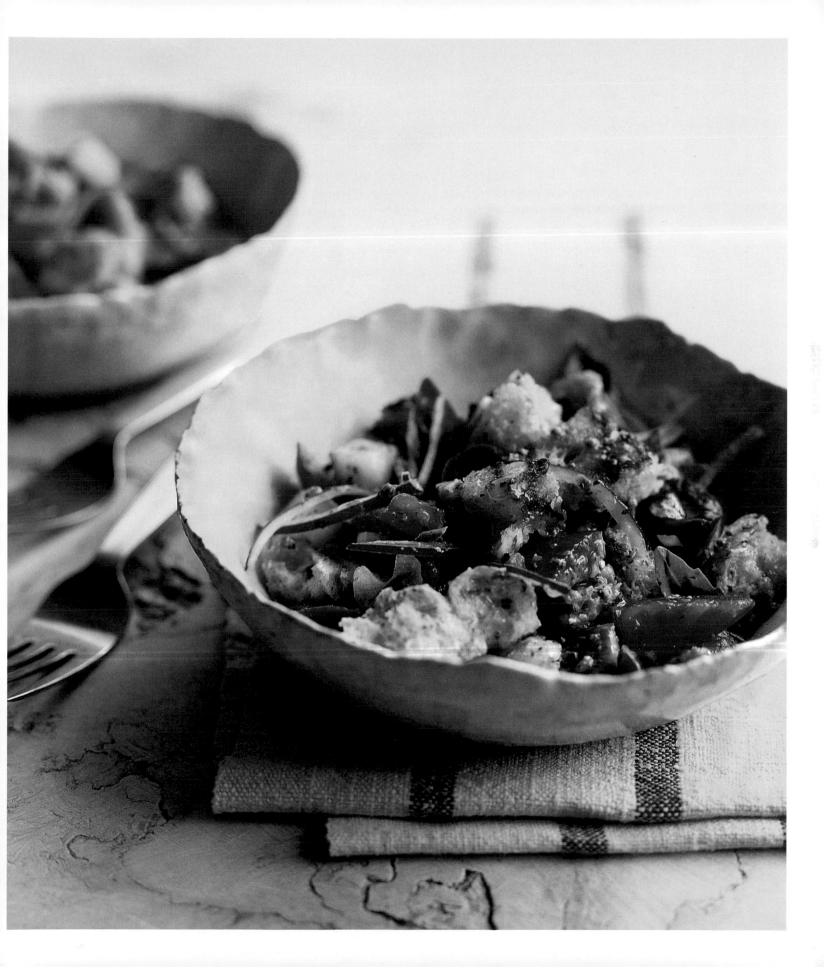

Cold Chicken and Two Cucumber Salad with Yogurt Dressing

This Scandivanian salad is good and summery and filled with popular flavours.

Serves 4
12 new potatoes, scrubbed and halved
450g cooked chicken, cut into bite-sized
pieces
1 cucumber, peeled, deseeded and diced
2 sour gherkins, sliced
salt and freshly ground black pepper

For the dressing
1 tablespoon grain mustard
2 teaspoons runny honey
½ small bunch of fresh dill, chopped
120g 0 per cent fat natural Greek yogurt
juice of ½ lemon

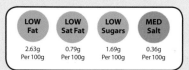

LOW Fat	LOW Sat Fat	LOW Sugars	MED Salt
2.63g Per 100g	0.79g Per 100g	1.69g Per 100g	0.36g Per 100g

1 This one is easy peasy: in one bowl mix all the dry ingredients together, then in a separate bowl combine all the dressing ingredients. Stir the dressing into the salad, season to taste, and serve.

Variation This works well with many meats or fish, but it works particularly well with cooked salmon.

Amount per portion
Energy 321 kcals, Protein 36.8g, Fat 9.3g, Saturated fat 2.8g, Carbohydrate 24.2g, Total sugars 6.0g, Salt 1.28g, Sodium 503mg

Tomato Salad with Sumac and Garlic Dressing

This ever-so-simple Middle Eastern salad is great as part of a meze buffet or with grilled fish – very garlicky, very delicious, with citrussy notes from the sumac. Serve with bread to mop up the juices.

Serves 4
6 garlic cloves
2 tablespoons 0 per cent fat natural
Greek yogurt
1 tablespoon extra virgin olive oil
3 beef tomatoes (I like the Jack Hawkins
variety), sliced
1 tablespoon sumac
1 teaspoon chopped fresh mint
freshly ground black pepper

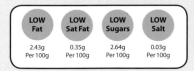

LOW Fat	LOW Sat Fat	LOW Sugars	LOW Salt
2.43g Per 100g	0.35g Per 100g	2.64g Per 100g	0.03g Per 100g

1 In a mini food processor blend together the garlic, yogurt and olive oil to a smooth dressing, and season with pepper.
2 Arrange the tomato slices on a flat plate, spread over the garlic dressing, and sprinkle with sumac and mint.

Variation If you like your dressing a little tart, add a squeeze of lemon juice.

Amount per portion
Energy 66 kcals, Protein 2.3g, Fat 3.5g, Saturated fat 0.5g, Carbohydrate 6.8g, Total sugars 3.8g, Salt 0.05g, Sodium 19mg

Greek Salad

There is something about a Greek salad that reminds me of sunshine and holidays. You'll never really get the true taste as the Greeks use the dried flower heads of the oregano, but this recipe is still great. This is best served as a side dish with some lean meat or fish.

Serves 4
4 plum tomatoes, each cut into 6 pieces
½ cucumber, peeled and cut into 1cm
    chunks
50g Kalamata olives, stoned
1 small red onion, thinly sliced
2 teaspoons fresh oregano leaves
85g feta cheese

For the dressing
1 tablespoon extra virgin olive oil
1 tablespoon aged red wine vinegar
1 teaspoon dried Greek oregano
1 garlic clove, finely chopped
freshly ground black pepper

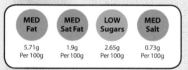

MED Fat	MED Sat Fat	LOW Sugars	MED Salt
5.71g Per 100g	1.9g Per 100g	2.65g Per 100g	0.73g Per 100g

1 Whisk all the dressing ingredients together and set aside for 30 minutes for the flavours to meld.
2 Mix all the salad ingredients except the feta into a large serving bowl. Shake the dressing, pour it over the salad and toss to coat. Pass the feta through a sieve to create a 'snow' effect over the salad.

Tip Delicious served with bread to mop up the fresh juices from the salad.

Amount per portion
Energy 138 kcals, Protein 4.9g, Fat 10.8g, Saturated fat 3.6g,
Carbohydrate 5.9g, Total sugars 5.0g,
Salt 1.38g, Sodium 547mg

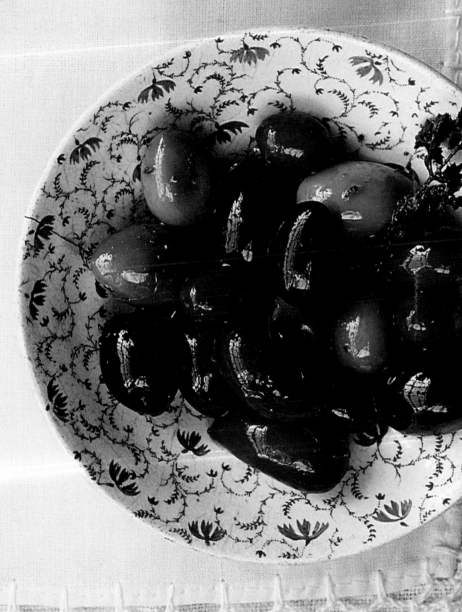

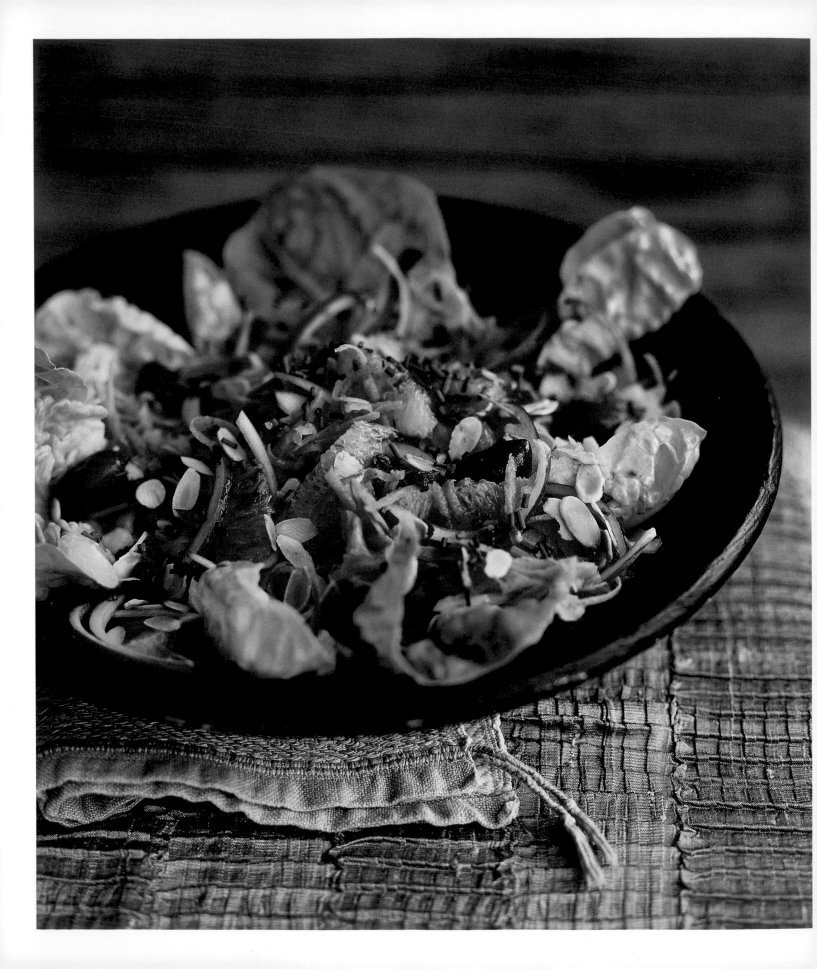

Orange, Cumin and Carrot Salad

A light refreshing African salad that is excellent on its own or with some seeded bread, tossed through some couscous or as an accompaniment to grilled meat or fish. If you want to impress, serve it in hollowed-out orange halves.

Serves 4

2 teaspoons cumin seeds
4 navel oranges, 1 zested,
    the remainder peeled
2 tablespoons extra virgin olive oil
1 tablespoon harissa chilli paste
2 carrots, grated
½ red onion, thinly sliced
50g black kalamata olives, stoned
50g toasted flaked almonds
1 tablespoon snipped fresh chives
salt and freshly ground black pepper
baby gem or cos lettuce, to serve

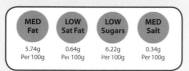

MED Fat	LOW Sat Fat	LOW Sugars	MED Salt
5.74g Per 100g	0.64g Per 100g	6.22g Per 100g	0.34g Per 100g

1 Heat a small frying pan then add the cumin seeds and toast until fragrant, then crush them with a mortar and pestle or in a small grinder.

2 Working over a bowl to catch the juices and using a small sharp knife, cut out the orange flesh by cutting between the membranes and drop the flesh into the bowl. Squeeze any juice remaining in the membranes into the bowl and discard any pips. To make the salad dressing, whisk together the olive oil, harissa and cumin, and set aside.

3 Just before serving mix the orange segments with the zest, carrots, onion, olives and almonds. Stir in the dressing, season to taste and sprinkle with the chives. Serve on baby gem or cos lettuce leaves.

Amount per portion
Energy 251 kcals, Protein 6g, Fat 17g, Saturated fat 1.9g, Carbohydrate 20g, Total sugars 18.4g, Salt 1.01g, Sodium 398mg

Spicy Lentil and Salmon Salad

This Middle Eastern-influenced salad is quick to put together and very nutritious, with lovely flavours and a spicy kick. I've used tinned lentils here but feel free to cook your own. Puy lentils are probably the best as they don't collapse easily. And there's nothing to stop you poaching your own salmon, but here I am trying to speed things up a little.

Serves 4

4 new potatoes, cut into ½ cm dice
1 x 400g tin brown lentils
120g 0 per cent fat natural Greek yogurt
1 tablespoon harissa chilli paste
1 garlic clove, crushed
1 small red onion, thinly sliced
leaves from 1 small bunch of fresh
    flat-leaf parsley
1 fresh red chilli, deseeded and thinly sliced
1 x 200g tin wild red Alaskan salmon, flaked
freshly ground black pepper

LOW Fat	LOW Sat Fat	LOW Sugars	MED Salt
2.39g Per 100g	0.46g Per 100g	1.37g Per 100g	0.61g Per 100g

1 Boil the potatoes in lightly salted water for 10 minutes or until tender, then drain. Meanwhile, gently heat the lentils in a saucepan.

2 Combine the yogurt with the harissa and garlic. Fold this dressing into the lentils, along with the onion, parsley leaves, chilli and potatoes. Season to taste. Spoon into a serving bowl, then scatter over the salmon flakes.

Amount per portion
Energy 177 kcals, Protein 17.0g, Fat 4.7g, Saturated fat 0.9g, Carbohydrate 17.8g, Total sugars 2.7g, Salt 1.21g, Sodium 475mg

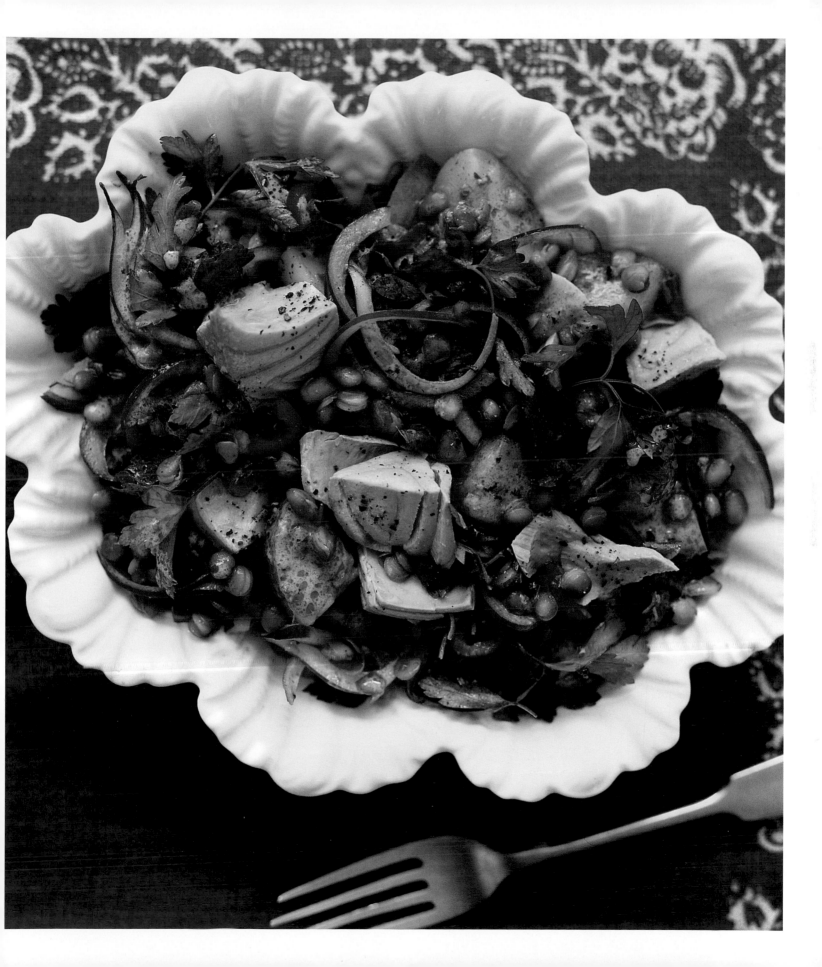

Posh Fried Rice

There's something particularly naughty-but-nice about fried rice, and it is the prefect dish for using up leftovers, a sort of Asian bubble and squeak. Ingredients can be varied to cater for personal taste or according to availability, but here is my suggestion.

Serves 4

2 x packets 2-minute brown rice
2 teaspoons sesame oil
100g shell-off tiger prawns, raw
1 tablespoon sunflower oil
2 eggs, beaten
1 garlic clove, finely chopped
1 hot chilli, deseeded and finely chopped
100g cooked chicken, shredded
100g French beans, cut into 1cm pieces,
    blanched briefly in boiling water
100g cooked cabbage or bok choi,
    shredded
1 carrot, cut into 1cm dice, blanched
    briefly in boiling water
3 spring onions, sliced
¼ teaspoon chilli powder
2 teaspoons soy sauce
1 teaspoon chicken stock granules
1 small can of Alaskan crabmeat, drained

To serve
chilli, spring onions and cucumber batons

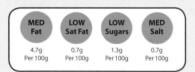

MED Fat	LOW Sat Fat	LOW Sugars	MED Salt
4.7g Per 100g	0.7g Per 100g	1.3g Per 100g	0.7g Per 100g

1 Microwave the rice according to the instructions on the packet. Set aside.

2 Heat the sesame oil in a wok to very hot and fry the prawns for 1 minute each side. Remove and set aside.

3 Add the sunflower oil to the wok then fry the beaten eggs along with the garlic and fresh chilli, breaking up the egg mixture with a wooden spoon. Remove and set aside.

4 Add the rice to the wok and fry until starting to crisp. Add the chicken, beans, cabbage, carrot and spring onions and toss to mix well. Mix in the prawns and eggs, along with the chilli powder, soy sauce and stock granules, and heat through briefly.

5 Arrange on individual warmed plates and scatter with crabmeat. Serve with fresh chilli, spring onion and cucumber batons.

Amount per portion
Energy 346 kcals, Protein 24.6g, Fat 12.5g, Saturated fat 1.9g, Carbohydrate 35.8g, Total sugars 3.6g, Salt 1.81g, Sodium 714mg

Saffron Pea Pilaf

Dishes mixing rice and peas are popular worldwide, and this one from Kashmir is particularly lovely. It has great colour and a lovely blend of spices, nuts and fruit. Serve it on its own, or as a partner to a stew or tagine.

Serves 4
225g basmati rice
1 tablespoon olive oil
25g flaked almonds
8 walnut halves, roughly chopped
2 tablespoons raisins
8 dried apricots, diced
4 cloves
2 cardamom pods
2.5cm cinnamon stick
12 black peppercorns
375g fresh or frozen peas
½ teaspoon saffron, soaked in
    1 tablespoon hot water
4 spring onions, finely sliced
600ml vegetable or chicken stock
3 tablespoons chopped fresh coriander
salt and freshly ground pepper

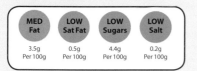

MED Fat — 3.5g Per 100g
LOW Sat Fat — 0.5g Per 100g
LOW Sugars — 4.4g Per 100g
LOW Salt — 0.2g Per 100g

1 Wash the rice and drain it well. Melt the butter in a saucepan and fry the almonds and walnuts until the nuts are golden brown and fry the raisins and apricots until they are plumped up. Remove and set aside.

2 To the same pan add the cloves, cardamom, cinnamon and peppercorns, and fry them over a low heat, stirring continuously, until they become aromatic. Stir in the peas, saffron and its soaking liquor, spring onions and rice, and cook for 2 minutes, stirring to ensure the rice is coated with butter.

3 Add the stock and bring to the boil, then reduce the heat, cover with a tightly fitting lid and simmer for about 20 minutes or until the rice has cooked. Stir in the coriander, nuts and fruit, and season to taste.

Amount per portion
Energy 440 kcals, Protein 14.6g, Fat 13.1g, Saturated fat 1.8g, Carbohydrate 70.4g, Total sugars 16.3g, Salt 1.03g, Sodium 406mg

Smashed Roast Butternut Salad with White Beans and Pine Nuts

I love butternut squash in many guises. This salad with the added GI value of the beans and pine nuts is perfect with some boiled ham, or simply spread on some toasted sesame bread.

Serves 4

1 teaspoon ground fennel
1 teaspoon ground coriander
1 teaspoon dried mint
½ teaspoon chilli flakes
1 butternut squash, unpeeled, halved
    lengthways, deseeded and each
    half cut into 4 wedges
spray olive oil
¼ teaspoon ground cinnamon
juice of 1 lemon
6 tablespoons 0 per cent fat natural
    Greek yogurt
2 teaspoons Dijon mustard
1 x 400g tin cannellini beans, drained
2 tablespoons toasted pine nuts
1 tablespoon snipped fresh chives,
    to garnish
salt and freshly ground black pepper

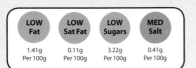

LOW Fat	LOW Sat Fat	LOW Sugars	MED Salt
1.41g Per 100g	0.11g Per 100g	3.22g Per 100g	0.41g Per 100g

1 Preheat the oven to 200°C/400°F/gas mark 6.

2 Mix together the ground fennel, ground coriander, dried mint and chilli. Spread the butternut squash wedges on to a roasting tin, spray them with olive oil then dust with the spice/herb mix, and then dust with cinnamon. Spray a sheet of greaseproof paper with olive oil and place oiled-side down over the butternut.

3 Roast in the oven for 30 minutes, then remove the greaseproof paper and roast for a further 20 minutes. Remove from the oven and leave to cool, then scrape the flesh off the skin into a bowl.

4 Meanwhile, combine the lemon juice, yogurt and Dijon mustard, then fold in the cannellini beans and pine nuts. Gently mix with the butternut so as not to break up the squash too much. Season to taste and garnish with chives.

Variation Substitute fresh mint for the chives if you prefer.

Amount per portion
Energy 205 kcals, Protein 10.8g, Fat 5.2g, Saturated fat 0.4g, Carbohydrate 30.9g, Total sugars 11.9g, Salt 1.53g, Sodium 602mg

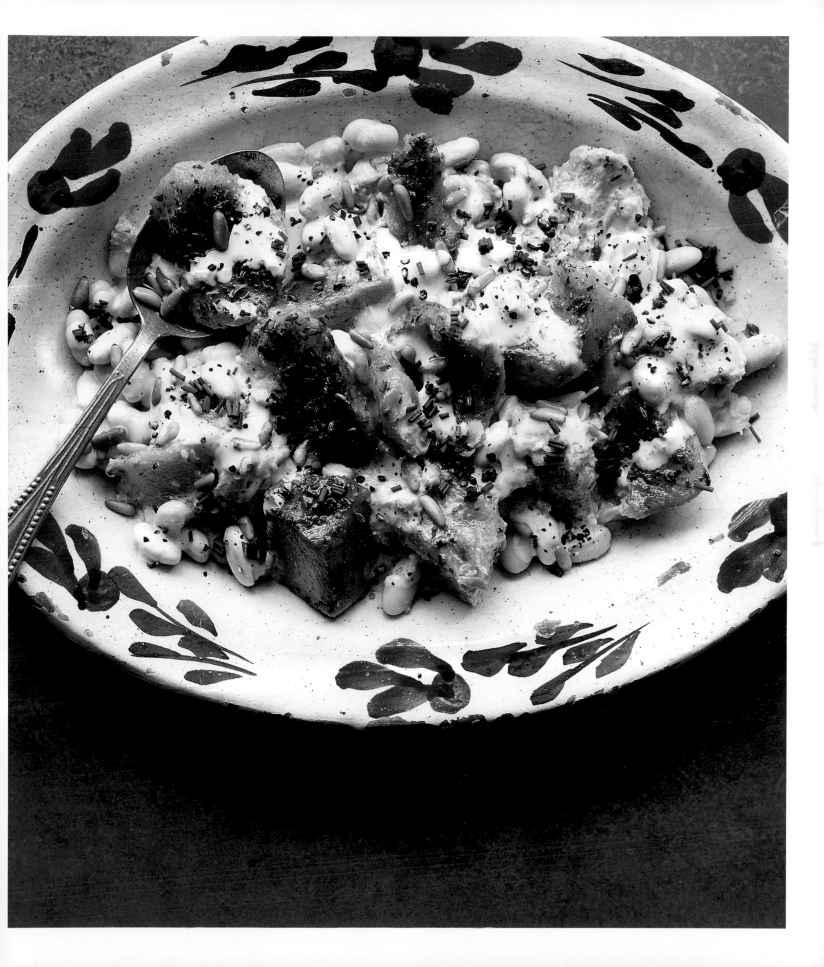

Roasted Carrots and Baby Onions

A delicious American sweet-and-sour carrot dish that goes perfectly with roast chicken.

Serves 4
spray sunflower oil
2 shallots, finely diced
2 garlic cloves, finely chopped
2 tablespoons orange juice
1 tablespoon raisins
1 tablespoon cider vinegar
1 tablespoon sunflower oil
grated zest of ½ orange
grated zest of ½ lemon
1 tablespoon black treacle
1 tablespoon tomato ketchup
1 teaspoon Coleman's English mustard
1 teaspoon Worcestershire sauce
1 teaspoon Tabasco sauce
450g carrots
225g baby onions
salt

To serve
¼ teaspoon fresh soft thyme leaves
1 tablespoon snipped fresh chives
1 tablespoon chopped fresh flat-leaf parsley
1 tablespoon toasted flaked almonds

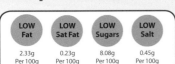

LOW Fat	LOW Sat Fat	LOW Sugars	LOW Salt
2.33g Per 100g	0.23g Per 100g	8.08g Per 100g	0.45g Per 100g

1 Preheat the oven to 180°C/350°F/gas mark 4. Spray a heavy-based saucepan with oil and place over a medium heat. Add the shallots and garlic and cook for 6 minutes to colour and soften.

2 Pour the orange juice into a food processor, add the raisins, vinegar and oil and blend until smooth. Add this mixture to the shallot mix in the saucepan, along with 300ml of water, the orange and lemon zests, treacle, ketchup, mustard, Worcestershire sauce, Tabasco and ¼ teaspoon of salt. Bring to a simmer and simmer for 10 minutes.

3 Put the carrots and onions in a roasting tin and pour over the hot sauce mixture, stirring to coat the vegetables. Roast for about 45 minutes or until the vegetables are tender, basting with the sauce mixture every 10 minutes. Just before serving, toss in the herbs and almonds.

Amount per portion
Energy 128 kcals, Protein 2.9g, Fat 5.1g, Saturated fat 0.5g, Carbohydrate 18.8g, Total sugars 17.7g, Salt 0.98g, Sodium 387mg

Charred Cauliflower with Tartare Flavours

Plain boiled cauliflower is not fun, cauliflower cheese is high in fat, so this French recipe zaps it up enough that you'll be glad to add it to your list of vegetable dishes. It also works as a delicious accompaniment to grilled salmon.

Serves 4

1 tablespoon non-pareille capers (baby capers)
3 cornichons (baby gherkins), sliced
1 shallot, diced
1 garlic clove, crushed to a paste with a little sea salt
1 hard-boiled egg, chopped
1 tablespoon chopped fresh parsley
2 teaspoons snipped fresh chives
2 teaspoons chopped fresh tarragon
1 tablespoon wholegrain Dijon mustard
1 tablespoon tarragon vinegar
60ml extra virgin olive oil
½ cauliflower, broken into florets, blanched in boiling water for 3 minutes
handful of baby spinach leaves
12 cherry tomatoes, halved
salt and freshly ground pepper

1 In a bowl, mix together the capers, cornichons, shallot, garlic, egg and herbs. In another bowl, whisk together the mustard and vinegar then slowly add two thirds of the oil. Mix this dressing with the flavoured egg mixture and season to taste.

2 Heat the remaining oil in a frying pan or griddle pan and over a fierce heat cook the cauliflower florets until charred on all sides – you may need to cook the florets in batches.

3 While the florets are still warm, mix them with the dressing, then fold in the spinach and tomatoes and adjust the seasoning to taste. Serve hot or at room temperature.

Amount per portion
Energy 210 kcals, Protein 8.3g, Fat 17.1g, Saturated fat 2.4g, Carbohydrate 6.2g, Total sugars 4.9g, Salt 1.31g, Sodium 518mg

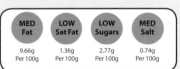

MED Fat	LOW Sat Fat	LOW Sugars	MED Salt
9.66g Per 100g	1.36g Per 100g	2.77g Per 100g	0.74g Per 100g

Spiced Chickpeas

I've prepared this recipe as a vegetable side dish. But it's also excellent at room temperature as a salad, and, once puréed and with more chickpeas added, it can be served on toasted seeded bread as a snack.

Serves 4

2 teaspoons sunflower oil
1 teaspoon aniseed
1 large onion, roughly chopped
2 garlic cloves, finely chopped
¼ small savoy cabbage, shredded
1 teaspoon mango powder
1 teaspoon chilli powder
½ teaspoon ground turmeric
½ teaspoon salt
1 teaspoon sugar
1 x 400g tinned chickpeas, drained and rinsed

1 Heat the oil in a saucepan or frying pan and fry the aniseed until it starts to pop. Add the onion and fry gently for 6 minutes. Add the remaining ingredients apart from the chickpeas and stir-fry for 5 minutes. Add the chickpeas and heat through for 2 minutes.

Tip Mango powder, also known as amchoor, is an Indian ingredient used in curries, pickles and chutneys and also used as a souring and tenderising agent.

Amount per portion
Energy 138 kcals, Protein 6.6g, Fat 4.5g, Saturated fat 0.3g, Carbohydrate 19.1g, Total sugars 7.1g, Salt 0.87g, Sodium 344mg

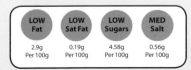

LOW Fat	LOW Sat Fat	LOW Sugars	MED Salt
2.9g Per 100g	0.19g Per 100g	4.58g Per 100g	0.56g Per 100g

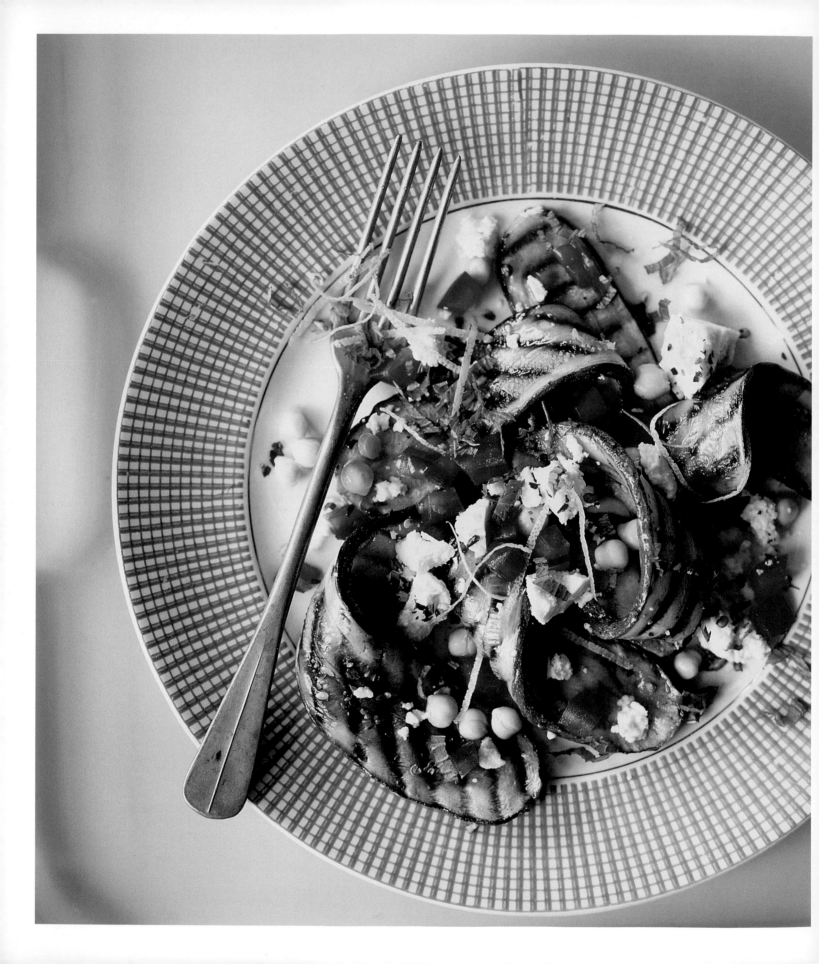

Griddled Courgettes with Chickpeas, Goat's Cheese and Mint

I file this fresh and vibrant magpie collection of Italy, Greece and the Middle East under 'Australia' because that's where I ate it. It's fantastically easy to make.

Serves 4
3 courgettes, each cut in 5 sliced lengthways
2 tablespoons extra virgin olive oil
50g crumbled goat's cheese
2 ripe tomatoes, deseeded and diced
400g tinned chickpeas, drained and rinsed
1 tablespoon chopped fresh mint
grated zest and juice of 1 lemon
½ teaspoon chilli flakes
salt and freshly ground black pepper

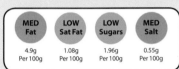

MED Fat	LOW Sat Fat	LOW Sugars	MED Salt
4.9g Per 100g	1.08g Per 100g	1.96g Per 100g	0.55g Per 100g

1 Preheat a griddle or frying pan, brush the courgette slices with some olive oil and cook for 1–2 minutes each side until grill-marked. Season to taste and arrange higgledy-piggledy onto a large platter.

2 Scatter the courgettes with the goat's cheese, tomatoes and chickpeas, and drizzle with the remaining olive oil. Sprinkle on the mint, lemon zest and chillies, then drizzle with the lemon juice and adjust the seasoning to taste.

Amount per portion
Energy 176 kcals, Protein 9g, Fat 10g, Saturated fat 2.2g, Carbohydrate 14g, Total sugars 4g, Salt 1.12g, Sodium 442mg

Fattoush

This lovely crunchy, herby salad is often served as part of Middle Eastern meze buffets. I've substituted a herby yogurt for the normal olive oil, and oven-cooked the pitta bread instead of frying it.

Serves 4

1 wholemeal pitta bread, halved horizontally and cut into small squares
1 baby gem lettuce
20 fresh mint leaves
1 small bunch of fresh parsley
1 small bunch of fresh coriander
2 beef tomatoes, deseeded and diced
6 French breakfast radishes, quartered
6 spring onions
1 small green pepper, deseeded and finely sliced
handful of watercress sprigs
1 small cucumber, deseeded and diced
juice and grated zest of 1 lemon
1 teaspoon sumac
3 tablespoons 0 per cent fat natural yogurt
salt and freshly ground black pepper

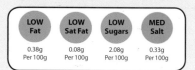

LOW Fat	LOW Sat Fat	LOW Sugars	MED Salt
0.38g Per 100g	0.08g Per 100g	2.08g Per 100g	0.33g Per 100g

1 Preheat the oven to 180°C/350°F/gas mark 4. Lay the pitta squares on a baking tray and toast them in the oven for 8–10 minutes until crisp. Remove and set aside.

2 Finely chop the lettuce, then finely chop the mint, then the parsley and then the coriander. Retain one teaspoon each of mint, parsley and coriander, and in a serving bowl mix the remaining herbs with the lettuce.

3 Add the tomatoes, radishes, spring onions, green pepper, watercress and cucumber. Toss in the lemon juice and zest, sumac, some salt and pepper and the pitta squares. Mix the yogurt with the reserved herbs, drizzle over the salad and mix.

Variation For a more substantial salad add a few hard-boiled eggs.

Amount per portion
Energy 73 kcals, Protein 4.0g, Fat 1.0g, Saturated fat 0.2g, Carbohydrate 12.7g, Total sugars 5.5g, Salt 0.87g, Sodium 342mg

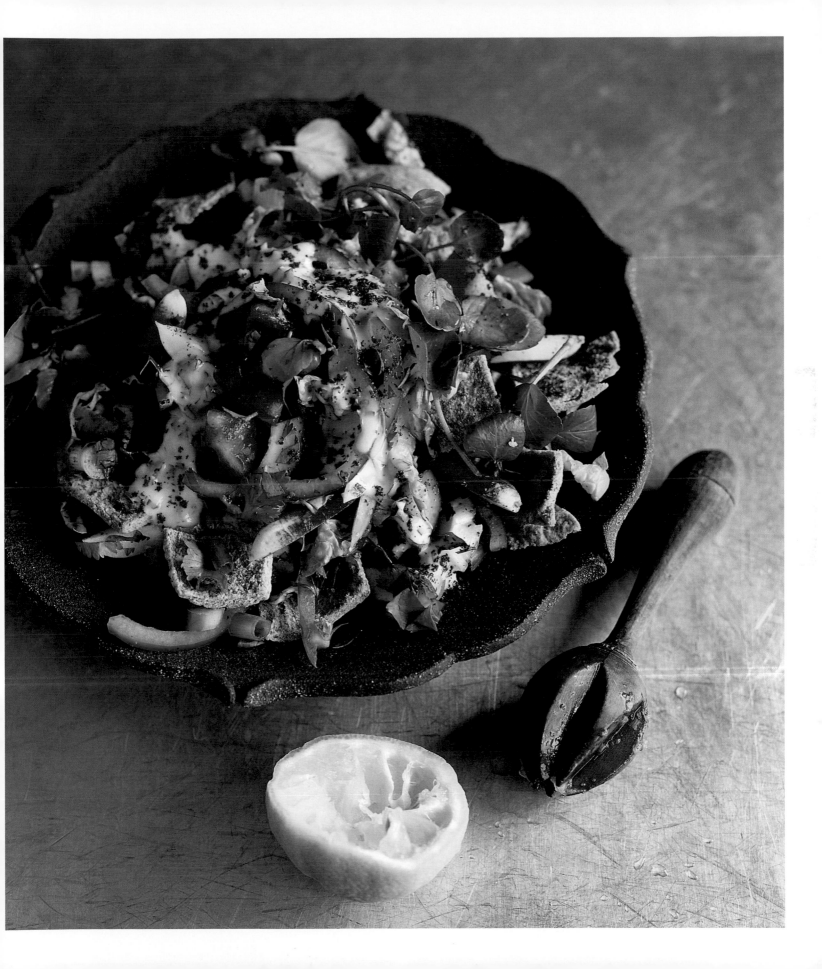

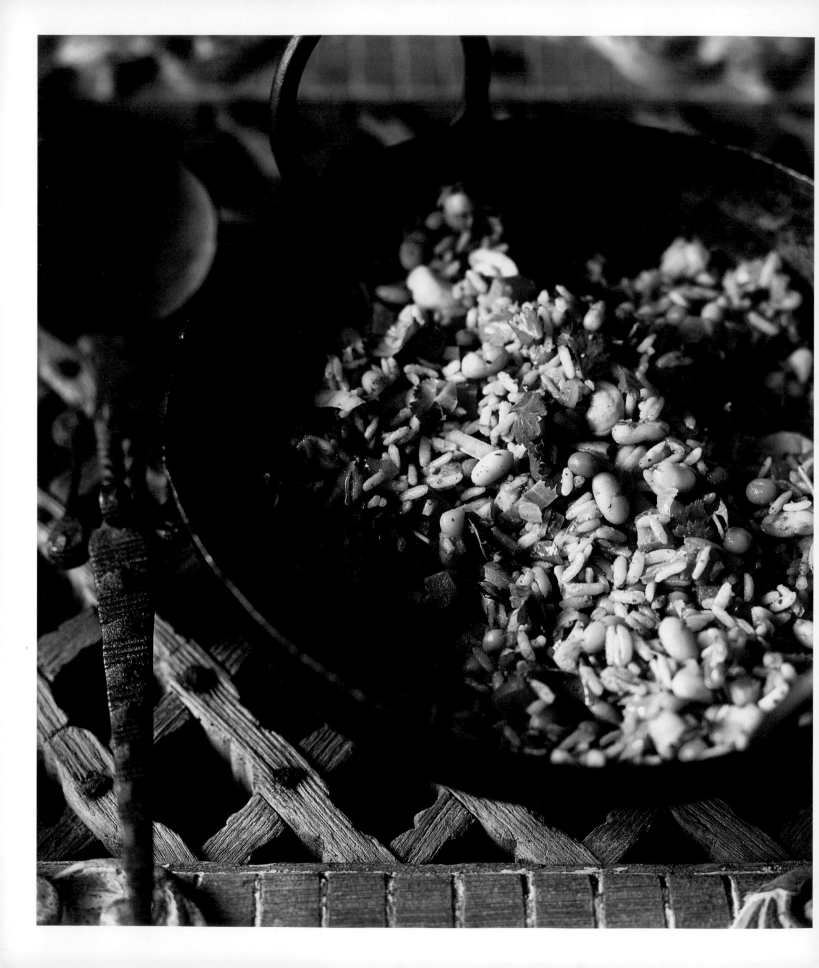

Spice and Rice

Let's face it, the word 'dull' often springs to mind in relation to brown rice, but not in this case. There are times when I could eat a bowl of this delicious Indian-style rice on its own. It's very filling and contains much of what we need in an all-round balanced diet. Here I've used a handy microwave rice; it's a little more expensive but for people in a hurry it's very useful.

Serves 4
2 teaspoons sunflower oil
½ teaspoon fenugreek seeds
¼ teaspoon asafoetida powder (optional)
2 hot red chillies, deseeded and finely diced
1 teaspoon ground coriander
2 teaspoons gram lentils (channa dal)
2 teaspoons tamarind paste, diluted
  in a little hot water
1 onion, finely diced
1 garlic clove, finely chopped
1 carrot, cut into ½ cm cubes
100g frozen peas, defrosted
1 x 400g tin haricot beans, drained
2 tablespoons roughly chopped
  cashew nuts
2 tablespoons chopped fresh coriander
2 x packets 2-minute brown rice
salt and freshly ground black pepper
salad, to serve

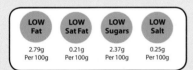

LOW Fat	LOW Sat Fat	LOW Sugars	LOW Salt
2.79g Per 100g	0.21g Per 100g	2.37g Per 100g	0.25g Per 100g

1 In a frying pan heat half the oil and stir in the fenugreek, asafoetida, chillies, ground coriander and lentils, and over a medium heat cook for 3 minutes, stirring continuously. Transfer the mixture to a mini food processor and blend until a smoothish paste, or grind with a mortar and pestle.

2 In a small pan, mix together the diluted tamarind and the spice paste, and cook until the paste is thick, about 2–3 minutes.

3 Meanwhile in a separate pan, heat the remaining oil and fry the onions for 8–10 minutes until lightly coloured, add the garlic and carrot and continue to cook gently, covered, for about 8 minutes until the carrot is starting to soften but still has a little bite. Add the tamarind paste, peas and beans and stir well.

4 Microwave the rice and fold it into the vegetable mix, then sprinkle over the cashews and coriander and season to taste. Serve piping hot, with a salad.

Amount per portion
Energy 303 kcals, Protein 11g, Fat 8g, Saturated fat 0.6g, Carbohydrate 50g, Total sugars 6.8g, Salt 0.73g, Sodium 289mg`

Dhal with Added Spice

Lentils are extremely nutritious, but there is a good reason for spicing them up: they are naturally rich in protein nitrogen compounds, which require much more effort to digest than the protein in meat, fish and dairy products. So the Indians learned to add certain digestion-friendly spices such as ginger.

Serves 4

250g red lentils, washed
1 tablespoon sunflower oil
5 garlic cloves, finely chopped
1 onion, finely chopped
2.5cm piece of fresh ginger, peeled and finely chopped
3 green chillies, deseeded and finely chopped
1 teaspoon ground coriander
1 teaspoon ground cumin
½ teaspoon chilli powder
1 teaspoon black mustard seeds (optional)
1 teaspoon ground turmeric
3 plum tomatoes, deseeded and diced
3 tablespoons chopped fresh coriander
2 teaspoons lime juice
salt and freshly ground black pepper

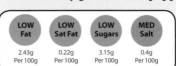

LOW Fat	LOW Sat Fat	LOW Sugars	MED Salt
2.43g Per 100g	0.22g Per 100g	3.15g Per 100g	0.4g Per 100g

1 Put 1.5 litres of water into a saucepan and bring to the boil. Add the lentils and cook for 15 minutes, stirring regularly at the beginning as the early period of cooking is when the lentils will stick together.

2 Meanwhile, melt the butter in a frying pan and add the garlic, onion, ginger and chillies, and cook over a medium heat for 10 minutes until the onion has softened. Add the spices and cook for a further 2 minutes. Fold this mixture into the lentils after they have cooked for 15 minutes.

3 Cook the dhal for a further 10–15 minutes until the lentils are very tender. Beat with a whisk until completely mashed, adjust the seasoning to taste, then fold in the tomatoes, fresh coriander and lime juice.

Amount per portion
Energy 267 kcals, Protein 16.8g, Fat 4.4g, Saturated fat 0.4g, Carbohydrate 42.6g, Total sugars 5.7g, Salt 0.72g, Sodium 284mg

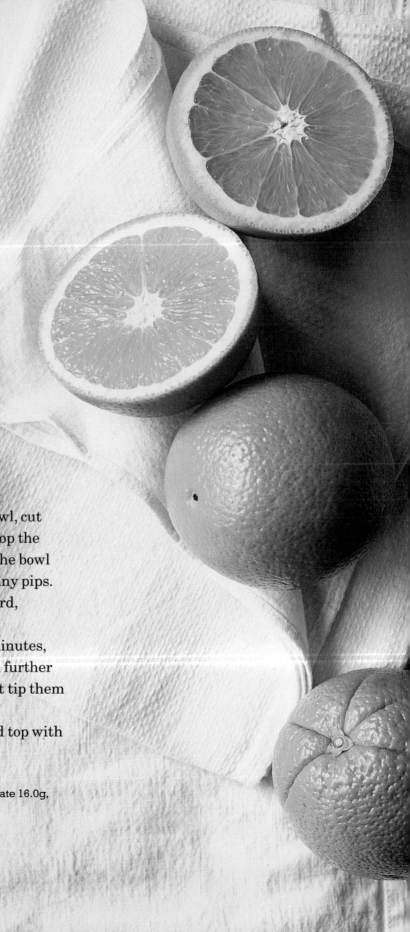

Green Vegetables with Almond and Orange

A pleasant little combo with its roots in Italy, that can be served as a salad as here, or hot as an accompaniment to grilled meat or fish.

Serves 4
2 oranges, peeled
45g toasted flaked almonds
1 garlic clove, finely chopped
1 tablespoon snipped fresh chives
1 teaspoon wholegrain mustard
1 shallot, finely diced
1 tablespoon extra virgin olive oil
1 tablespoon walnut or hazelnut oil
200g French beans, topped and cut into
    3cm pieces
200g sugar snap peas
100g edamame beans, fresh or frozen
a few handfuls of rocket leaves
salt and freshly ground black pepper

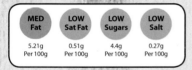

MED Fat	LOW Sat Fat	LOW Sugars	LOW Salt
5.21g Per 100g	0.51g Per 100g	4.4g Per 100g	0.27g Per 100g

1 With a small sharp knife and working over a large bowl, cut out the orange segments from their membranes and drop the segments into the bowl. Squeeze the membranes over the bowl to release any juices, and discard the membranes and any pips. To the segments add the almonds, garlic, chives, mustard, shallot and two oils. Whisk and season to taste.
2 Cook the French beans in boiling salted water for 3 minutes, add the sugarsnaps and edamame beans and cook for a further 2 minutes. Drain well. While the vegetables are still hot tip them into the nutty orange dressing and stir.
3 Scatter some rocket leaves on to individual plates and top with the salad.

Amount per portion
Energy 221 kcals, Protein 10.0g, Fat 13.4g, Saturated fat 1.3g, Carbohydrate 16.0g, Total sugars 11.3g, Salt 0.70g, Sodium 278mg

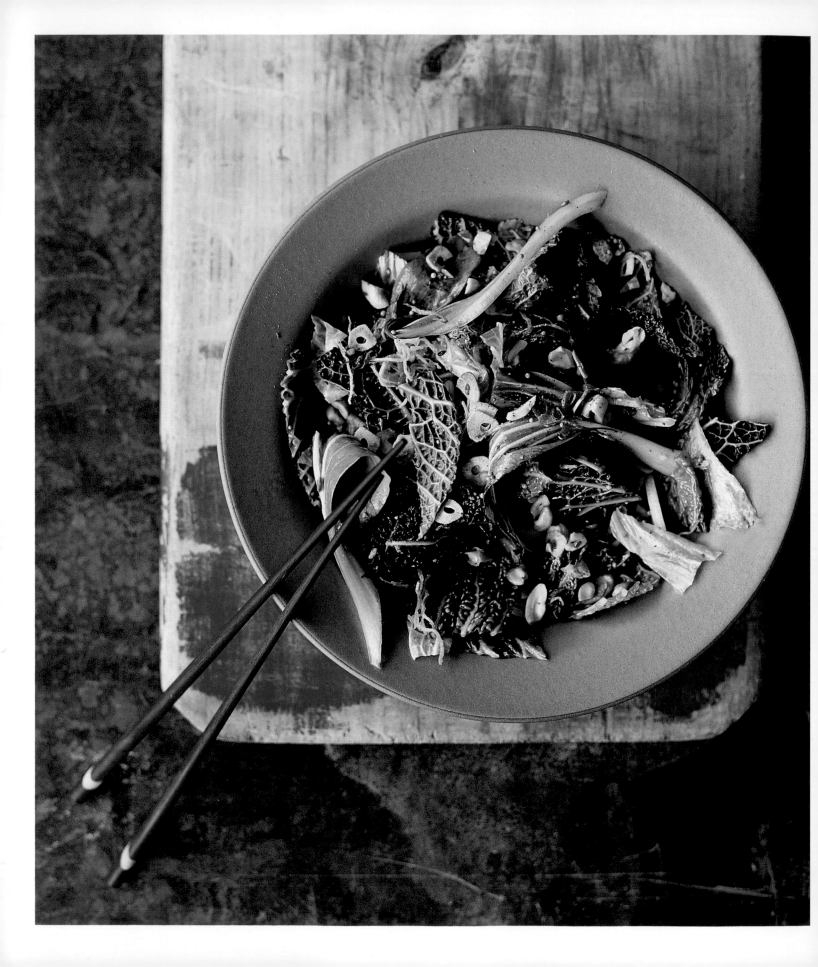

Stir-Fried Greens with Mustard Seeds and Cashews

A wonderful way to zap up your greens. I could eat these on their own without feeling the need for protein.

Serves 2–4

1 tablespoon rapeseed oil
1.5cm piece of fresh ginger, peeled and
    cut into small matchsticks
2 garlic cloves, thinly sliced
2 teaspoons yellow mustard seeds
450g greens (spring greens, bok choi, Savoy
    cabbage), cut into bite-sized pieces
1 tablespoon reduced-salt soy sauce
1 tablespoon chopped unsalted cashew nuts

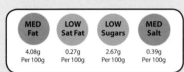

MED Fat	LOW Sat Fat	LOW Sugars	MED Salt
4.08g Per 100g	0.27g Per 100g	2.67g Per 100g	0.39g Per 100g

1 Heat the oil in a wok and fry the ginger until it just starts to colour, then add the garlic and mustard seeds and continue to fry until the seeds start to pop.

2 Add the greens, increase the heat and cook until they start to wilt. Fold in the soy sauce and cashews and serve immediately.

Tip Serve tossed through some rice noodles.

Amount per portion (for 2)
Energy 163 kcals, Protein 7.5g, Fat 10.4g, Saturated fat 0.7g, Carbohydrate 10.7g, Total sugars 6.8g, Salt 1g, Sodium 395mg

Amount per portion (for 4)
Energy 82 kcals, Protein 3.8g, Fat 5.2g, Saturated fat 0.3g, Carbohydrate 5.3g, Total sugars 3.4g, Salt 0.5g, Sodium 198mg

Butter beans with Chillies and Asian Influence

Butter beans are not often used in Asia but I had this Asian-influenced dish with a grilled swordfish steak in Adelaide, and it was a good combination. Butter beans have a wonderful silky creamy texture, but unless you're a really keen cook I wouldn't suggest using dried beans.

Serves 4

2 x 400g tins butter beans, drained
2 tablespoons chopped fresh coriander
2 teaspoons chopped fresh mint

For the Asian mix

4 garlic cloves, crushed to a paste
    with a little salt
1cm piece of fresh ginger, peeled and grated
1 hot green chilli, deseeded and finely
    chopped
2 mild green chillies, deseeded and
    thinly sliced
1 red pepper, deseeded and diced
2 shallots, thinly sliced
2 tablespoons sweet chilli sauce
1 tablespoon sesame oil
2 tablespoons reduced-salt soy sauce
2 tablespoons lime juice
3 spring onions, sliced

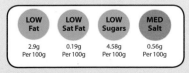

LOW Fat	LOW Sat Fat	LOW Sugars	MED Salt
2.9g Per 100g	0.19g Per 100g	4.58g Per 100g	0.56g Per 100g

1 In a bowl, mix together all the ingredients for the Asian mix and leave for 30 minutes to allow the flavours to develop.

2 Heat the butter beans in boiling water for 2 minutes. Drain, mix them into the Asian mix and then sprinkle with coriander and mint. Serve hot or at room temperature.

Amount per portion
Energy 153 kcals, Protein 8.2g, Fat 3.6g, Saturated fat 0.4g, Carbohydrate 23.3g, Total sugars 8.7g, Salt 2.42g, Sodium 956mg

LEFT Stir-Fried Greens with
Mustard Seeds and Cashews

rry A Potato and Butter Bean Curry with Cottage Cheese B
eans Stuffed Peppers with Braised Potatoes Ratatouille Cak
Spinach and Sweet Potato Stew Chickpea and Lentil Curry
g – Indonesian Fried Rice Stuffed Green Top Onions Courge
Texan Spinach and Bean Bake One Pot Cauli Herby Green
occoli Frittata Stuffed Aubergines with Tamarind Stuffed Ca
kes Simple Spaghetti with Raw Tomato and Cauliflower A M
y Three Bean Stew with Grated Feta Watercress and Mushr
e Cakes Baked Eggs in Spiced Mushrooms Slow Cooked C
reen Pilaf Rice Rich but Sinless Vegetable Curry A Potato a

Vegetarian

d Cabbage Leaves with Tomatoes and Beans Stuffed Peppe
editerranean Artichoke Stew Chickpea, Spinach and Swee
room Pancakes Vegetarian Nasi Goreng – Indonesian Fried
d Green Polenta with Mediterranean Veg Texan Spinach an
ter Bean Curry with Cottage Cheese Broccoli Frittata Stuffe
pers with Braised Potatoes Ratatouille Cakes Simple Spaghe
eet Potato Stew Chickpea and Lentil Curry Three Bean Stew
an Fried Rice Stuffed Green Top Onions Courgette Cakes B
pinach and Bean Bake One Pot Cauli Herby Green Pilaf Ric
occoli Frittata Stuffed Aubergines with Tamarind Stuffed Ca

Stuffed Green Top Onions

So, I admit this American recipe requires a little work but it can be prepared ahead of time. It makes an impressive vegetarian dish, with its mix of creamy and crunchy textures.

Serves 4
4 large onions
1 small sweet potato, cut into 1cm dice
1 x 400g tin white haricot beans, drained
   and rinsed
1 garlic clove, crushed to a paste with
   a little salt
a pinch of chilli flakes
125g cooked fresh spinach (or defrosted
   frozen spinach), chopped
2 tablespoons 0 per cent fat Greek yogurt
1 teaspoon Dijon mustard
¼ teaspoon salt
¼ teaspoon grated nutmeg
2 tablespoons seeded breadcrumbs
salad and new potatoes, to serve

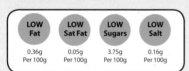

LOW Fat	LOW Sat Fat	LOW Sugars	LOW Salt
0.36g Per 100g	0.05g Per 100g	3.75g Per 100g	0.16g Per 100g

1 Peel the onions without damaging the inner layers, and cut a cross in the root end. Cook, along with the sweet potato, in boiling water for 6 minutes. Drain and set the sweet potato aside.

2 When the onions are cool enough to handle, cut a third off the top. With your fingers or a teaspoon, remove the insides of the onions, leaving the 2 outer layers intact; you will now have four onion containers. Chop a third of the removed onion and place in a bowl with the sweet potato and discard the remaining two thirds of the onions. Add half the beans, the garlic, chilli and spinach. Mix well.

3 Mash the remaining beans with the yogurt, mustard, salt and nutmeg. Mix this with the sweet potato and spinach mix, and spoon the mixture into the onion shells, piling it high. (The recipe can be made ahead to this point.)

4 Preheat the oven to 200°C/400°F/gas mark 6. Place the onions in a lightly oiled baking tray, scatter the tops with breadcrumbs and bake for 25 minutes. Serve with salad and new potatoes.

Amount per portion
Energy 179 kcals, Protein 9.7g, Fat 1.4g, Saturated fat 0.2g, Carbohydrate 35.1g, Total sugars 14.6g, Salt 0.61g, Sodium 242mg

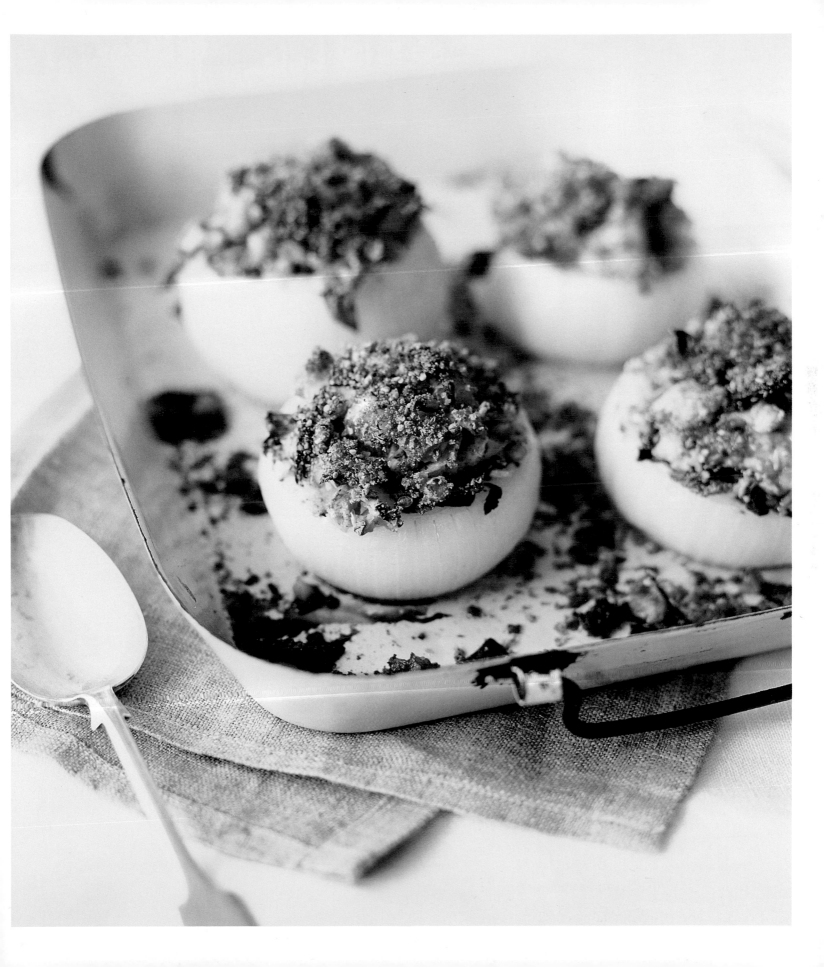

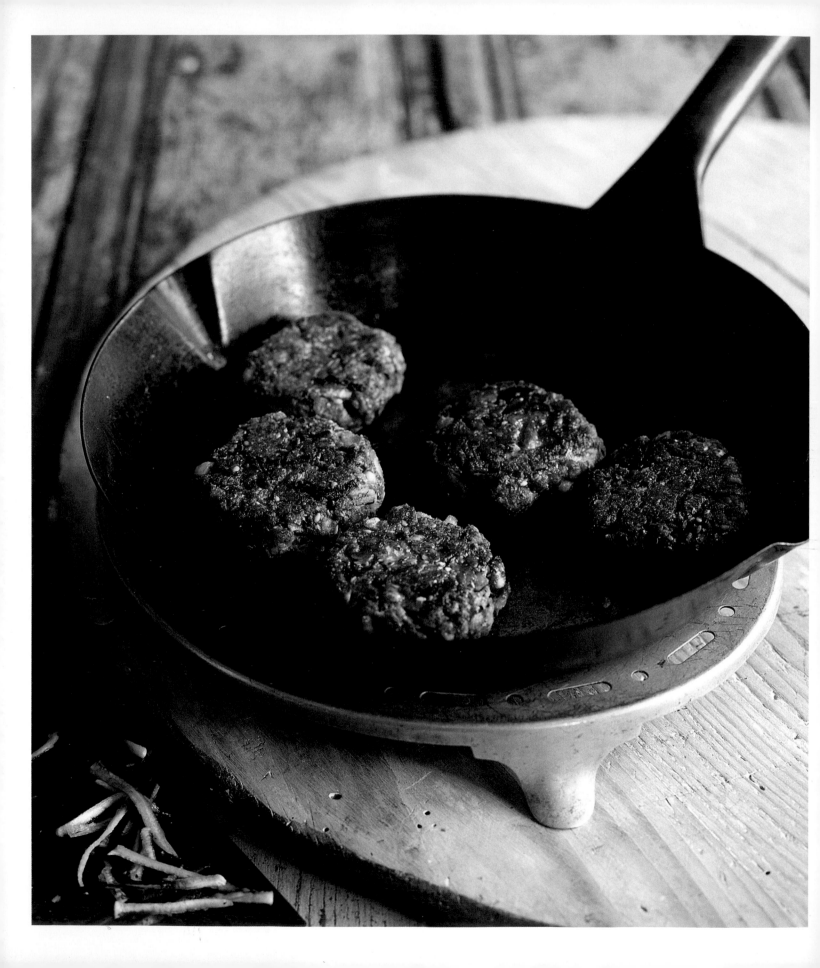

Courgette Cakes

Great with a poached egg, as part of a vegetarian buffet or served with a spicy tomato sauce or tzatziki.

Serves 4
225g courgettes
2 pickled jalapeño chillies, chopped
2 shallots, finely diced
1 garlic clove, finely chopped
1 teaspoon curry powder
2 teaspoons sesame seeds
1 tablespoon extra virgin olive oil
175g wholemeal flour
½ teaspoon baking powder
1 tablespoon sunflower oil, for cooking
salt

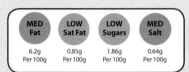

MED Fat	LOW Sat Fat	LOW Sugars	MED Salt
6.2g Per 100g	0.85g Per 100g	1.86g Per 100g	0.64g Per 100g

1 Grate the courgettes into a colander, sprinkle with about 1 teaspoon of salt and stir, then leave for 20 minutes to release the liquid. Squeeze out the excess moisture.

2 In a bowl, mix together the grated courgette with the remaining ingredients except the sunflower oil, and 1 tablespoon of water. With floured hands, shape the mixture into 8 rounds and flatten them slightly.

3 In a large frying pan heat the sunflower oil then cook the cakes on one side for 1 minute until golden. Gently flip them over, reduce the heat to low and cook the cakes for 12–15 minutes, turning once again halfway through. (Depending on the size of your frying pan, you may need to cook in two batches, in which case keep the first batch warm in a low oven while you cook the next.)

Amount per portion
Energy 214 kcals, Protein 7.2g, Fat 8.0g, Saturated fat 1.1g, Carbohydrate 30.2g, Total sugars 2.4g, Salt 0.83g, Sodium 328mg

Baked Eggs in Spiced Mushrooms

Mushrooms are relatively calorie-free, but the modern mushroom is also free of good flavour so here's a French recipe that will zap it up. The mushroom mix can be prepared ahead of time and cooked later.

Serves 4
3 tomatoes, roughly chopped
1 teaspoon coriander seeds, crushed
2 teaspoons tomato purée
½ teaspoon thyme leaves
1 bay leaf
2 tablespoons olive oil
25g sultanas
20g toasted pine nuts
juice of ½ lemon
250g button mushrooms, quartered
4 eggs
1 tablespoon 0 per cent fat Greek yogurt
freshly ground black pepper

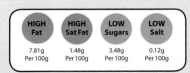

HIGH Fat	HIGH Sat Fat	LOW Sugars	LOW Salt
7.81g Per 100g	1.48g Per 100g	3.48g Per 100g	0.12g Per 100g

1 In a saucepan place the tomatoes, coriander, tomato purée, thyme and bay leaf. Add the oil and season generously with pepper. Add 150ml of water and simmer gently for 8 minutes. Increase the heat and add the sultanas, pine nuts, lemon juice and mushrooms, and cook for a further 5 minutes. (The dish can be prepared ahead up to this point.)

2 Preheat the oven to 180°C/350°F/gas mark 4. Spoon the mushroom mixture into individual large ramekins and make a well in the centre of each one. Break an egg into each indent and top with a dollop of yogurt. Bake for 9 minutes if the mushrooms are hot or 12 if cold.

Amount per portion
Energy 220 kcals, Protein 10.7g, Fat 16.4g, Saturated fat 3.1g, Carbohydrate 7.9g, Total sugars 7.3g, Salt 0.26g, Sodium 104mg

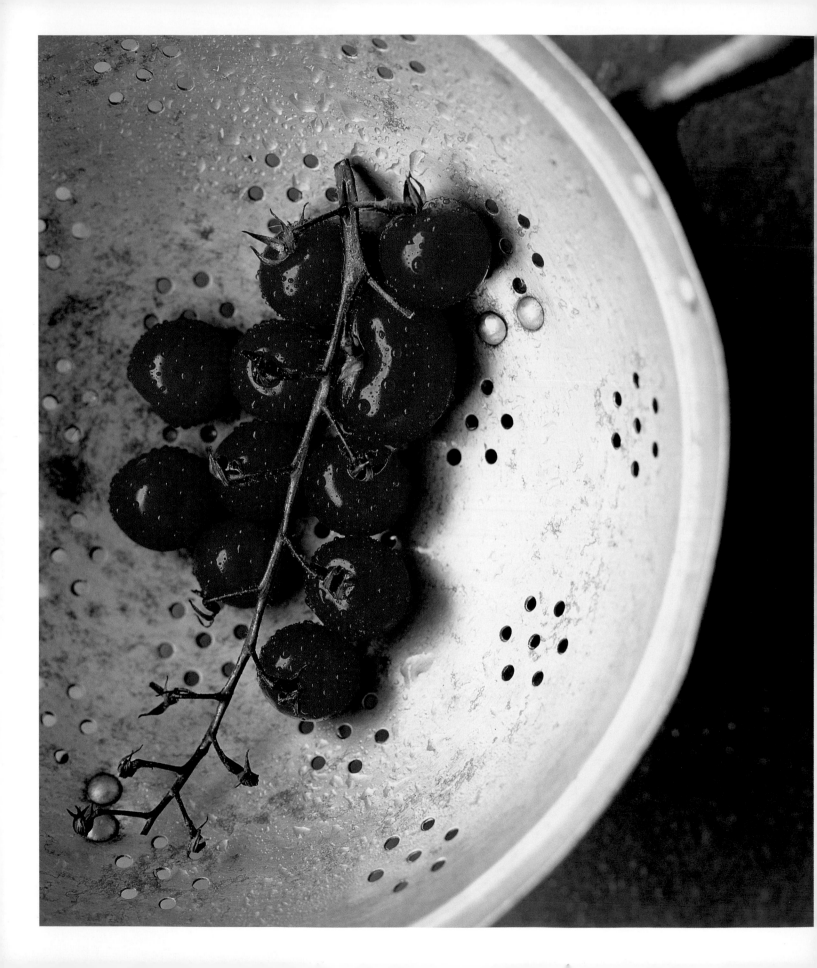

Slow-Cooked Green Polenta with Mediterranean Veg

It's a divided camp when it comes to polenta. Many of us love this creamy cornmeal dish, a staple food throughout much of Northern Italy. If you're one of those who aren't very keen on it, I'd like you to give this dish a chance – it's packed full of goodness, but best of all it tastes delicious.

Serves 4

1 litre vegetable stock
300g 'real' polenta (see Tip below)
2 tablespoons olive oil
4 garlic cloves, sliced
1 onion, roughly chopped
1 red pepper, deseeded and cut into
    2.5cm pieces
1 small aubergine, cut into 2.5cm pieces
2 courgettes, cut into 2.5cm pieces
12 cherry tomatoes
200g spring greens or dark cabbage,
    roughly chopped
2 handfuls of spinach, central stems
    removed
1 x 400g tin chickpeas, drained and rinsed
40g grated Parmesan cheese
salt and freshly ground pepper

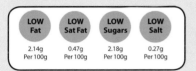

LOW Fat	LOW Sat Fat	LOW Sugars	LOW Salt
2.14g Per 100g	0.47g Per 100g	2.18g Per 100g	0.27g Per 100g

1 In a large saucepan bring the stock to the boil, then pour in the polenta a little at a time, whisking furiously to prevent lumps. Reduce the heat to low and cook gently, stirring every 3–4 minutes to ensure every part of the polenta is moved about to prevent catching. The polenta will need to cook for about 40 minutes but follow the instructions on the packet.

2 Meanwhile, in a large frying pan heat the olive oil, then add the garlic, onion, red pepper and aubergine, and cook over a low heat until the vegetables are tender. Add the courgettes and tomatoes and cook for a further 5 minutes, then season to taste.

3 At the same time cook the spring greens or cabbage in boiling water for 3 minutes, then stir in the spinach and cook for a further 1 minute. With a slotted spoon, transfer the green veg straight into a food processor, with water clinging. Blitz to a smooth purée and season to taste.

4 Just before serving, fold the green purée into the polenta, stir, then fold in the mediterranean veg, the chickpeas and Parmesan, and adjust the seasoning if needed. Serve piping hot.

Tip You can use instant or quick-cook polenta, they're never as good but are convenient. If you do use either, prepare your veg and greens first so you're ready to fold everything together.

Amount per portion
Energy 503 kcals, Protein 20.4g, Fat 14.6g, Saturated fat 3.2g, Carbohydrate 77.4g, Total sugars 14.9g, Salt 1.84g, Sodium 723mg

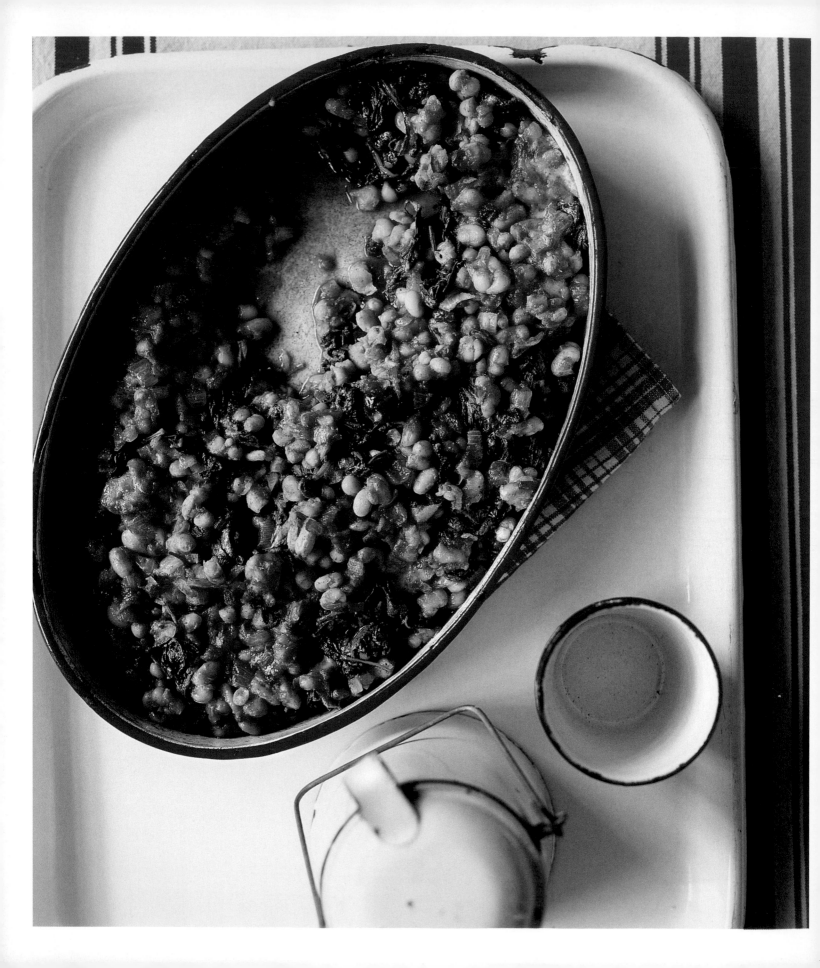

Texan Spinach and Bean Bake

It's not exactly beans around the campfire but it's heading in that direction. A good dish that can be prepared ahead.

Serves 4
1 tablespoon olive oil
1 onion, chopped
1 garlic clove, finely chopped
1 hot red chilli, deseeded and
    finely chopped
1 tablespoon smoked paprika
1 tablespoon tomato ketchup
½ teaspoon salt
300g cooked or frozen leaf spinach,
    defrosted, squeezed and chopped
2 tablespoons sultanas
2 x 400g tins pinto or haricot beans, drained
50g grated cheddar cheese
4 tablespoons vegetable stock
salad, to serve

1 Preheat the oven to 200°C/400°F/gas mark 6. Heat the olive oil in a saucepan and cook the onion until soft and translucent, about 8 minutes. Add the garlic, chilli, paprika, ketchup, salt, spinach, sultanas, beans and cheddar. Mix well then moisten with the stock.

2 Spoon the mixture into a baking dish and cook for 25 minutes in the preheated oven. Serve with salad.

Amount per portion
Energy 302 kcals, Protein 17.1g, Fat 9.1g, Saturated fat 3.1g, Carbohydrate 40.6g, Total sugars 9.8g, Salt 1.08g, Sodium 000mg

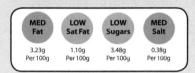

MED Fat	LOW Sat Fat	LOW Sugars	MED Salt
3.23g Per 100g	1.10g Per 100g	3.48g Per 100g	0.38g Per 100g

One Pot Cauli

This Spanish dish makes a lovely vegetarian supper in its own right but I've also included chorizo and bacon as optional extras to make it flexible for any occasion.

Serves 4
2 tablespoons extra virgin olive oil
1 cauliflower, broken into florets
1 x 400g tin chick peas, drained
1 x 200g tin chopped tomatoes
6 spring onions, sliced
2 garlic cloves, crushed to a paste
    with a little salt
85g chorizo sausage, diced (optional)
2 rashers smoked bacon, cut into lardons
    (optional)
25g sultanas
15g toasted pine nuts
2 teaspoons smoked paprika
salt and freshly ground black pepper

1 Put all the ingredients in a saucepan, stir, cover and cook over a gentle heat for 15–20 minutes, shaking the pan from time to time – try to resist lifting the lid as you don't want the steam to escape. Season to taste and serve.

Amount per portion
Energy 325 kcals, Protein 18.0g, Fat 18.9g, Saturated fat 4.1g, Carbohydrate 22.1g, Total sugars 10.3g, Salt 2.14g, Sodium 844mg

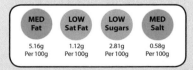

MED Fat	LOW Sat Fat	LOW Sugars	MED Salt
5.16g Per 100g	1.12g Per 100g	2.81g Per 100g	0.58g Per 100g

LEFT Texan Spinach
and Bean Bake

Herby Green Pilaf Rice

This Middle Eastern rice dish is excellent on its own, or for non-vegetarians it makes a great accompaniment to grilled meats and fish.

Serves 4

1 tablespoon sunflower oil
1 onion, finely chopped
1 garlic clove, finely chopped
4 cardamom pods, crushed
2cm cinnamon stick
3 cloves
½ teaspoon ground black pepper
½ teaspoon ground turmeric
225g long-grain rice
500ml hot vegetable stock
2 tablespoons chopped fresh parsley
1 tablespoon chopped fresh coriander
5 spring onions, chopped
2 handfuls of watercress, chopped
2 handfuls of baby spinach leaves
2 tablespoons toasted flaked almonds
2 tablespoons raisins
salt

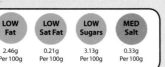

LOW Fat	LOW Sat Fat	LOW Sugars	MED Salt
2.46g Per 100g	0.21g Per 100g	3.13g Per 100g	0.33g Per 100g

1 Heat the oil in a large lidded saucepan, add the onion and cook gently until soft, about 6–8 minutes. Add the garlic, cardamom, cinnamon stick, cloves and pepper and turmeric, and cook for 2 minutes. Add the rice, mix well and cook for 1 minute, then add the hot stock. Bring to the boil and reduce the heat to medium. Cover and cook for 15 minutes.

2 Turn off the heat but leave the rice untouched, covered, for 5 minutes. Fluff up the rice, return to a low heat and add all the herbs and greens, almonds and raisins, and season to taste with salt. Serve hot.

Amount per portion
Energy 317 kcals, Protein 7g, Fat 7g, Saturated fat 0.6g, Carbohydrate 60g, Total sugars 8.9g, Salt 0.93g, Sodium 365mg

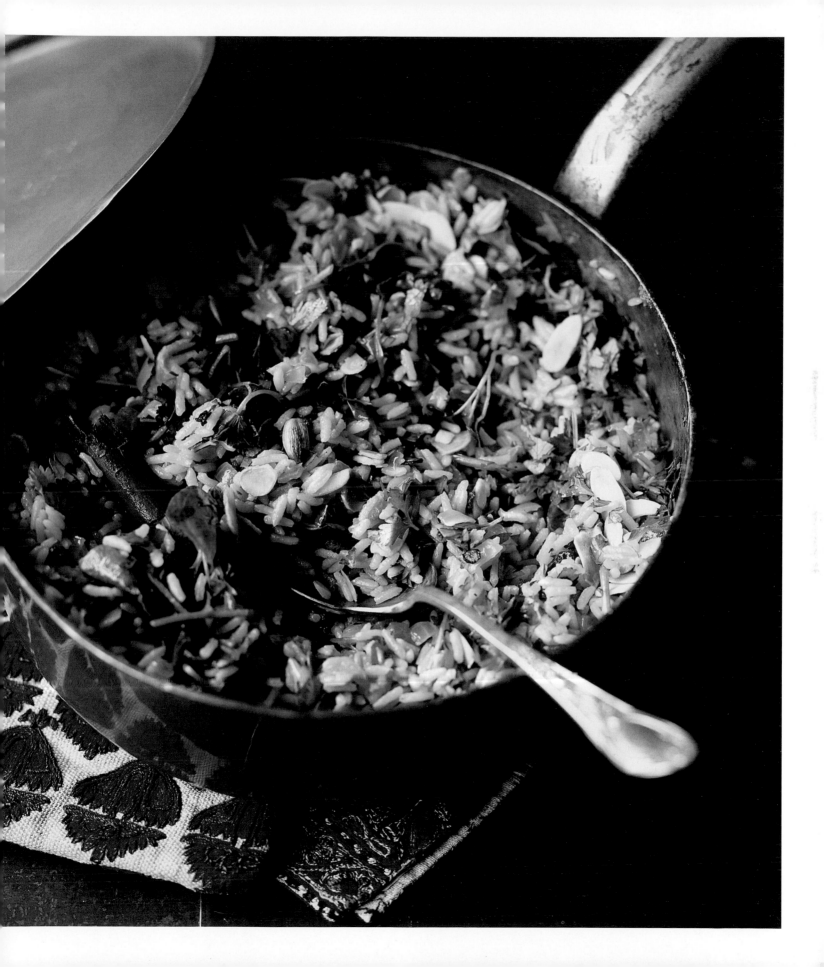

Rich but Sinless Vegetable Curry

There's loads going on here, but it's certainly a fantastic way of contributing to your five a day. This Indian-influenced dish is very much korma in style, even meat eaters will love it.

Serves 4
2 large onions, roughly chopped
1 teaspoon lazy garlic
1 tablespoon lazy ginger
1 teaspoon ground turmeric
1 teaspoon chilli powder
1 teaspoon ground cumin
1 teaspoon ground coriander
2 tablespoons sunflower oil
1 x 400g tin chopped tomatoes
1 teaspoon caster sugar
180g 0 per cent fat Greek yogurt
4 tablespoons ground almonds
2 large carrots, diced
1 x 400g tin chickpeas, drained and rinsed
8 new potatoes, halved
½ cauliflower, broken into small florets
¼ savoy cabbage, shredded
100g French beans, cut into 1cm lengths
2 tablespoons dried cherries, chopped
2 tablespoons sunflower seeds
1 tablespoon chopped fresh coriander
1 tablespoon garam masala
salt and freshly ground pepper
rice, to serve

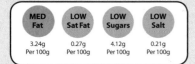

MED Fat	LOW Sat Fat	LOW Sugars	LOW Salt
3.24g Per 100g	0.27g Per 100g	4.12g Per 100g	0.21g Per 100g

1 In a food processor, blend together the onions, garlic, ginger and spices to a smooth purée.

2 Heat the oil in a saucepan and over a gentle heat cook the spiced onion purée until all the moisture has evaporated. Stir in the tomatoes and cook for a further 5 minutes. Add the sugar and yogurt and bring to a simmer. Reduce the heat and add the almonds, carrots, chickpeas and potatoes, cover and cook for 15 minutes. Add the cauliflower, cabbage and beans and cook for a further 6 minutes.

3 Fold in the cherries, sunflower seeds, fresh coriander and garam masala. (If the curry is thicker than you like, add a little water to thin.) Adjust the seasoning to taste. Serve with rice.

Tip You can find lazy garlic and ginger in most supermarkets these days – a jar of already chopped/crushed garlic and ginger to make our lives easier.

Amount per portion
Energy 491 kcals, Protein 22.5, Fat 21.2g, Saturated fat 1.8g, Carbohydrate 56.0g, Total sugars 27.0g, Salt 1.39g, Sodium 551mg

A Potato and Butter Bean Curry with Cottage Cheese

In normal circumstances I would use paneer in this Indian-influenced dish. Low-fat cottage cheese makes a good replacement, acting as a great vehicle for picking up and absorbing all these wonderful flavours.

Serves 4
2 tablespoons sunflower oil
2 teaspoons mustard seeds
1 pinch asafoetida powder (optional)
1 onion, roughly chopped
1 large carrot, cut into 2cm chunks
1 sweet potato, cut into 2cm dice
1 teaspoon ground turmeric
1 teaspoon chilli powder
1 teaspoon ground coriander
325g new potatoes, halved
50g desiccated coconut
1 x 400g tin butter beans, drained
3 tablespoons roughly chopped fresh coriander
1 teaspoon finely chopped fresh mint leaves
175g low-fat cottage cheese
salt

1 Heat the oil in a saucepan and cook the mustard seeds until they start to pop, then add the asafoetida and onion and fry gently for 8 minutes. Add the carrot, sweet potato, turmeric, chilli powder, ground coriander and potatoes. Season with salt and add 200ml water and stir, then cover and cook gently until the vegetables are tender, about 20 minutes.

2 Fold in the coconut, butter beans, coriander and mint, adjust the seasoning to taste and heat until warmed through. Divide between individual warmed bowls and dot with spoonfuls of cottage cheese. Serve with brown rice.

Amount per portion
Energy 354 kcals, Protein 13.8g, Fat 14g Saturated fat 8.0g, Carbohydrate 34.3g, Total sugars 9.4g, Salt 1.6g, Sodium 626mg

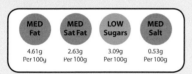

MED Fat	MED Sat Fat	LOW Sugars	MED Salt
4.61g Per 100g	2.63g Per 100g	3.09g Per 100g	0.53g Per 100g

Broccoli Frittata

This excellent Italian frittata is a useful standby as a simple main course or for fridge snacking. Non-vegetarians could add a little bacon with the onion for extra flavour.

Serves 4
2 tablespoons olive oil
2 onions, finely chopped
2 garlic cloves, finely chopped
450g small broccoli florets, blanched
    in boiling water for 2 minutes
1 teaspoon thyme leaves
175g cooked brown rice
¼ teaspoon chilli flakes
6 eggs, beaten
spray oil
115g low-fat ricotta or cream cheese
salt and freshly ground white pepper
salad and new potatoes, to serve

1 Heat the oil in a frying pan and gently cook the onions until soft and translucent, about 8 minutes. Add the garlic, broccoli and thyme and stir-fry for 2 minutes. Fold in the rice and chilli, and season to taste with salt and pepper. Tip the mixture into a bowl and leave to cool. Meanwhile, preheat the oven to 160°C/325°F/gas mark 3.

2 Fold the cooled rice mixture into the eggs. Spray a non-stick, ovenproof pan with a light coating of oil and heat the pan over a medium heat. Pour in the egg mixture and dot the surface with nuggets of ricotta. Cook over a low heat for 5 minutes, then transfer to the preheated oven for 15–20 minutes, depending on the thickness of the frittata – when ready, the eggs should be set but not dry. Serve with salad and new potatoes.

Amount per portion
Energy 337 kcals, Protein 21.0g, Fat 18.8g, Saturated fat 4.7g, Carbohydrate 22.2g, Total sugars 6.0g, Salt 1.04g, Sodium 412mg

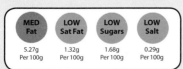

MED Fat	LOW Sat Fat	LOW Sugars	LOW Salt
5.27g Per 100g	1.32g Per 100g	1.68g Per 100g	0.29g Per 100g

Stuffed Aubergines with Tamarind

I'm an aubergine fan, but it needs to be thoroughly cooked otherwise it resembles tasteless shoe leather. That can't be said about this fantastic Indian recipe.

Serves 4

2 large aubergines, cut in half lengthways
2 tablespoons sunflower oil
1 large onion, finely chopped
2 garlic cloves, finely chopped
4 cloves
2 tablespoons coriander seeds
1 tablespoon cumin seeds
40g desiccated coconut
3 tomatoes, deseeded and diced
1 tablespoon toasted pine nuts
2 tablespoons chopped cashew nuts
1 teaspoon chilli powder
1 teaspoon ground turmeric
2 teaspoons tamarind paste
175g frozen spinach, defrosted, squeezed
    and chopped
8 cooked new potatoes, diced
1 teaspoon caster sugar
4 tablespoons 0 per cent fat Greek yogurt
salt and freshly ground pepper

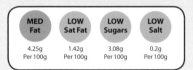

MED Fat	LOW Sat Fat	LOW Sugars	LOW Salt
4.25g Per 100g	1.42g Per 100g	3.08g Per 100g	0.2g Per 100g

1 Preheat the oven to 190°C/375°F/gas mark 5. When it has come up to temperature, brush the cut surfaces of the aubergine with a little oil, sprinkle with a touch of salt and place cut-side down on a baking tray. Transfer to the preheated oven and roast for 30 minutes.

2 Meanwhile, heat the remaining oil in a pan, add the onions and cook over a gentle heat until softening and turning colour, about 8 minutes. Remove half and set aside. To the remaining onions, add the garlic, cloves, coriander seeds, cumin seeds and a dash of pepper, and fry for 1 minute. Add the coconut and continue to cook until the coconut has turned a pale brown colour.

3 Process the spicy coconut onion mix in a food processor, adding a little water if necessary. Spoon this mixture into a bowl, then add the reserved softened onions and all the remaining ingredients. Season to taste.

4 When the aubergines are cooked, remove them from the oven but do not turn the oven off. Hollow out the aubergine shells, taking care not to split them. Chop the flesh and add it to the savoury mix. Heap the mixture back into the shells, return to the oven and cook for 20 minutes.

Tip These can be made ahead of time and refrigerated for up to a couple of days until you're ready to heat them through. They'll take 30–35 minutes at 190°C/375°F/gas mark 5 to heat through from cold.

Amount per portion
Energy 336 kcals, Protein 10.4g, Fat 19.7g, Saturated fat 6.6g, Carbohydrate 31.2g, Total sugars 14.3g, Salt 0.93g, Sodium 367mg

Stuffed Cabbage Leaves with Tomatoes and Beans

As a child my mother would regularly make a Polish recipe for stuffed cabbage which usually involved minced pork. Here's an excellent vegetarian version from Greece.

Serves 4

12 leaves savoy cabbage, large rib trimmed
2 tablespoons good-quality olive oil
2 red onions, finely chopped
3 garlic cloves, finely chopped
2 celery stalks, finely sliced
225g carrot, finely sliced
2 bay leaves
110g easy-cook brown rice
1 teaspoon smoked paprika
2 tomatoes, chopped
1 tablespoon each chopped fresh chives,
  parsley and basil
1 x 400g tin chopped tomatoes
1 x 400g tin borlotti beans, drained
  and rinsed
½ tablespoon dried oregano
salt and freshly ground black pepper

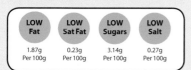

LOW Fat	LOW Sat Fat	LOW Sugars	LOW Salt
1.87g Per 100g	0.23g Per 100g	3.14g Per 100g	0.27g Per 100g

1 Cook the cabbage leaves in boiling salted water for 3 minutes, then remove, drain and refresh under cold running water, and drain and pat dry. Lay the leaves outside-down on a work surface.

2 Using two frying pans, heat half the olive oil in each, then add half the onion and garlic in each. Allow the onions to soften under a medium heat, about 5–8 minutes. To one pan add the celery, carrot and bay and cook gently for 8 minutes.

3 Meanwhile, to the other pan add the rice and paprika and cook for 5 minutes, stirring frequently. Add the fresh chopped tomatoes and half the fresh herbs, season to taste and leave to cool.

4 To the vegetable pan add the tinned tomatoes, borlotti beans and dried oregano, then stir in 300ml of water and simmer gently. Set a heaped teaspoon of the rice stuffing on each cabbage leaf and loosely wrap to allow the rice to expand during cooking. Place the stuffed leaves on the bean and tomato stew, cover and simmer gently for 20–25 minutes.

5 Arrange 3 stuffed leaves on each warmed plate. Add the remaining fresh herbs to the tomato and bean stew and season to taste, then spoon the stew around the stuffed leaves.

Amount per portion
Energy 286 kcals, Protein 11g, Fat 8g, Saturated fat 1g, Carbohydrate 46g,
Total sugars 13.4g, Salt 1.17g, Sodium 459mg

Stuffed Peppers with Braised Potatoes

Peppers make useful containers for some delicious fillings, such as this Greek rice filling. With the potatoes on the side as here, this makes quite a substantial dish, and an excellent vegetarian meal.

Serves 4
4 large red or yellow peppers
1 tablespoon olive oil
1 onion, finely chopped
2 garlic cloves, crushed to a paste
     with a little salt
2 tomatoes, chopped
2 tablespoons sultanas
1 tablespoon toasted pine nuts
1 tablespoon chopped fresh mint
100g long-grain brown rice
450g new potatoes, sliced
150ml tomato passata
salad, to serve

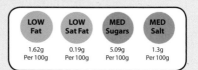

LOW Fat	LOW Sat Fat	MED Sugars	MED Salt
1.62g Per 100g	0.19g Per 100g	5.09g Per 100g	1.3g Per 100g

1 Preheat the oven to 180°C/350°F/gas mark 4. Slice one-third off the top of each pepper, then scoop out the seeds and pith and discard, but retain the top.

2 Heat the olive oil in a frying pan, add the onion and garlic and cook gently for 10 minutes. Add the tomatoes, sultanas, pine nuts and mint and cook for a further 5 minutes. Stir in the rice.

3 Fill the lower sections of the peppers with the rice mix – do not overfill as the rice will expand on cooking. Replace the pepper tops and set the peppers on a baking tray. Scatter the potato slices around the peppers, drizzle with a little olive oil then pour the passata over the potatoes.

4 Bake, uncovered, for about 45 minutes, checking towards the end that they are not burning or collapsing. Serve hot or at room temperature, with salad.

Amount per portion
Energy 318 kcals, Protein 7g, Fat 7g, Saturated fat 0.8g, Carbohydrate 61g, Total sugars 22.1g, Salt 0.26g, Sodium 102mg

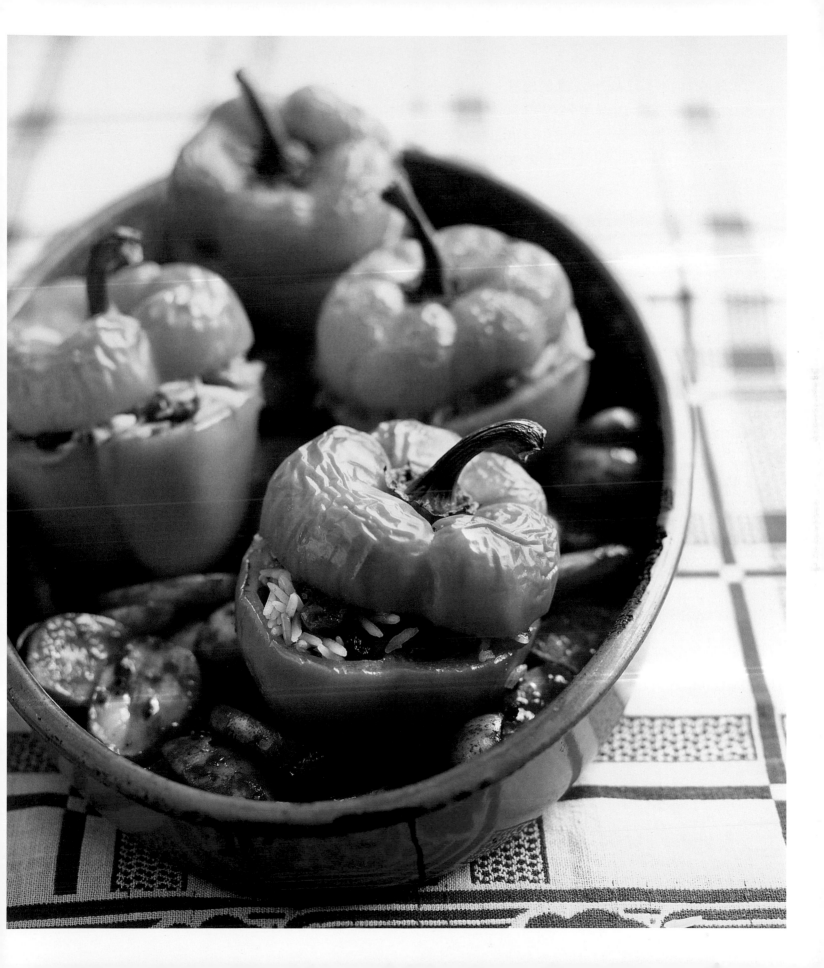

Ratatouille Cakes

Accompanied by a salad, this delicious Australian dish makes a great vegetarian main course, but served as a starter I'm sure it would also appeal to carnivores.

Serves 4

1 medium aubergine
1 tablespoon olive oil
1 small onion, finely chopped
1 garlic clove, finely chopped
½ teaspoon fresh thyme leaves
1 tablespoon tomato purée
½ green pepper, deseeded and cut into
   5mm dice
1 courgette, cut into 5mm dice
1 tomato, deseeded and diced
2 tablespoons chopped fresh
   flat-leaf parsley
1 tablespoon chopped fresh basil
1 egg, beaten
2 tablespoons freshly grated
   Parmesan cheese
½ teaspoon baking powder
4 tablespoons fresh seeded breadcrumbs
spray oil, for frying
salt and freshly ground black pepper
salad or tomato sauce, to serve

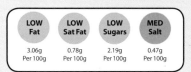

LOW Fat	LOW Sat Fat	LOW Sugars	MED Salt
3.06g Per 100g	0.78g Per 100g	2.19g Per 100g	0.47g Per 100g

1 Preheat the oven to 220°C/425°F/gas mark 7. Prick the aubergine in several places with a fork, place it on a baking tray and roast in the oven for 30–40 minutes or until the aubergine is very soft and on the point of collapsing. Remove from the oven and set aside to cool slightly.

2 Meanwhile, heat the oil in a large frying pan and over a medium heat cook the onion, garlic and thyme until the onion is softening but without colouring, about 6 minutes. Add the tomato purée, green pepper and courgette, increase the heat and cook for a further 5 minutes. Leave to cool slightly.

3 Cut the aubergine in half lengthways and scoop out the flesh; discard the skin. Mash the aubergine flesh to a purée with a fork, or use a food processor. Mix the purée with the fried vegetables and all the remaining ingredients except the spray oil, and add salt and pepper to taste. If the mix is very soft, add extra breadcrumbs.

4 Heat a frying pan and spray with a light coating of oil. Take tablespoonfuls of the aubergine mixture and drop on to the frying pan – do not overcrowd the pan. Cook until brown on both sides, about 4–5 minutes. Keep the cakes warm in the oven on kitchen paper while cooking the remaining cakes. Serve with a salad or your favourite tomato sauce.

Amount per portion
Energy 124 kcals, Protein 6.3g, Fat 6.7g, Saturated fat 1.7g, Carbohydrate 10.4g, Total sugars 4.8g, Salt 1.04g, Sodium 411mg

Simple Spaghetti with Raw Tomato and Cauliflower

I'm sure your initial reaction to the title of this Italian dish will be to give one big yawn, but there will be times when your body demands simplicity, and this quick-and-easy recipe will satisfy that craving.

Serves 4
375g dried spaghetti
4 garlic cloves
1 bunch of fresh basil leaves
¼ teaspoon salt
¼ teaspoon dried chilli flakes
2 tablespoons extra virgin olive oil
4 tomatoes, roughly chopped
    (save any juices)
2 tablespoons chopped hazelnuts
¼ cauliflower, finely chopped
50g low-fat ricotta or cottage cheese
freshly ground black pepper
green salad, to serve

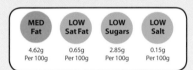

MED Fat	LOW Sat Fat	LOW Sugars	LOW Salt
4.62g Per 100g	0.65g Per 100g	2.85g Per 100g	0.15g Per 100g

1 Cook the spaghetti in boiling salted water for 1 minute less than the packet instructions.

2 Meanwhile, in a food processor or with a mortar and pestle purée the garlic, basil, salt and chilli flakes together until smooth. Add the oil a little at a time, whisking continuously, then dilute with 2 tablespoons of water. In a bowl, mix together the tomatoes, hazelnuts and cauliflower, then stir in the garlic and basil sauce.

3 Drain the spaghetti and tip it on to the tomato mixture, toss well and season with pepper to taste. Spoon into individual bowls and dot the surface with dollops of cheese. Serve with a green salad.

Amount per portion
Energy 452 kcals, Protein 15.6g, Fat 12.0g, Saturated fat 1.7g, Carbohydrate 75.0g, Total sugars 7.4g, Salt 0.38g, Sodium 150mg

Mediterranean Artichoke Stew

I've cheated a little on your behalf in this Italian dish. I believe artichokes are a vegetable too far for the domestic cook: you get spiked, your hands turn black, the artichoke turns black and what are you left with – a pile of inedible leaves, leaving you thinking, why did I bother? So, my solution is to buy jars of wood-roasted artichokes; delicious and so simple.

Serves 4
8 new potatoes
12 baby onions
8 baby carrots
3 garlic cloves
grated zest and juice of 1 lemon
4 sage leaves
3 tablespoons olive oil
300ml vegetable stock
100g frozen peas
2 tomatoes, deseeded and diced
1 x jar wood-roasted artichokes, drained
salt and freshly ground pepper

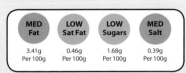

MED Fat	LOW Sat Fat	LOW Sugars	MED Salt
3.41g Per 100g	0.46g Per 100g	1.68g Per 100g	0.39g Per 100g

1 In a gratin dish, mix together the potatoes, onions, carrots, garlic, lemon zest and juice, sage and some pepper. Add the olive oil and mix well so that all the ingredients are coated, and pour in the stock. Leave to marinate for 30 minutes. Meanwhile, preheat the oven to 180°C/350°F/gas mark 4.

2 Cover the gratin dish with greaseproof paper and then some aluminium foil. Transfer the dish to the preheated oven and cook for 35–45 minutes. Discard the covering and add the peas, tomatoes, artichokes and some salt, and cook for a further 5 minutes. Serve either hot or at room temperature.

Amount per portion
Energy 216 kcals, Protein 4.7g, Fat 14.2g, Saturated fat 1.9g, Carbohydrate 18.4g, Total sugars 7.0g, Salt 1.62g, Sodium 642mg

Chickpea, Spinach and Sweet Potato Stew

This Middle Eastern-influenced dish offers a great balance of carbs, protein (the soya beans) and wonderful flavours. This is perfect served with couscous or Saffron Pea Pilaf (see page 117).

Serves 4

For the sweet potatoes
350g sweet potatoes, cut into 1cm dice
1 tablespoon olive oil
2 tablespoons runny honey
1 teaspoon finely chopped fresh rosemary
½ teaspoon each salt and freshly ground
    black pepper
100g 0 per cent fat Greek yogurt
1 garlic clove, crushed to a paste with
    a little salt
grated zest and juice of 1 orange

For the stew
1 tablespoon olive oil
1 large onion, chopped
1 teaspoon ground cumin
1½ teaspoons ground coriander
1 tablespoon harissa chilli paste
1 tablespoon tomato purée
1 x 400g tin chopped tomatoes
150g frozen edamame beans
1 x 400g tin chickpeas, drained and rinsed
100g frozen peas
100g baby spinach
2 tablespoons chopped fresh coriander
salt and freshly ground black pepper
couscous or rice, to serve

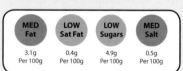

MED Fat	LOW Sat Fat	LOW Sugars	MED Salt
3.1g Per 100g	0.4g Per 100g	4.9g Per 100g	0.5g Per 100g

1 Put the sweet potatoes in a saucepan along with 500ml of water, oil, honey and rosemary, cover and cook gently for 30–35 minutes until very little liquid remains and the potatoes have developed a nice sheen. If too much liquid remains, remove the lid and cook until little remains.

2 Meanwhile, prepare the stew: in a separate saucepan heat the oil and cook the onion together with the cumin and coriander until soft, about 8 minutes. Stir in the harissa and tomato purée, then add the tomatoes and cook for a further 15 minutes or until thick. Add the soya beans, chickpeas, peas and spinach and cook for a further 8 minutes. Fold in the coriander and adjust the seasoning to taste.

3 To make the sauce for the sweet potatoes, mix together the salt and pepper, yogurt, garlic and orange zest and juice. Fold in the sweet potato. Spoon the chickpea stew into individual warmed bowls then top with the sweet potato mix. Serve with couscous or rice.

Amount per portion
Energy 385 kcals, Protein 17.3g, Fat 13.2g, Saturated fat 1.8g, Carbohydrate 52.5g, Total sugars 20.6g, Salt 2.04g, Sodium 803mg

Chickpea and Lentil Curry

This Indian staple is a great curry base for vegetarians, and others, with the option of adding any vegetables you fancy.

Serves 4
200g yellow lentils (toor dal), soaked
    in water for 30 minutes and drained
1 tablespoon sunflower oil
2 large onions, roughly chopped
2 small carrots, sliced
1 teaspoon cumin seeds
¼ teaspoon asafoetida powder (optional)
1 teaspoon chopped garlic
1 teaspoon lazy ginger (see Tip on
    page 144)
2 mild green chillies, deseeded
    and chopped
4 tomatoes, chopped
1 teaspoon chilli powder
1 teaspoon ground turmeric
200g 0 per cent low-fat yogurt
1 teaspoon garam masala
1 x 400g tin chickpeas, drained and rinsed
2 tablespoons chopped fresh coriander
salt and freshly ground pepper
1 tablespoon fresh pomegranate seeds,
    to garnish
brown rice, to serve

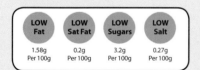

LOW Fat	LOW Sat Fat	LOW Sugars	LOW Salt
1.58g Per 100g	0.2g Per 100g	3.2g Per 100g	0.27g Per 100g

1 Cook the lentils in fresh water until tender. Drain well and season with salt to taste.

2 Meanwhile heat the oil in a frying pan then add the onions and carrots, together with the cumin, asafoetida, garlic, ginger and green chillies, and cook gently until the onions are soft, about 10 minutes.

3 Stir in the tomatoes, chilli powder, turmeric, yogurt and garam masala. Tip in the lentils, then add the chickpeas and coriander and adjust the seasoning to taste. Spoon into individual bowls and garnish with pomegranate seeds. Serve with brown rice.

Amount per portion
Energy 364 kcals, Protein 21.4g, Fat 6.4g, Saturated fat 0.8g, Carbohydrate 50.1g, Total sugars 13.0g, Salt 1.1g, Sodium 420mg

Three Bean Stew with Grated Feta

No meat, no fish, just beans with flavour, with or without the feta 'snow' – your choice. This Greek stew also makes a good partner to roast or grilled meats.

Serves 4

1 tablespoon olive oil
2 onions, roughly chopped
2 carrots, roughly sliced
2 celery stalks, finely sliced
3 garlic cloves, sliced
1 teaspoon dried Greek oregano
350ml tomato passata
1 tablespoon tomato purée
1 x 400g tin red kidney beans, drained
    and rinsed
1 x 400g tin butter beans, drained
    and rinsed
175g runner beans, de-strung and sliced
85g feta cheese
freshly ground black pepper

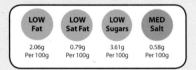

LOW Fat	LOW Sat Fat	LOW Sugars	MED Salt
2.06g Per 100g	0.79g Per 100g	3.61g Per 100g	0.58g Per 100g

1 Warm the olive oil in a large saucepan over a moderate heat, then add the onions, carrots, celery and garlic and cook for 10 minutes. Add the oregano, passata and tomato purée. Cover and cook for 45 minutes, topping up with water as necessary.

2 Now add the tinned beans and runner beans and cook for 20 minutes or until the sauce is thick and the vegetables are cooked. Spoon into warm bowls, then pass the feta through a fine sieve over the bowls to create a 'snow' effect over the stew.

Variation Like more spice? Then zap the stew with a little chopped chilli or season with Tabasco.

Amount per portion
Energy 265 kcals, Protein 14.2g, Fat 8.4g, Saturated fat 3.2g, Carbohydrate 35.3g, Total sugars 14.7g, Salt 2.37g, Sodium 933mg

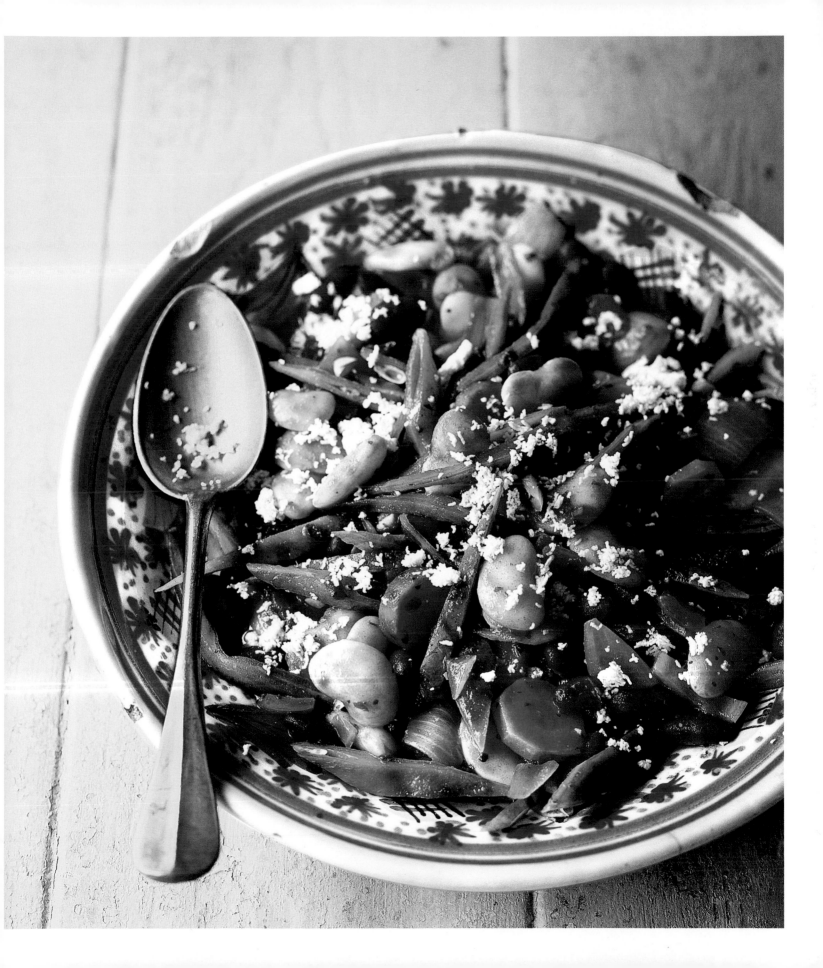

Watercress and Mushroom Pancakes

The Americans love a good pancake or two. Theirs tend to be more like our drop scones but in this case it is thin pancakes we're aiming for. You can play with the filling if you like but in the first instance get used to the pancake recipe before experimenting.

Serves 4

For the pancake batter
1 shallot, finely diced
8 button mushrooms, sliced
2 tablespoons watercress leaves
1 tablespoon sunflower oil
80g plain flour
¼ teaspoon each salt and freshly
    ground black pepper
1 egg, beaten
180ml skimmed milk
spray oil, for frying

For the filling
100g button mushrooms, sliced
2 spring onions, sliced
2 tomatoes, deseeded and diced
1 x 400g tin cannellini beans, drained
    and rinsed
200g 0 per cent fat Greek yogurt
1 tablespoon lemon juice
¼ teaspoon each salt and freshly ground
    black pepper
3 tablespoons roughly chopped
    watercress leaves
1 teaspoon chopped fresh oregano leaves

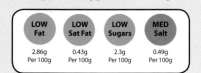

LOW Fat	LOW Sat Fat	LOW Sugars	MED Salt
2.86g Per 100g	0.43g Per 100g	2.3g Per 100g	0.49g Per 100g

1 To make the pancake batter, heat half the oil in a frying pan, add the shallot and mushrooms, and cook over a medium heat for 3 minutes, stirring regularly. Leave to cool slightly.

2 In a food processor, blend together the mushroom mix, the watercress, flour, salt and pepper, egg, milk and 2 tablespoons of water; blend for about 2 minutes, scraping down the sides from time to time. Pour into a jug and leave to rest for 15 minutes.

3 Make the filling by mixing together all the filling ingredients. Set aside.

4 To cook the pancakes, heat a non-stick pan, spray with oil, remove from the heat and pour in about 3 tablespoons of batter, tilting the pan in all directions to cover the base thinly. Return the pan to the heat and cook until the edges of the pancake start to brown, about 1 minute. Flip the pancake over and cook for 1–2 minutes. Tip on to a plate and repeat until all the mixture has been used.

5 Preheat the oven to 180°C/350°F/gas mark 4. Lightly grease a baking sheet. Set 1 pancake on a work surface and spoon about 1 tablespoon of the filling down one half, then roll it up, tucking the ends in, and set it on the baking sheet. Repeat with the remaining pancakes.

6 Cover the baking sheet in foil, transfer to the preheated oven and heat through for 10–12 minutes. Serve with salad.

Amount per portion
Energy 269 kcals, Protein 16.7g, Fat 8.8g, Saturated fat 1.3g, Carbohydrate 32.9g, Total sugars 7.0g, Salt 1.49g, Sodium 589mg

Vegetarian Nasi Goreng – Indonesian Fried Rice

This delicious dish is traditionally served for breakfast and usually includes fish or prawns. This vegetarian version is just as tasty and very easy to put together

Serves 4

150g mixed fresh mushrooms, such as shiitake, button mushrooms and oyster mushrooms, chopped
2 garlic cloves, finely chopped
2.5cm piece of fresh root ginger, peeled and grated
2 fresh red chillies, deseeded and finely chopped
3 shallots, finely chopped
1 tablespoon sunflower oil
375g cold cooked brown rice
1 egg, lightly beaten
1 tablespoon ketjap manis (Indonesian sweet soy sauce)
1 tablespoon light soy sauce
1 tablespoon soy bean paste
115g frozen petit pois
handful of mangetout, topped and tailed and shredded
4 spring onions, finely chopped
½ small bunch of fresh coriander, leaves picked
juice of ½ lime
salt and freshly ground black pepper
lime cheeks, to garnish

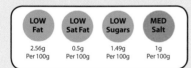

LOW Fat	LOW Sat Fat	LOW Sugars	MED Salt
2.56g Per 100g	0.5g Per 100g	1.49g Per 100g	1g Per 100g

1 Preheat the oven to 200°C/400°F/gas mark 6. Toss the mushrooms with the garlic, ginger, chillies, shallots and a little of the oil and season with salt and black pepper. Spread the mixture out on a baking tray, and bake in the oven for 10 minutes until the mushroom and shallots have started to caramelise.

2 Break up the rice with a fork so that the grains are separated. (it is best to use cold leftover rice as if the rice is warm, it absorbs too much oil. If cooking rice just for this dish, cool it as quickly as possible; rice that is kept warm for a long time is prone to dangerous bacteria). Lightly grease a non-stick frying pan with a couple of drops of oil. Fry the beaten egg to make a thin egg pancake, allow to cool, then roll up and cut into thin shreds. Set aside.

3 Heat a wok over a high heat. Add the rTemaining oil and baked mushroom mixture – make sure you get any juices from the bottom of the pan. Add the rice, ketjap manis, light soy sauce and soybean paste, and stir fry for 2 minutes. Add the peas and mangetout. Stir constantly for 4–5 minutes until the rice is heated all the way through and the green vegetables are cooked, but still have a bite.

4 Add the spring onion, coriander, and shredded omelette and then add the lime juice. Check the seasoning – it should be sweet, rich and earthy; hot from the chilli and salty from the soy sauce. Serve with lime wedges.

Amount per portion
Energy 229 kcals, Protein 8.6g, Fat 6.2g, Saturated fat 1.2g, Carbohydrate 37.0g, Total sugars 3.6g, Salt 2.42g, Sodium 953mg

and Coriander Asian Prawn Cakes Chermoula Grilled Sea
ns Chermoula Grilled Tuna on a Salad of Green White Bean
ackerel Grilled Sea Bass, Spiced Cabbage Grilled Sardines
Polpette di Sarde – Sardine Cakes Scallops and Bacon on S
on, Tomatoes and Olives Crab and Tomato Linguini Penne w
Cannellini Bean Stew Prawn Linguini Fragrant Prawns with
d Sour Sauce New Potatoes and Smoked Mackerel with Avo
n Chowder-style Broth Barley Risotto with Greens and Prawn
d Spices Sweet-and-Sour Prawns Sweet Potato with Crab,
Crabcakes with Asian Coleslaw Spicy Stew of Red Lentils,

Green Salad and Sweet-and-Sour Dressing Omega 3 Plaki
mbs Seared Tuna with a Sicilian Tomatoey Potato Salad Tun
Fillets of Sea Bass with Aniseed Scented Tomatoes Roast C
Tomato Pasta with Anchovies, Pine Nuts and Sultanas Roast
Lemon and Basil Stuffing Paella Asian Surf and Turf Balls in S
Poached Haddock with Eggs and Spinach Cotriade Roast
Fish Parcels Spicy Goan Fish Curry Sardines filled with Bu
r Asian Prawn Cakes Chermoula Grilled Sea Bass Tandoor
la Grilled Tuna on a Salad of Green White Beans Pan-Fried
Grilled Sea Bass, Spiced Cabbage Grilled Sardines with

Fish
and shellfish

Spicy Asian Mussels

Mussels represent excellent value as a shellfish, but there are times when moules marinière has to stand aside for more robust flavours. Serve this Thai-influenced dish with some crusty seeded bread and a salad … be warned, it's hot!

Serves 4

2 tablespoons sunflower oil
1 stalk lemongrass, bruised
2cm piece of fresh galangal, bruised
2cm piece of fresh ginger, peeled and
   bruised
2 shallots, roughly chopped
4 bird's-eye chillies, deseeded and
   roughly chopped
4 garlic cloves
2 tablespoons oyster sauce
1 tablespoon Tabasco sauce
2 teaspoons curry paste
1.5kg mussels, cleaned, any open ones
   discarded

To garnish

3 spring onions, sliced
1 tablespoon chopped fresh coriander

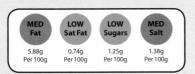

MED Fat	LOW Sat Fat	LOW Sugars	MED Salt
5.88g Per 100g	0.74g Per 100g	1.25g Per 100g	1.38g Per 100g

1 In a wok, heat half the oil and stir-fry the lemongrass and galangal together for 3 minutes.

2 Meanwhile, in a mini food processor blend together the ginger, shallots, chillies, garlic and the remaining oil. Add this paste to the wok and cook for 3 minutes over a medium heat. Stir in the oyster sauce, Tabasco and curry paste, then add 150ml of water, increase the heat and tip in the mussels. Cover and boil for 5 minutes, tossing the mix from time to time.

3 Spoon into individual warmed bowls, discarding any mussels that have not opened. Pour over the spicy liquor, then scatter with spring onion and coriander.

Amount per portion

Energy 155 kcals, Protein 15g, Fat 8g, Saturated fat 1g, Carbohydrate 6g, Total sugars 1.7g, Salt 1.87g, Sodium 736mg

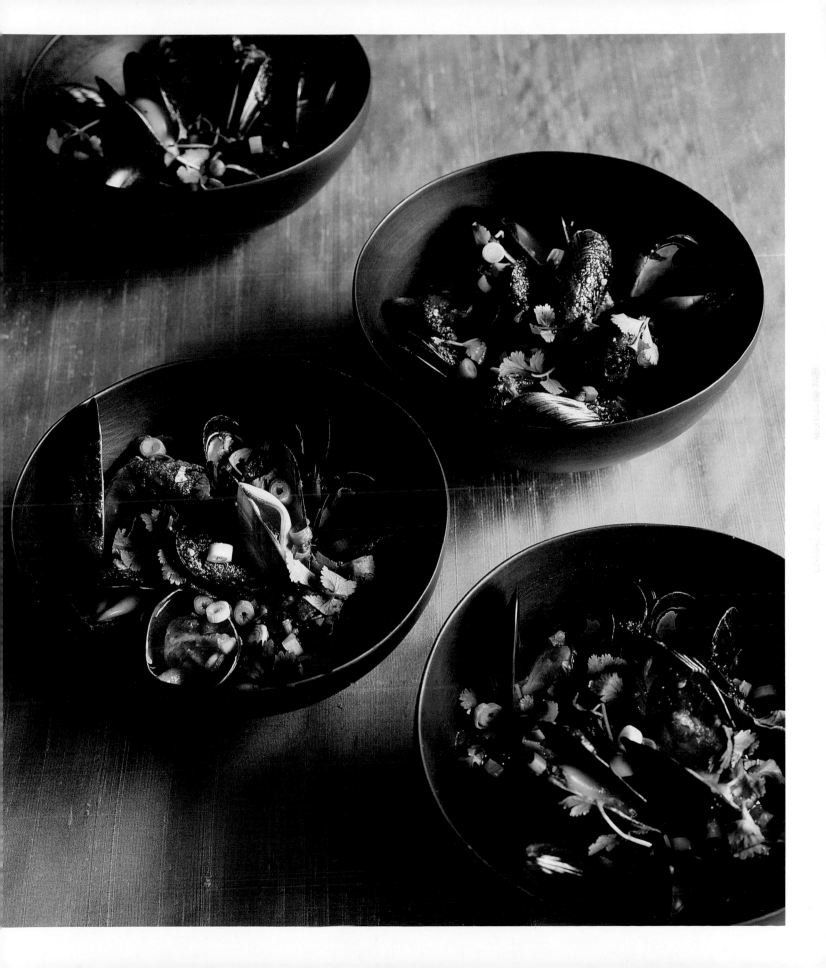

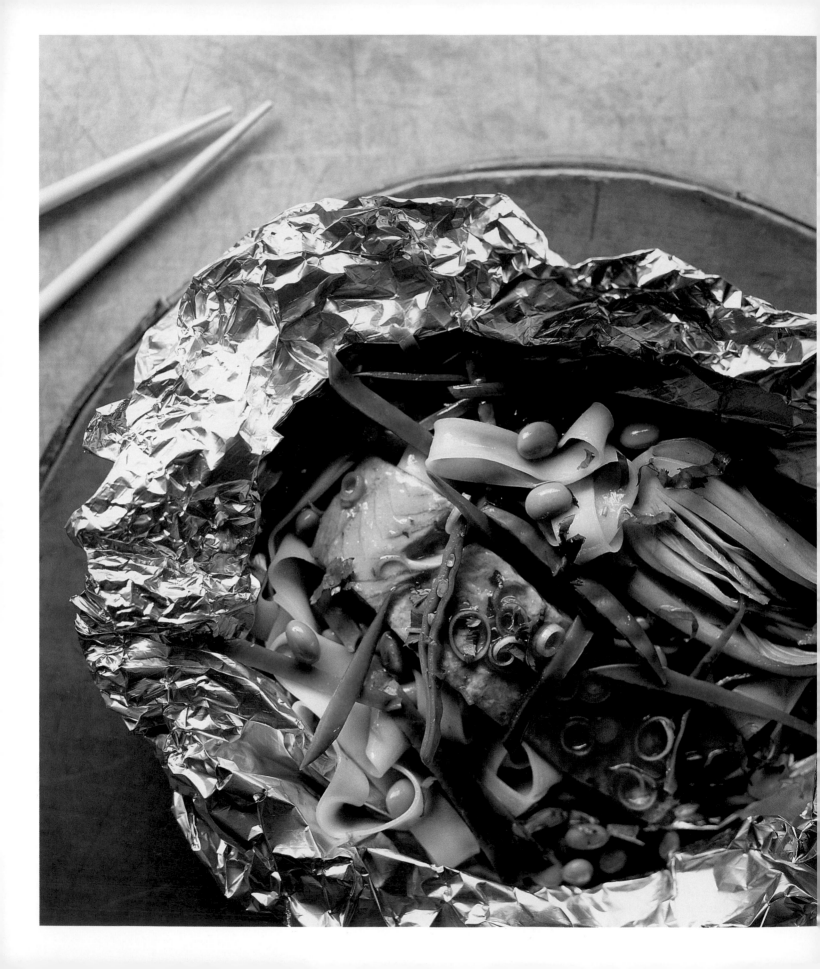

Aromatic Fish Parcels

A fantastic Asian dish that is really easy to do for a dinner party and can be prepared well in advance. What sweet flavours …

Serves 4

150g thick rice noodles
1 teaspoon reduced-salt soy sauce
1 teaspoon fish sauce (nam pla)
1 tablespoon sweet chilli sauce
juice and zest of 1 lime
2 teaspoons finely chopped lemongrass
2 heads of bok choi, halved lengthways
4 salmon fillets (about 150g each), skinned
100g frozen edamame beans
100g mangetout, thinly sliced lengthways
1 tablespoon chopped fresh coriander,
   to garnish

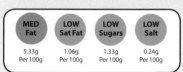

MED Fat	LOW Sat Fat	LOW Sugars	LOW Salt
5.33g Per 100g	1.06g Per 100g	1.33g Per 100g	0.24g Per 100g

1 Preheat the oven to 220°C/425°F/gas mark 7. Place the noodles in a large bowl and cover with boiling water. Stand until tender, about 2 minutes, then drain well.

2 Combine the three sauces, lime juice and zest and lemongrass, and leave to stand for 30 minutes to allow the flavours to develop.

3 Set four large pieces of foil on the work surface. Divide the noodles between the sheets, top with bok choi then with the salmon, scatter over the edamame beans and mangetout, and drizzle with the sauce.

4 Bring up the edges of the foil to seal the parcel, place on a baking tray and cook in the oven for 12 minutes. Open the parcels at the table and sprinkle with coriander.

Amount per portion
Energy 451 kcals, Protein 36.9g, Fat 17.6g, Saturated fat 3.5g, Carbohydrate 38.6g, Total sugars 4.4g, Salt 0.8g, Sodium 316mg

Spicy Goan Fish Curry

This dry curry has airs of vindaloo about it. It packs a punch but has great depth of flavour.

Serves 4

For the spice paste
1 teaspoon ground cumin
1 teaspoon ground coriander
1 teaspoon ground turmeric
3 garlic cloves
2.5cm piece of fresh ginger, peeled and grated
4 dried red chillies, deseeded and soaked in hot water
2 tablespoons lemon juice

For the fish
½ teaspoon salt
½ teaspoon ground turmeric
4 cod or haddock fillets, about 175g each

For the vegetable curry
2 tablespoons sunflower oil
12 new potatoes, halved
2 large onions, roughly chopped
1 aubergine, cut into 2cm pieces
3 cloves
1 teaspoon freshly ground black pepper
115g button mushrooms, quartered
6 cardamom pods, lightly crushed
4 medium green chillies, split lengthways and deseeded
1 teaspoon caster sugar
brown rice, to serve

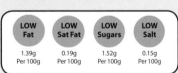

LOW Fat	LOW Sat Fat	LOW Sugars	LOW Salt
1.39g Per 100g	0.19g Per 100g	1.52g Per 100g	0.15g Per 100g

1 In a food processor blend together all the spice paste ingredients to a reasonably smooth paste. Prepare the fish: mix together the salt and turmeric and rub on to the fish, then leave to marinate.
2 Meanwhile, make the vegetable curry. Heat the oil in a large saucepan and fry the potatoes until golden. Remove and set aside. In the same oil, fry the onions and aubergine so that they take on a little colour, about 8 minutes. Add the cloves, pepper, mushrooms and cardamom, and cook for a further 1 minute, stirring.
3 Add the potatoes, chillies and sugar, and cook for a further 2 minutes. Add the spice paste, cover and cook over a gentle heat until the potatoes are half cooked.
4 Place the fish on top of the vegetable curry, cover and continue to cook over a gentle heat for a further 15 minutes. Serve hot, with steaming brown rice.

Variation You can use chicken instead of fish if you like, just add it at the beginning with the onions and aubergine.

Amount per portion
Energy 341 kcals, Protein 37.4g, Fat 8.8g, Saturated fat 1.2g, Carbohydrate 29.9g, Total sugars 9.6g, Salt 0.94g, Sodium 371mg

Sardines filled with Bulgar and Spices

Fresh sardines represent good value, and this oily fish is packed full of all the right omegas. This Middle Eastern recipe will help towards the weekly two portions of oily fish those with diabetes should be eating.

Serves 4
8–12 fresh sardines, scaled, headed, gutted, boned and butterflied
spray oil, for cooking
salt and freshly ground black pepper

For the spiced bulgar mix
185g quick-cook bulgar wheat
2 spring onions, thinly sliced
grated zest and juice of 1 lemon
8 dried apricots, chopped
25g pistachio nuts, chopped
25g dried cranberries
4 tablespoons chopped fresh parsley
2 teaspoons chopped fresh mint
1 tablespoon chopped fresh coriander
¼ teaspoon ground cinnamon
½ teaspoon ground allspice
2 tablespoons pomegranate molasses
2 tablespoons extra virgin olive oil

To serve
4 lime wedges, to serve
new potatoes
salad

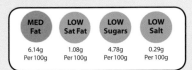

MED Fat	LOW Sat Fat	LOW Sugars	LOW Salt
6.14g Per 100g	1.08g Per 100g	4.78g Per 100g	0.29g Per 100g

1 To make the bulgar mix, tip the bulgar wheat into a bowl, cover with cold water and soak for 20 minutes. Drain then squeeze dry. Meanwhile, preheat the oven to 200°C/400°F/gas mark 6.

2 Mix together the bulgar wheat and the remaining mix ingredients. Season with a little salt and lots of black pepper.

3 Lay the sardines skin-side down on a work surface. Spoon a little bulgar mix on to the middle of each fish, bring the head end over the stuffing and then fold the tail end over. Secure with a cocktail stick – some mixture will fall out, don't worry as there should be surplus left over to serve with the sardines.

4 Lightly oil a baking tray and arrange the sardines on it tail-side up. Transfer to the preheated oven and roast for 8 minutes. Serve with lime wedges and the surplus spiced bulgar mix, along with new potatoes and salad.

Tip Pomegranate molasses is a rich, sticky reduction of pomegranate juice often found in Middle Eastern shops. You can make your own, however, by combining 1 litre of pomegranate juice with 50g of sugar and 60ml lemon juice in a medium saucepan. Bring to a boil, stirring to dissolve the sugar, over a medium heat. Reduce the heat and simmer, stirring occasionally. The molasses are ready when the liquid has reduced by about three-quarters and is thick and syrupy.

Amount per portion
Energy 536 kcals, Protein 33.8g, Fat 22.1g, Saturated fat 3.9g, Carbohydrate 53.9g, Total sugars 17.2g, Salt 1.06g, Sodium 420mg

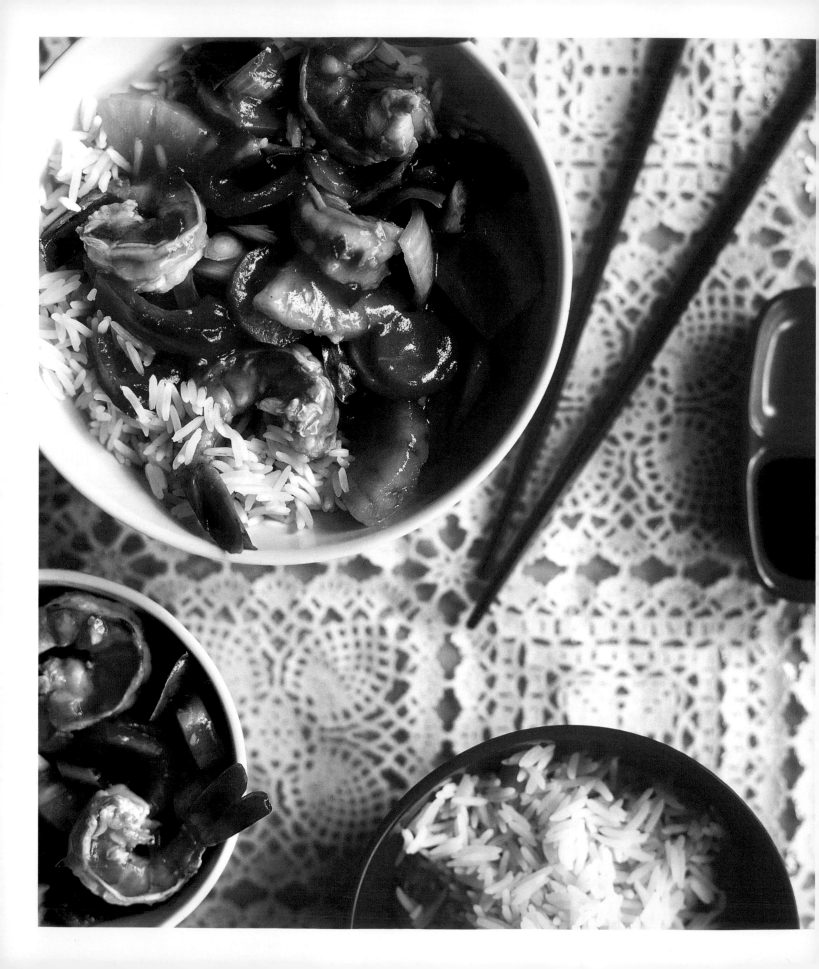

Sweet-and-Sour Prawns

An all-time favourite – this Chinese westernised dish is loved by children and adults alike.

Serves 4

juice of 1 lemon

½ teaspoon salt

24 raw tiger prawns with tail on, head
   and shells removed

2 spring onions, finely sliced at an angle

1 white onion, roughly chopped

1 carrot, thinly sliced

1 red pepper, chopped into 2.5cm pieces

1 green pepper, chopped into 2.5cm pieces

1 x small tin water chestnuts, drained
   and sliced

1 x small tin pineapple pieces, drained

steamed rice, to serve

For the sauce

2 garlic cloves, finely chopped

2.5cm piece of fresh ginger, peeled
   and grated

1 fresh red chilli, deseeded and
   finely chopped

150ml pineapple juice

1 tablespoon light soy sauce

2 tablespoons white wine vinegar

1 tablespoon tomato purée

1 tablespoon tomato ketchup

1 tablespoon sugar or low-calorie
   granulated sweetener

1 tablespoon cornflour mixed to a paste
   with 3 tablespoons cold water

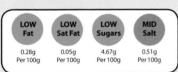

LOW Fat	LOW Sat Fat	LOW Sugars	MID Salt
0.28g Per 100g	0.05g Per 100g	4.67g Per 100g	0.51g Per 100g

1 In a large bowl, mix together the lemon juice and salt. Add the prawns and stir well to coat, then set aside to marinate.

2 To make the sauce, in a pan sweat the garlic, ginger and chilli then reduce the heat and cook for 5 minutes. Add the remaining sauce ingredients except for the cornflour paste, bring to the boil and cook for 3 minutes.

3 Meanwhile in a large pan sweat the onions, carrots and peppers. Stir in the water chestnuts and pineapple pieces and cook just long enough to heat through. Add the prawns and cook for a further 1 minute.

4 Add the cooked sauce and the cornflour paste, and cook until thickened and glossy, about 2 minutes. Serve with steamed rice on the side.

Amount per portion (low-calorie sweetener)
Energy 174 kcals, Protein 18.3g, Fat 1.1g, Saturated fat 0.2g, Carbohydrate 24.4g, Total sugars 18.2g, Salt 1.99g, Sodium 783mg

Amount per portion (sugar)
Energy 188 kcals, Protein 18.3g, Fat 1.1g, Saturated fat 0.2g, Carbohydrate 28.2g, Total sugars 22.0g, Salt 1.99g, Sodium 784mg

Sweet Potato with Crab, Red Snapper and Coriander

To this fantastic rustic West Indian stew brimming with freshness and flavour, I've added some black-eyed peas – not necessarily traditional for this type of dish, but it's good for you. Scotch bonnets are about the hottest chillies, hence the reason West Indians use them whole in cooking: the chillies can be easily removed when the dish has reached the preferred intensity of heat.

Serves 4

1 tablespoon sunflower oil
2 onions, chopped
5 garlic cloves, crushed
2 Scotch bonnet chillies (use gloves)
2 sweet potatoes, cut into 1cm dice
1.2 litres reduced-salt fish or chicken stock
175g brown crabmeat
325g red snapper fillets, pin-boned
    and cut into 2.5cm pieces
175g white crabmeat
juice of 2 limes
2 tablespoons chopped fresh coriander
1 x 400g tin black-eyed peas, drained
warm seeded bread, to serve

1 Heat the oil in a large saucepan, then add the onion and garlic and cook over a gentle heat for 8–10 minutes until the onion has softened. Add the Scotch bonnets whole, the sweet potatoes and the stock and simmer for 10 minutes.

2 Stir in the brown crabmeat, cook for 2 minutes to create a sauce, then add the snapper and cook for a further 3 minutes. Add the remaining ingredients and cook for a further for 2 minutes, without allowing the stew to boil. Eat with warm seeded bread.

Amount per portion

Energy 392 kcals, Protein 40.6g, Fat 10.7g, Saturated fat 1.3g, Carbohydrate 35.7g, Total sugars 9.5g, Salt 2.12g, Sodium 837mg

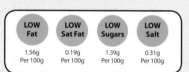

LOW Fat — 1.56g Per 100g | LOW Sat Fat — 0.19g Per 100g | LOW Sugars — 1.39g Per 100g | LOW Salt — 0.31g Per 100g

Asian Prawn Cakes

This luxurious little number can be served as a canapé, starter or main course, depending on the size of the prawn cakes. For a main course, serve them with Stir-fried Greens with Mustard Seeds and Cashews (see page 131), rice and a dipping sauce (see page 107).

Serves 4

350g raw tiger prawns, shell-off
    and deveined
1cm piece ginger, peeled and chopped
1 garlic clove
2 tablespoons chopped fresh coriander
3 spring onions, sliced
2 teaspoons fish sauce (nam pla)
1 egg white
4 tablespoons chopped water chestnuts
4 tablespoons sweetcorn niblets
1 tablespoon chopped cashew nuts
1 hot red chilli, deseeded and finely diced
spray oil, for frying

1 In a food processor, blend together the prawns, ginger, garlic, coriander, spring onions, fish sauce and egg white to a smooth paste. Decant into a bowl, fold in the remaining ingredients except the oil and mix well.

2 With wet hands, shape the mixture into 8 small 'burgers' or cakes. Refrigerate them to firm up – for about 2 hours if possible.

3 Spray a large frying pan with oil and over a medium heat cook the cakes for 2–3 minutes on each side.

Amount per portion

Energy 97 kcals, Protein 17.5g, Fat 1.1g, Saturated fat 0.2g, Carbohydrate 4.7g, Total sugars 1.2g, Salt 0.98g, Sodium 389mg

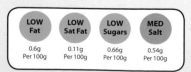

LOW Fat — 0.6g Per 100g | LOW Sat Fat — 0.11g Per 100g | LOW Sugars — 0.66g Per 100g | MED Salt — 0.54g Per 100g

RIGHT Sweet Potato with Crab, Red Snapper and Coriander

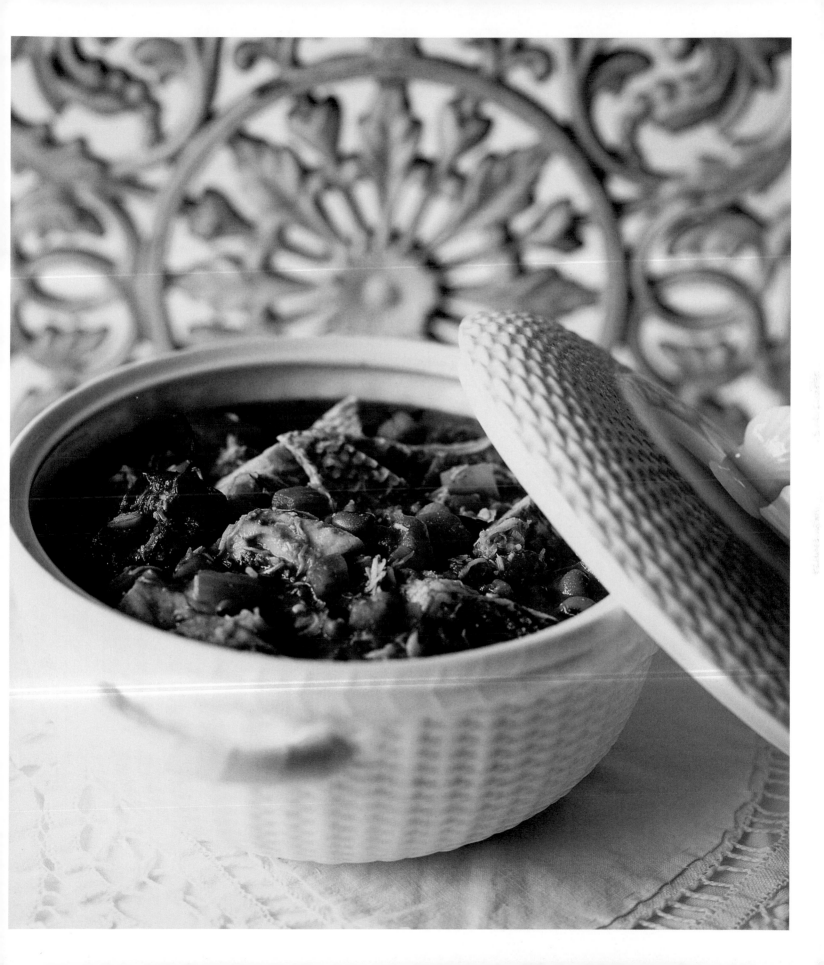

Chermoula Grilled Sea Bass

In this recipe, I'm using a variation of the North African chermoula marinade as a vegetable flavouring as well as a delicious fish marinade.

Serves 4
4 sea bass fillets, about 175g each
16 new potatoes, quartered
½ cauliflower, broken into small florets
100g French beans, cut into 2.5cm pieces
200ml tomato passata
1 x 400g tin chickpeas, drained and rinsed
salt and freshly ground black pepper
lime wedges, to serve

For the chermoula marinade
6 garlic cloves
2 bunches fresh coriander, roughly
    chopped
1 tablespoon ground cumin
1 teaspoon dried chilli flakes
1 tablespoon paprika
2 lemons – grated zest of 1, juice of 2
60ml extra virgin olive oil

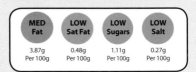

MED Fat	LOW Sat Fat	LOW Sugars	LOW Salt
3.87g Per 100g	0.48g Per 100g	1.11g Per 100g	0.27g Per 100g

1 To make the chermoula, in a food processor, purée together the garlic, coriander, cumin, chilli, paprika, lemon zest and juice. When smooth, add the olive oil, running the machine slowly. Season with salt and pepper. Put three-quarters of the chermoula into a saucepan and set aside. Scrape the remaining quarter of chermoula into a bowl, add the sea bass and stir well to coat both sides of the fillets. Set aside.

2 Cook the potatoes in boiling water for 15 minutes, then add the cauliflower and beans and cook for a further 5 minutes. Drain, then transfer the vegetables to the pan containing the chermoula. Fold in the chickpeas and heat gently.

3 When the vegetables are hot, grill the fish for 2 minutes each side. Spoon the vegetables on to warmed plates, top with the fish fillets, and serve with lime wedges.

Amount per portion
Energy 532 kcals, Protein 45.9g, Fat 22.4g, Saturated fat 2.8g, Carbohydrate 39.3g, Total sugars 6.4g, Salt 1.59g, Sodium 627mg

Tandoori-Style Fish

I've used fish for this Indian classic, but the marinade works well with chicken as well. Serve with brown rice and some spiced chickpeas (see page 121).

Serves 4

4 mackerel or herring fillets,
　　pin bones removed
juice of 1 lime
½ teaspoon salt
4 shallots, roughly chopped
1 teaspoon ground cumin
½ teaspoon ground turmeric
2 teaspoons chilli powder
1 teaspoon garlic powder
4 tablespoons 0 per cent fat Greek yogurt
1 tablespoon sunflower oil, plus extra
　　for greasing
1 teaspoon paprika
½ teaspoon ground cardamom
spray oil, to grease

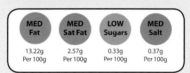

MED Fat	MED Sat Fat	LOW Sugars	MED Salt
13.22g Per 100g	2.57g Per 100g	0.33g Per 100g	0.37g Per 100g

1 Preheat the oven to 220°C/425°F/gas mark 7. With a small sharp knife, make 3–4 shallow incisions on both sides of the fish fillets. Mix together the lime juice and salt, rub into the fish and leave for 10 minutes to marinate.

2 In a food processor blend together the shallots, spices and yogurt. Rub this mixture over the fish on both sides, then leave to marinate for a further 20 minutes.

3 Mix together the oil, paprika and cardamom and set aside. Lightly grease a roasting tin, place the fish skin-side up in the tin and brush with the flavoured oil. Transfer to the oven and roast for 10 minutes.

Amount per portion
Energy 501 kcals, Protein 39.9g, Fat 36.5g, Saturated fat 7.1g, Carbohydrate 3.4g, Total sugars 0.9g, Salt 1.03g, Sodium 406mg

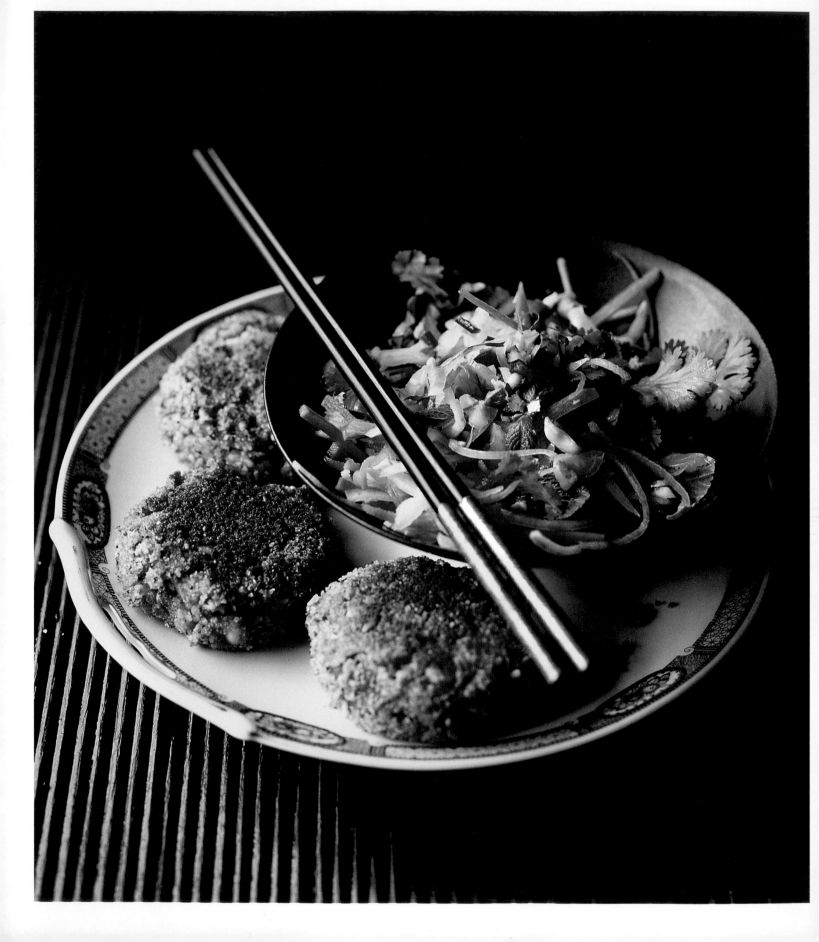

Crabcakes with Asian Coleslaw

There's something very satisfying about crabcakes, and whenever I'm in America I always try out their different versions. This one, like many dishes from the US West Coast, owes much to Asian influences.

Serves 4
2 spring onions, finely chopped
1 fresh red chilli, deseeded and finely chopped
1 tablespoon chopped fresh coriander
1 tablespoon snipped fresh chives
½ tablespoon chopped fresh mint
1½ tablespoons low-fat mayonnaise
½ teaspoon English mustard powder
½ teaspoon wasabi powder
1 egg yolk
450g fresh white crabmeat
50g seeded breadcrumbs (see Tips)
spray sunflower oil

For the coating
115g seasoned plain flour
2 eggs, beaten
115g seeded breadcrumbs

For the coleslaw
225g bok choi, shredded
125g carrots, julienned
4 shallots, sliced
½ tablespoon grated fresh ginger
2 tablespoons shredded basil leaves
2 tablespoons coriander leaves
1 tablespoon mint leaves
1 clove garlic, chopped
1 fresh hot chillies, de-seeded and finely chopped
grated zest of 1 orange
juice of 1 orange
juice of 2 limes
1 tablespoon Asian fish sauce
½ teaspoon sugar
4 tablespoons peanut oil
salt and freshly ground black pepper, to taste

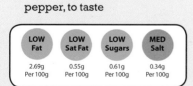

LOW Fat	LOW Sat Fat	LOW Sugars	MED Salt
2.69g Per 100g	0.55g Per 100g	0.61g Per 100g	0.34g Per 100g

1 To make the Asian Coleslaw, mix the bok choi in a bowl with the carrots, shallots, ginger, basil, coriander, mint, garlic, chilli and orange zest. In a small bowl, whisk together the orange juice, lime juice, Asian fish sauce and sugar. Slowly whisk in the oil until emulsified. Add the dressing to the cabbage and toss well. Season with salt and pepper. Chill, covered for 2–6 hours.

2 In a bowl combine the spring onion, chilli and herbs. In another bowl whisk together the mayonnaise, mustard, wasabi and egg yolk, then add the herb mixture to the mayo. Fold this mixture into the crabmeat, then add enough breadcrumbs to bind efficiently. Shape into 4 patties, then chill to firm up on an oiled plate, uncovered, for an hour but ideally overnight.

3 Preheat the grill to high. Lay out 3 plates to prepare the coating: one for the flour, one for the beaten egg and one for the breadcrumbs. Dip the crab cakes into the flour, then the egg (making sure all floury bits are covered) and then the breadcrumbs.

4 Spray the surface of each crabcake with sunflower oil, pop under the grill and cook for 3–4 minutes each side, ensuring they do not burn. Serve with Asian Coleslaw.

Tip When coating the cakes in breadcrumbs, only coat the surface not the sides, as you won't be deep-frying, will you?
To make seeded breadcrumbs, dry some seeded bread slices in a low oven (no higher than 130°C/275°F/gas mark 1) until brittle enough to snap. Break them up into pieces, pop in a food processor and blitz into crumbs. Do not pass the bread through a sieve as you want to retain a little texture.

Amount per portion
Energy 387 kcals, Protein 33.0g, Fat 10.2g, Saturated fat 2.1g, Carbohydrate 43.4g, Total sugars 2.3g, Salt 1.3g, Sodium 911mg

Spicy Stew of Red Lentils, Cod and Prawns

Indian food has so much depth of flavour, and it's all about spices, not necessarily about chilli. The lentil base here can play host to so many other ingredients. This recipe features lots of ingredients but most of them should already be in your store-cupboard.

Serves 4

1 tablespoon sunflower oil
1 onion, finely chopped
4 garlic cloves, crushed
1 carrot, roughly chopped
1 red pepper, deseeded and cut into
   2.5cm pieces
½ cinnamon stick
1 teaspoon grated ginger
1 teaspoon ground turmeric
2 teaspoons ground cumin
2 teaspoons ground coriander
2 teaspoons yellow mustard seeds
1 teaspoon ground cardamom
2 bay leaves
1 tablespoon chopped fresh coriander
   stalk or root
175g red lentils, washed
1 x 200g tin chopped tomatoes
225g cod fillet, skinned and cut into
   2.5cm pieces
275g raw tiger prawns, shell-off
juice of ½ lemon
3 tablespoons chopped fresh coriander
salt and freshly ground black pepper
brown rice, to serve

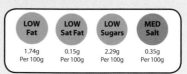

LOW Fat	LOW Sat Fat	LOW Sugars	MED Salt
1.74g Per 100g	0.15g Per 100g	2.29g Per 100g	0.35g Per 100g

1 In a large saucepan heat the oil, then add the onion, garlic, carrot, red pepper and ginger and cook over a medium heat for 10–12 minutes until the vegetables have softened.

2 Add all spices, bay leaves and coriander stalks and stir to combine. Cook gently for a further 2 minutes. Add the lentils, tomatoes and 600ml of cold water. Bring to the boil, reduce the heat and simmer gently until the lentils start to break down – this can take from 45 minutes to 1 hour 30 minutes depending on the heat and the lentils.

3 Remove the cinnamon stick, fold in the cod, prawns, lemon juice and chopped coriander and cook for a further 6 minutes. Season to taste and serve, ideally with brown rice.

Variation This works really well as a vegetarian dish. Simply omit the fish and fold in a host of green vegetables.

Amount per portion
Energy 333 kcals, Protein 36.0g, Fat 5.9g, Saturated fat 0.5g, Carbohydrate 36.2g, Total sugars 7.8g, Salt 1.2g, Sodium 471mg

Chermoula Grilled Tuna on a Salad of Green White Beans

North African chermoula sauce is a great marinade for fish. It requires a certain amount of store-cupboard ingredients but it's worth the effort.

Serves 4

For the chermoula marinade
1 bunch fresh coriander, roughly chopped
leaves from 1 bunch fresh flat-leaf parsley
4 garlic cloves
1 fresh red chilli, deseeded
3 spring onions, roughly chopped
2 teaspoons turmeric
2 teaspoons ground cumin
2 teaspoons chilli powder
2 teaspoons sweet paprika
juice and grated zest of 1 lemon
1 tablespoon olive oil
salt

For the fish
4 fresh tuna steaks, about 150g each
spray olive oil
2 x 400g tins cannellini beans, drained
    and rinsed
lemon wedges, to serve
green salad, to serve

1 In a food-processor, blend all the marinade ingredients together to a paste. Coat the tuna with half the marinade and set aside. Preheat the grill to high.

2 Heat a frying pan, spray it lightly with oil and cook the remaining marinade for 2 minutes. Add the beans and a splash of water, cook for 3 minutes to heat through and season to taste.

3 Grill the tuna for 2 minutes each side. Serve on the beans, with lemon wedges and a green salad.

Amount per portion
Energy 399 kcals, Protein 47.1g, Fat 12.4g, Saturated fat 2.1g, Carbohydrate 26.8g, Total sugars 3.5g, Salt 2.17g, Sodium 855mg

LOW Fat	LOW Sat Fat	LOW Sugars	MED Salt
4.07g Per 100g	0.69g Per 100g	1.15g Per 100g	0.71g Per 100g

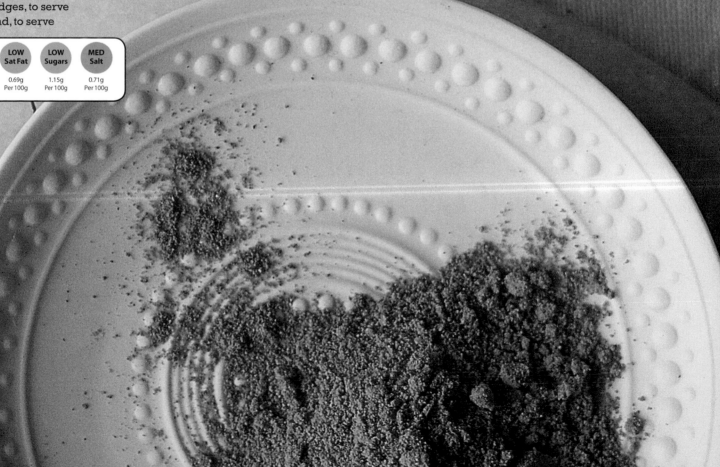

Pan-fried Sea Bass with Green Salad and Sweet-and-Sour Dressing

Lots of Asian influences going on here, although their choice of fish would be different. Fresh and tangy, it's the perfect light meal.

Serves 4
60g plain flour
½ teaspoon each sea salt and freshly
    ground white pepper
4 firm white fish fillets (sea bass, pollack)
50ml sunflower oil
lime wedges, to serve

For the zesty vegetable salad
¼ Savoy cabbage, shredded
20 mangetout, finely sliced
2 large fresh red chillies, deseeded
    and sliced on the diagonal.
15g fresh coriander leaves
12 fresh mint leaves
4 shallots, finely sliced
zest of 1 lime

For the sweet-and-sour dressing
1 tablespoon sugar
2 tablespoons fish sauce (nam pla)
2 tablespoons lime juice

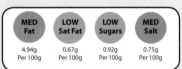

MED Fat	LOW Sat Fat	LOW Sugars	MED Salt
4.94g Per 100g	0.67g Per 100g	0.92g Per 100g	0.75g Per 100g

1 Stir the flour, salt and pepper together in a bowl, and use to coat the skin side of the fish fillets. Heat the oil in a large non-stick frying pan over a medium to high heat. Add the fish, skin-side down, and cook for 6 minutes. Turn over, remove the pan from the heat and allow the fish to cook in the residual heat of the pan for 1 minute until the fish is cooked.

2 Meanwhile, make the salad. In a pan of lightly salted boiling water cook the cabbage and mangetout together for 2 minutes. Drain and set aside. Into a large bowl mix the chilli, coriander, mint and shallots, then stir in the cabbage and mangetout and the lime zest.

3 To make the dressing, stir the sugar and 2 tablespoons of water in a small pan over a low heat until the sugar has dissolved. Remove from the heat, add the fish sauce and lime juice and stir to combine.

4 Serve the fish on top of the salad and dribble on some sweet-and-sour dressing, and accompany with lime wedges.

Amount per portion
Energy 326 kcals, Protein 32.7g, Fat 15.5g, Saturated fat 2.1g, Carbohydrate 14.8g, Total sugars 2.9g, Salt 2.37g, Sodium 933mg

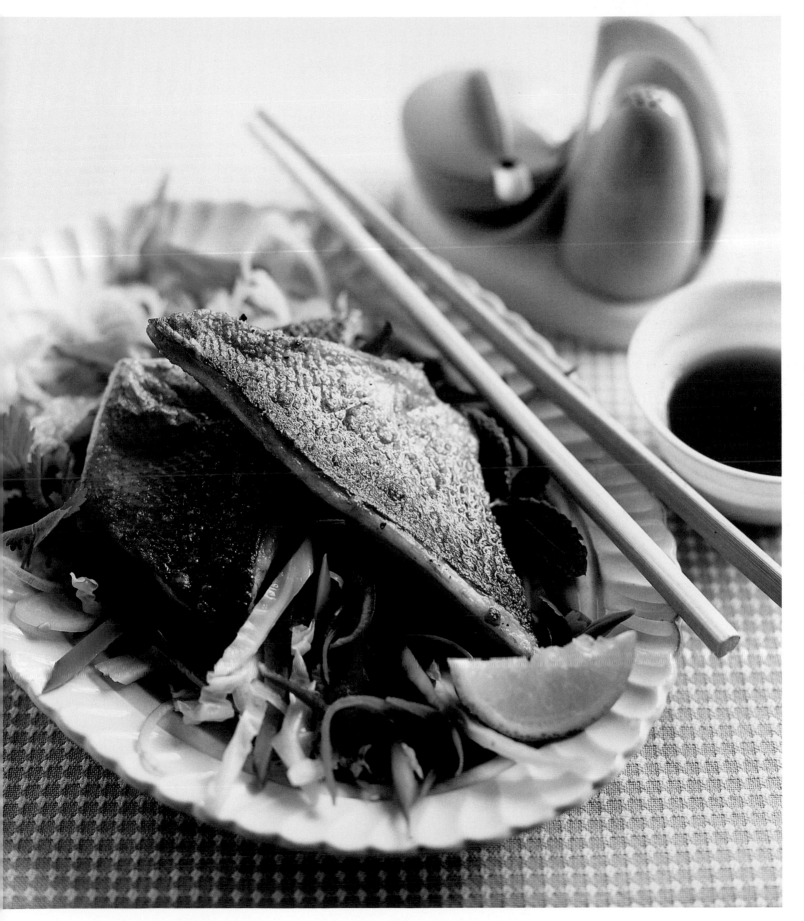

Omega 3 Plaki – Baked Mackerel

On average, we eat less than 1 portion of fish per week. But we all know we should be eating at least two portions of oily fish a week. Here's a delicious and nutritious Greek alternative to that same old boring piece of grilled fish.

Serves 4

8 mackerel or herring fillets, about
   100g each
2 tomatoes, each sliced into 4
2 tablespoons extra virgin olive oil
salt and fresh ground black pepper
1 tablespoon chopped fresh parsley,
   to garnish

For the vegetable 'sauce'

2 carrots, sliced
2 onions, sliced
1 celery stalk, sliced
3 garlic cloves, crushed to a paste with
   a little salt
1 sprig of fresh thyme
2 bay leaves
1 x 400g tin chopped tomatoes
100ml dry white wine
1 x 400g tinned chickpeas, drained
   and rinsed
brown rice and salad, to serve

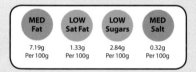

MED Fat	LOW Sat Fat	LOW Sugars	MED Salt
7.19g Per 100g	1.33g Per 100g	2.84g Per 100g	0.32g Per 100g

1 Preheat the oven to 180°C/350°F/gas mark 4. Combine all the 'sauce' ingredients and tip into a lightly oiled deep roasting tin or casserole dish. Cover with foil and cook for 20 minutes. Remove the dish from the oven but do not turn the oven off.

2 Season the fish fillets and place them on top of the 'sauce'. Top each fillet with 2 slices of tomato, drizzle with olive oil and season to taste. Return to the oven, uncovered, and bake for 15 minutes. Sprinkle with parsley and serve with brown rice and a salad.

Amount per portion
Energy 636 kcals, Protein 44.6g, Fat 40.0g, Saturated fat 7.4g, Carbohydrate 24.0g, Total sugars 11.8g, Salt 1.46g, Sodium 578mg

Grilled Sea Bass with Spiced Cabbage

Lovely fresh sea bass cooked until the skin is crispy, served with a tamarind relish and spicy cabbage – loads of flavour but pretty quick to prepare.

Serves 4

4 sea bass fillets, about 175g each,
 bones removed
¼ teaspoon each salt and ground
 white pepper
¼ teaspoon ground turmeric
juice of 1 lime
spray cooking oil
rice or new potatoes, to serve

For the salsa relish

2 shallots, finely sliced
1 red bird's eye chilli, deseeded and
 finely chopped
1 medium hot chilli, deseeded and
 finely sliced
2 tomatoes, deseeded and chopped
1 tablespoon shrimp paste (blachan)
1 teaspoon grated ginger
100ml tamarind juice
1 teaspoon caster sugar
pinch of salt
1 tablespoon chopped fresh mint leaves

For the cabbage

½ savoy cabbage, shredded
1 medium hot red chilli, deseeded and
 roughly chopped
½ teaspoon shrimp paste (blachan)
2 shallots, roughly chopped
1 teaspoon caster sugar
¼ teaspoon salt
1 tablespoon sunflower oil
2 sweet potatoes, cut into 1cm dice
 and cooked

LOW Fat	LOW Sat Fat	LOW Sugars	MED Salt
2.46g Per 100g	0.39g Per 100g	4.73g Per 100g	0.54g Per 100g

1 In a shallow dish, season the fish with salt, pepper, turmeric and lime juice, and leave to marinate for 20 minutes. Meanwhile, combine all the ingredients for the salsa relish in a bowl and leave to stand for at least 15 minutes.

2 Blanch the cabbage in boiling salted water for 3 minutes, then drain well. In a mini food processor, blend together the chilli, shrimp paste, shallots, sugar and salt to a smooth paste. Heat the oil in a frying pan and cook the paste for 3 minutes, stirring regularly. Add the blanched cabbage and sweet potatoes, heat through and keep warm.

3 Heat a large flat griddle or frying pan, spray with oil, and over a high temperature cook the sea bass skin-side down for 6 minutes. Turn the fish over, remove the pan from the heat and allow the fish to cook in the residual heat of the pan for 2 minutes until the fish is cooked.

Amount per portion
Energy 354 kcals, Protein 39.8g, Fat 8.2g, Saturated fat 1.3g, Carbohydrate 32.3g, Total sugars 15.8g, Salt 1.79g, Sodium 705mg

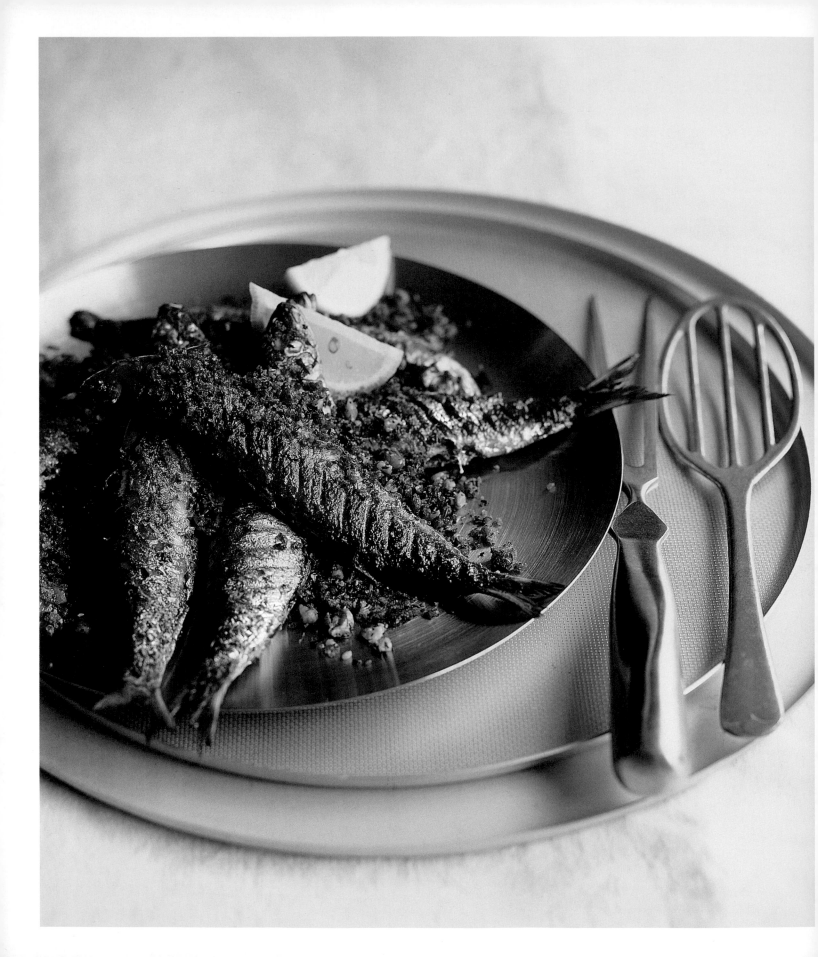

Grilled Sardines with Walnut and Chilli Crumbs

This dish could have been invented anywhere – it's got a touch of Portugal, a sprinkling of the Middle East and even a touch of the UK – but I ate it in a restaurant in Sydney, so I must give them the credit. Just like in the USA and now even the UK, they are culinary magpies in Australia.

Serves 4

3 slices seeded bread, crusts removed, shredded
3 garlic cloves
3 spring onions, roughly chopped
1 hot fresh red chilli, deseeded
1 teaspoon fresh thyme leaves
2 tablespoons fresh curly parsley leaves
2 tablespoons extra virgin olive oil
grated zest of 1 lemon
40g walnut halves, toasted
12 large fresh sardines, cleaned and gutted
spray olive oil
salt and freshly ground black pepper
lemon wedges and salad, to serve

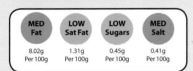

MED Fat	LOW Sat Fat	LOW Sugars	MED Salt
8.02g Per 100g	1.31g Per 100g	0.45g Per 100g	0.41g Per 100g

1 Put the bread in a food processor along with the garlic, spring onions, chilli, thyme, parsley, olive oil and lemon zest. Blitz until crumb-like and green, then add the walnuts and, using a pulse action, break up the walnuts – you need to retain texture. Season to taste, then tip the mixture into a dry frying pan and cook the crumbs over a low to medium heat, shaking the pan regularly, until golden. This requires careful attention.

2 Meanwhile, heat a griddle pan on a high heat. Season the sardines with black pepper and spray lightly with olive oil. Cook for 2–3 minutes each side depending on their size. Scatter the crumbs over the sardines and serve with lemon wedges and salad.

Tip This is wonderful when the sardines are cooked on a charcoal barbecue, adding a lovely smokiness. It's also great served with a tomato and onion salad and some bread to mop up all the juices.

Amount per portion
Energy 478 kcals, Protein 38.7g, Fat 28.7g, Saturated fat 4.7g, Carbohydrate 17.2g, Total sugars 1.6g, Salt 1.48g, Sodium 581mg

Seared Tuna with a Sicilian Tomatoey Potato Salad

A really summery number with lots of Mediterranean flavours, this is a perfect dish for outdoor eating.

Serves 4

650g waxy salad potatoes, quartered
2 tablespoons olive oil
2 garlic cloves, sliced
2 onions, finely sliced
1 teaspoon dried wild oregano
1 fresh chilli, deseeded and finely chopped
4 anchovy fillets, roughly chopped
1 x 400g tin plum tomatoes
juice of ½ lemon
1 teaspoon sugar
12 cherry tomatoes
4 fresh tuna steaks, about 150g each
salt and freshly ground black pepper
1 tablespoon snipped fresh chives, to
    garnish

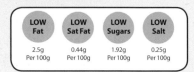

LOW Fat	LOW Sat Fat	LOW Sugars	LOW Salt
2.5g Per 100g	0.44g Per 100g	1.92g Per 100g	0.25g Per 100g

1 Cook the potatoes in boiling salted water for 15–20 minutes or until tender but still intact. Drain and set aside.

2 Heat 1½ tablespoons of the olive oil in a saucepan, add the garlic, onion, oregano, chilli and anchovies and cook for 5 minutes. Tip the tinned tomatoes into a sieve over a bowl to collect the juices and set the tomatoes aside. Add the juices to the onion mix, then the lemon juice and sugar. Cook until the sauce is thick then season to taste.

3 Crush the tinned tomatoes between your fingers to create small pieces and add to the sauce, along with the potatoes and the cherry tomatoes. Cook for 5 minutes.

4 Brush a griddle pan with the remaining olive oil and heat the pan to very hot, season the tuna then cook for 1 minute each side. Set the tuna on top of the potato salad and sprinkle with chives.

Tip I urge you not to overcook the tuna, otherwise you may as well open a tin. This salad is equally good eaten the next day at room temperature, maybe this time using flakes of tinned tuna.

Amount per portion
Energy 427 kcals, Protein 41.5g, Fat 13.7g, Saturated fat 2.4g, Carbohydrate 36.7g, Total sugars 10.5g, Salt 1.36g, Sodium 536mg

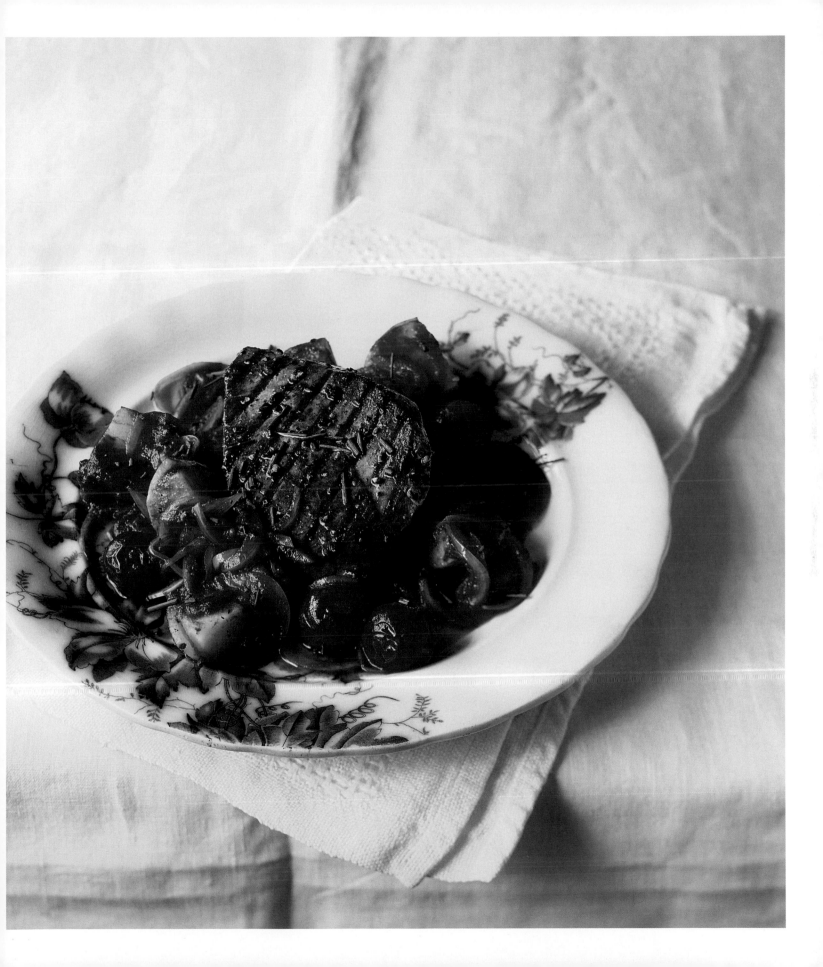

Tunisian Fish Stew

North African fisherfolk make this dish with the fish from their catch that is unsuitable for more simple cooking, so traditionally a variety of rock fish would be used. You can use any non-oily fish, normally a white fish. I've made this dish more GI-friendly by adding new potatoes instead of floury ones, more vegetables than would normally be the case and white beans.

Serves 4

2 tablespoons olive oil
2 onions, finely diced
1 bird's eye chilli, deseeded and finely
    chopped
4 garlic cloves, finely chopped
1 tablespoon harissa chilli paste
2 teaspoons ground cumin
pinch of saffron
1 bulb fennel, outer leaves removed, diced
12 new potatoes, halved
juice of 2 lemons
1.5 litre reduced-salt fish or vegetable stock
1 x 400g tin chopped tomatoes
1 teaspoon salt
2 courgettes, cut into 2cm rounds
115g French beans, cut into 2cm lengths
1 x 400g tin white haricot or cannellini
    beans, drained and rinsed
600g white fish fillets, skinned, cut into
    bite-sized pieces
½ bunch fresh coriander, roughly chopped
1 lemon, cut into wedges, to serve

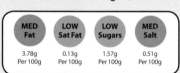

MED Fat	LOW Sat Fat	LOW Sugars	MED Salt
3.78g Per 100g	0.13g Per 100g	1.57g Per 100g	0.51g Per 100g

1 Heat the olive oil in a large saucepan, then add the onions, chilli and garlic and cook gently for 8–10 minutes. Add the harissa, cumin, saffron, fennel, potatoes, lemon juice and stock. Bring to the boil then cover and reduce the heat, and simmer for 15 minutes.

2 Add the tomatoes and salt and simmer for a further 10 minutes. Add the vegetables, beans and fish and simmer for 10 minutes more. Stir in the coriander and serve with lemon wedges on the side for a citrus kick.

Amount per portion
Energy 700 kcals, Protein 47.6g, Fat 32.6g, Saturated fat 1.1g, Carbohydrate 57.6g, Total sugars 13.5g, Salt 4.36g, Sodium 1718mg

Scallops and Bacon on Sweet-and-Sour Cabbage

Scallops, bacon and cabbage, I'm in heaven! It's the perfect threesome and so easy for such a treat. Serve with new potatoes.

Serves 4

1 Savoy cabbage, shredded
1 egg yolk
½ onion, finely diced
3 teaspoons sugar or low-calorie
    granulated sweetener
85ml cider vinegar
150g 0 per cent fat natural Greek yogurt
2 teaspoons Dijon mustard
1 bunch fresh dill, finely chopped
12 large shucked scallops
4 rashers streaky bacon
salt and freshly ground black pepper

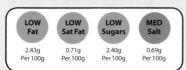

LOW Fat	LOW Sat Fat	LOW Sugars	MED Salt
2.43g Per 100g	0.71g Per 100g	2.40g Per 100g	0.69g Per 100g

1 Preheat the grill to high. Cook the cabbage in boiling salted water for about 8 minutes.

2 Meanwhile, in a large saucepan over a low heat, whisk together the egg yolk, onion, sugar or sweetener and vinegar until the mixture begins to thicken; do not allow the mixture to boil. Remove from the heat and fold in the yogurt, mustard and dill. Drain the cabbage thoroughly and fold into the sauce. Season to taste.

3 Grill the scallops and bacon together for 2 minutes each side. Serve the scallops and bacon on top of the cabbage.

Tip If you prefer to cook your scallops a little underdone in the centre, grill them for a little less than 2 minutes each side.

Amount per portion (low-calorie sweetener)
Energy 273 kcals, Protein 40.4g, Fat 8.5g, Saturated fat 2.5g, Carbohydrate 9.5g, Total sugars 8.4g, Salt 2.4g, Sodium 945mg

Amount per portion (sugar)
Energy 286 kcals, Protein 40.4g, Fat 8.5g, Saturated fat 2.5g, Carbohydrate 13.0g, Total sugars 11.9g, Salt 2.4g, Sodium 945mg

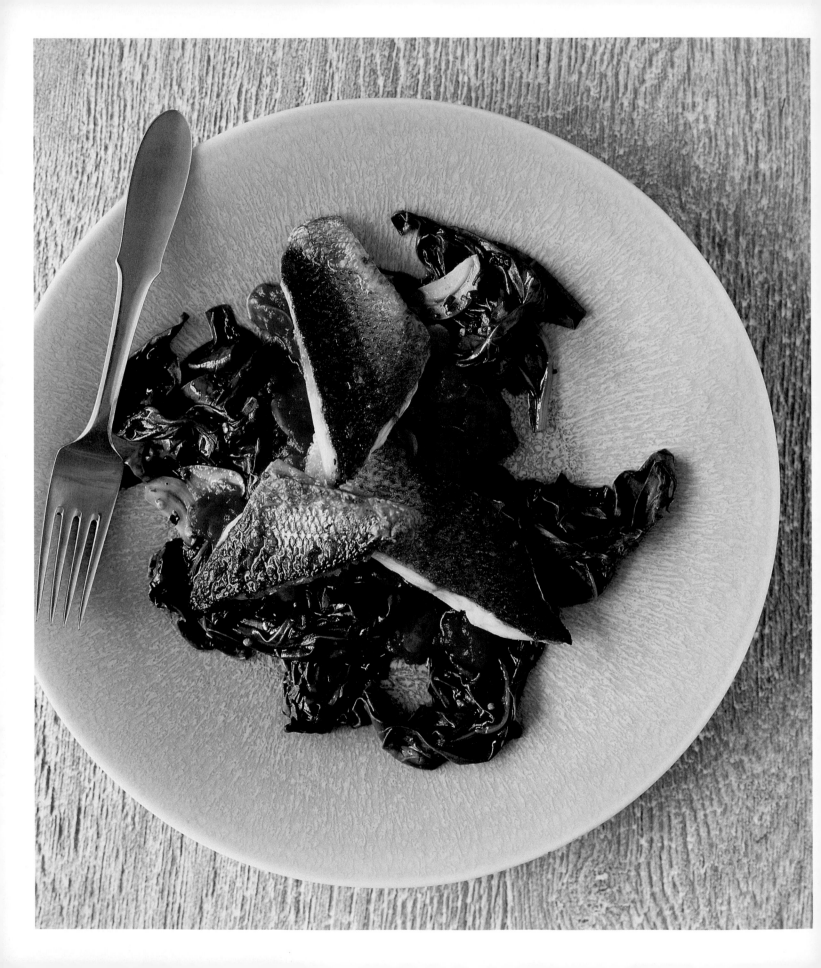

Fillets of Sea Bass with Aniseed Scented Tomatoes

This is the sort of dish you would die for when sitting in a Greek taverna overlooking the sea. Unfortunately it's usually just roast or barbecued sea bass with a wedge of lemon but this is what I dream of.

Serves 4

2 tablespoons extra virgin olive oil
3 garlic cloves, thinly sliced
pinch of dried chilli flakes
1kg spinach, tough stems removed,
    shredded
pinch of grated nutmeg
4 fillets of sea bass, about 175g each, skin
    on, each fillet cut in 3 crossways
3 tablespoons aniseed-flavoured liqueur
    (ouzo, sambuca, Pernod)
3 tablespoons dry white wine
1 x 400g tin chopped tomatoes
1 tablespoon flaked almonds
1 teaspoon chopped fresh tarragon
salt and freshly ground black pepper
new potatoes or brown rice, to serve

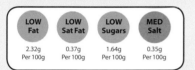

LOW Fat	LOW Sat Fat	LOW Sugars	MED Salt
2.32g Per 100g	0.37g Per 100g	1.64g Per 100g	0.35g Per 100g

1 Heat half the oil in a large saucepan, add the garlic and, over a gentle heat, cook until the garlic turns golden. Add the chilli flakes then the spinach and cook until wilted, about 5 minutes. Sprinkle on some nutmeg and season to taste with salt and pepper.

2 Set a colander over a bowl and drain the spinach well, pressing to remove as much liquid as possible. Retain the liquor and set aside, and keep the spinach warm.

3 Meanwhile, in a frying pan heat the remaining oil and cook the fish skin-side down over a medium heat for 4 minutes until the skin is golden and the flesh has nearly cooked through. Turn the fish over then add the aniseed liqueur and white wine and cook until the liquid has almost evaporated, about 2 minutes. Remove the fish and keep warm.

4 To the fish pan, add the spinach liquor and boil vigorously to reduce, add the tomatoes, flaked almonds and tarragon and cook for 15 minutes until slightly thickened. Return the fish to the pan briefly to warm through.

5 Divide the spinach between individual warmed plates and top each with 3 pieces of fish, then spoon over the sauce. Serve with new potatoes or brown rice.

Amount per portion
Energy 361 kcals, Protein 43g, Fat 13g, Saturated fat 2.1g, Carbohydrate 11g, Total sugars 9.2g, Salt 1.95g, Sodium 768mg

Roast Cod with Lemon, Tomatoes and Olives

The Italians would use whole red mullet for this simple, delicious dish – lovely, but home cooks are not generally fans of bony, head-on fish. I've used cod fillets, but use whatever fish you prefer, adjusting the cooking time accordingly.

Serves 4
450g new potatoes, left unpeeled
12 garlic cloves
spray olive oil
4 thick cod fillets, about 175g each
1 tablespoon smoked or sweet paprika
1 lemon, zested and finely sliced
325g cherry tomatoes
1 yellow pepper, deseeded and cut into
    2.5cm pieces
handful of stoned black olives
6 anchovy fillets, chopped
handful of ripped fresh basil leaves,
    to garnish
freshly ground black pepper
green salad, to serve

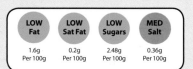

LOW Fat	LOW Sat Fat	LOW Sugars	MED Salt
1.6g Per 100g	0.2g Per 100g	2.48g Per 100g	0.36g Per 100g

1 Preheat the oven to 230°C/450°F/gas mark 8. Put the potatoes and garlic in a pan of boiling water and cook for 15 minutes until tender. Drain and transfer to a roasting tin, spray with oil and season with black pepper, and pop into the preheated oven. Cook for 15 minutes.

2 Meanwhile, spray the fish fillets with olive oil, dust with paprika and lemon zest, then set aside.

3 Remove the roasting tin from the oven and add the lemon slices, tomatoes, yellow pepper, olives and anchovies, and stir to combine. Place the cod on top and return to the oven for 15 minutes. Arrange on to individual warmed plates, scatter with basil and serve with a green salad.

Variation If you prefer crispier potatoes, ignore the boiling stage in Step 1 and roast the potatoes for 40 minutes before adding the other ingredients.

Amount per portion
Energy 296 kcals, Protein 38.4g, Fat 4.7g, Saturated fat 0.6g, Carbohydrate 26.7g, Total sugars 7.3g, Salt 1.07g, Sodium 422mg

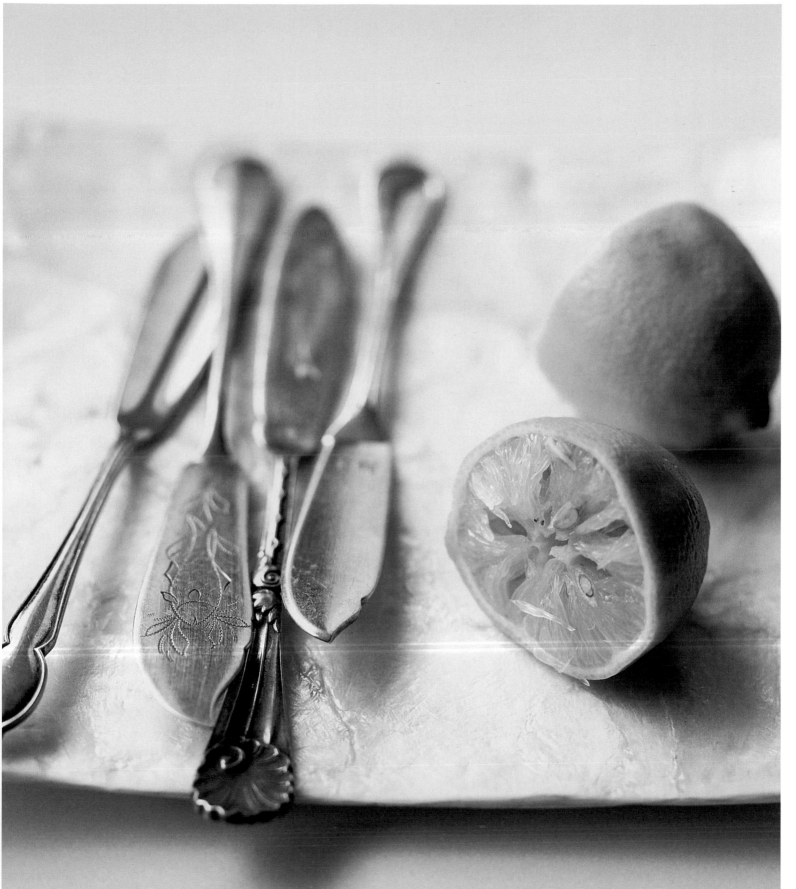

Crab and Tomato Linguini

I love crab – fresh, ideally, but rarely can I be bothered with the hassle of boiling and picking a whole crab. Decent crabmeat is on offer in many fishmongers and supermarkets, but failing that I'm a bit of a fan of Alaskan canned crab; it's certainly much better than the frozen stuff. In this Italian-influenced dish, it makes a great partner to pasta.

Serves 4
1 tablespoon olive oil
3 garlic cloves, sliced
1 small onion, finely chopped
2 mild fresh chillies, deseeded
    and chopped
1 bay leaf
300ml tomato passata
20 cherry tomatoes, halved
325g dried linguini
325g fresh or tinned white crabmeat
100g brown crabmeat (optional)
salt and freshly ground black pepper

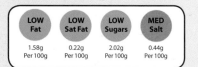

LOW Fat	LOW Sat Fat	LOW Sugars	MED Salt
1.58g Per 100g	0.22g Per 100g	2.02g Per 100g	0.44g Per 100g

1 Heat the oil in a large frying pan and over a medium heat cook the garlic, onion, chillies and bay leaf until the onion has softened. Add the passata and cook for 8–10 minutes until thickened. Add the cherry tomatoes and cook for a further 5 minutes.

2 Meanwhile, cook the linguini in boiling salted water for 1 minute less than the manufacturers' recommendation. Drain.

3 Fold the crabmeat into the sauce, then fold in the pasta with a little cooking water still clinging to it. Stir to combine, check the seasoning and serve.

Variations You can ring the changes on this one – try it with prawns or cubes of white fish or salmon. And you can add a few peas or chopped beans, at the same time as the cherry tomatoes.

Amount per portion
Energy 412 kcals, Protein 27.4g, Fat 5.8g, Saturated fat 0.8g, Carbohydrate 66.9g, Total sugars 7.4g, Salt 1.6g, Sodium 628mg

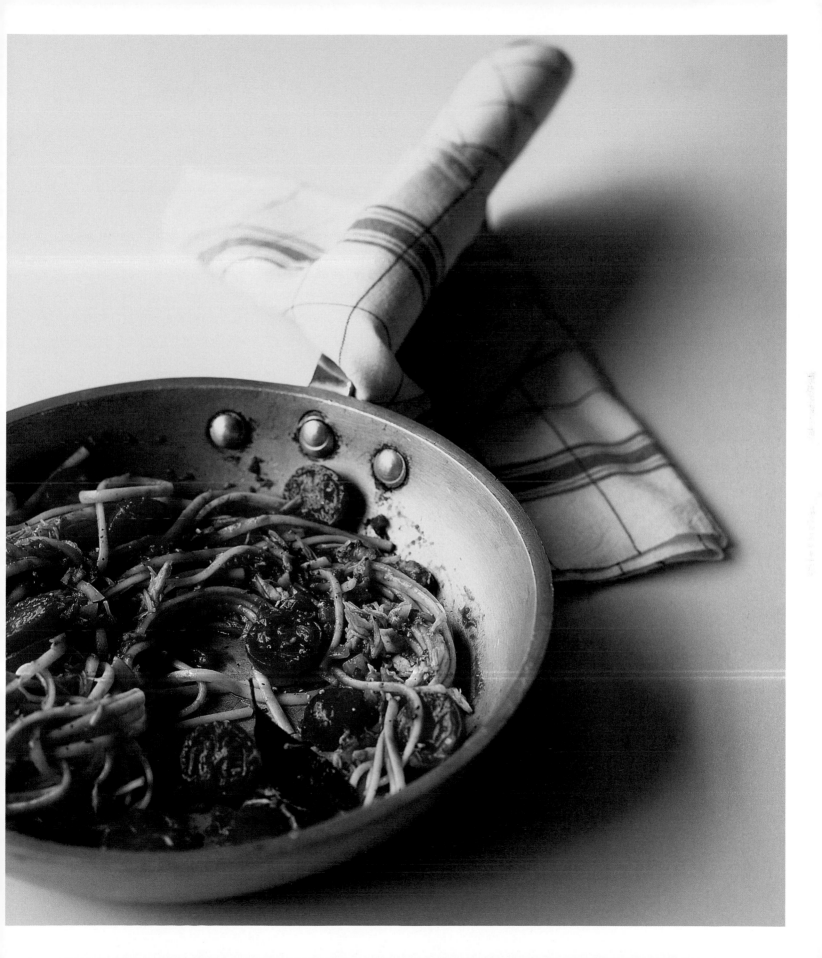

Penne with Salmon, Beans, Mint and Tomato

The Italians don't normally mix cheese and fish, but in this Sicilian recipe they make an exception, usually using mozzarella. I'm not a fan of low-fat mozzarella so I've substituted low-fat cottage cheese, which is added at the end of the recipe.

Serves 4
2 tablespoons olive oil
2 garlic cloves
1 x 200g tin chopped tomatoes
1 bunch of fresh mint leaves, chopped
1 red chilli, deseeded and sliced
120ml dry white wine
325g salmon fillet, skinned and cut into 1cm dice
1 x 400g tin borlotti beans, drained and rinsed
325g dried penne
85g low-fat cottage cheese
salt and freshly ground black pepper
green salad, to serve

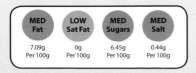

1 Heat the oil in a frying pan, add the garlic and cook over a medium heat until pale golden. Add the tomatoes, half the mint, all the chilli and white wine and simmer for 5 minutes. Remove the garlic and discard.

2 Add the salmon and beans to the tomato sauce and return to the boil, then reduce the heat and cook for a further 3 minutes.

3 Meanwhile, cook the penne in boiling salted water for 1 minute less than the packet instructions. Drain the pasta briefly and add it, along with a little of its cooking water and the remaining mint, to the sauce. Toss to combine and season to taste.

4 Divide between individual warmed bowls, then dot the surface with cottage cheese. Serve with a green salad.

Amount per portion
Energy 580 kcals, Protein 34.1g, Fat 16.8g, Saturated fat 2.8g, Carbohydrate 75.4g, Total sugars 5.2g, Salt 1.25g, Sodium 496mg

Pasta with Anchovies, Pine Nuts and Sultanas

Simplicity is often best, as in this energy-giving Sicilian dish. It's got lovely flavours, as long as you enjoy anchovies, and loads of different textures.

Serves 4
450g dried spaghetti
50g sultanas, soaked in 2 tablespoons of Pernod or ouzo
2 tablespoons olive oil
1 fennel bulb, very finely sliced
2 garlic cloves, finely sliced
50g pine nuts
8 anchovies in oil, drained and chopped
1 tablespoon chopped fresh oregano or marjoram
115g toasted seeded breadcrumbs (see page 173)

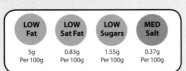

1 Cook the spaghetti in plenty of boiling salted water for 1 minute less than specified on the packet instructions, then drain, retaining a little of its cooking water, and keep warm.

2 Meanwhile, heat the oil in a pan, add the fennel and garlic and cook gently for 8–10 minutes until softened without colouring. Add the sultanas with their liquid, pine nuts, anchovies and oregano and cook until the anchovies break down.

3 Add the pasta with a little of its cooking water and toss to mix well. Divide between individual plates and scatter with crunchy seeded breadcrumbs.

Amount per portion
Energy 668 kcals, Protein 20.5g, Fat 17.8g, Saturated fat 00g, Carbohydrate 109.0g, Total sugars 16.2g, Salt 1.11g, Sodium 440mg

Roast Cod on a Cannellini Bean Stew

Inspired by Italy but created by Australians – they're great at flavours and this marriage of ingredients shows off this talent to the full.

Serves 4

1 tablespoon olive oil
115g chorizo, sliced and diced
1 large onion, finely diced
2 carrots, cut into 1cm dice
2 celery stalks, cut into 1cm dice
3 garlic cloves, crushed to a paste
    with a little salt
1 teaspoon fresh thyme leaves
1 bay leaf
4 jarred artichoke hearts in oil, drained
    and quartered
pinch of saffron
1 medium red chilli, deseeded and diced
300ml reduced-salt chicken stock
1 x 400g tin cannellini beans, drained
    and rinsed
1 tablespoon freshly grated Parmesan
    cheese
1 tablespoon chopped fresh parsley
4 fillets of cod, about 175g each, skin on
spray oil, for cooking
salt and freshly ground black pepper

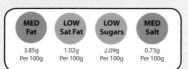

MED Fat	LOW Sat Fat	LOW Sugars	MED Salt
3.85g Per 100g	1.02g Per 100g	2.09g Per 100g	0.73g Per 100g

1 Preheat the oven to 220°C/425°F/gas mark 7. Heat the oil in a saucepan or frying pan and cook the chorizo for 2–3 minutes to release fats and crispen the sausage. Remove and set aside.

2 In the chorizo fat cook the onion, carrots, celery, garlic, thyme and bay leaf for 8 minutes. Add the artichokes, saffron, chilli, stock and cannellini beans and continue cooking gently until most of the liquid has evaporated. Fold in the Parmesan, parsley and the cooked chorizo. Adjust the seasoning to taste.

3 Meanwhile season the cod fillets, spray with oil and place them in a lightly sprayed roasting tin. Transfer to the preheated oven and cook for 12–15 minutes. Spoon the beans on to individual plates, then top with the oven-roasted cod.

Amount per portion
Energy 411 kcals, Protein 45.7g, Fat 16.2g, Saturated fat 4.3g, Carbohydrate 21.9g, Total sugars 8.8g, Salt 3.09g, Sodium 1217mg

Prawn Linguini

Pasta with a touch of class, a bestseller in Italian restaurants – and it's easy to make and pretty quick. Feel free to substitute a firm white fish for the prawns.

Serves 4
325g dried linguini
spray olive oil
1 tablespoon non-pareille capers
   (baby capers), rinsed and drained
4 anchovy fillets, sliced
4 garlic cloves, sliced
½ teaspoon dried chilli flakes
24 raw prawns, shell-off
60ml dry white wine (optional)
150ml fish or chicken stock
150ml tomato passata
4 spring onions, roughly sliced
12 cherry tomatoes, halved
handful of rocket leaves
handful of baby spinach
1 teaspoon chopped fresh oregano
salt and freshly ground black pepper

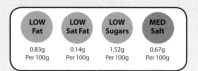

LOW Fat	LOW Sat Fat	LOW Sugars	MED Salt
0.83g Per 100g	0.14g Per 100g	1.52g Per 100g	0.67g Per 100g

1 In a large pan of boiling salted water, cook the pasta for a minute less than the manufacturer recommends. Drain and keep warm.

2 Meanwhile, spray a saucepan with a little oil then over a low heat gently cook the capers, anchovies, garlic and chilli flakes until the anchovies start to break down. Add the prawns, increase the temperature and cook for a further 3 minutes. Remove the prawns and keep warm.

3 To the pan add the wine if using, stock and passata, and boil until reduced by half. Add the spring onions and tomatoes and cook for 3 minutes. Add the rocket, baby spinach, oregano and prawns and continue cooking until the greens have wilted. Add the pasta, toss to combine and season to taste.

Variation For a more intense sauce, buy shell-on raw prawns and peel them before you start cooking. Add the shells to the capers and anchovies in Step 2. After you have reduced the sauce in Step 3, remove the shells and blend them, then pass them through a sieve, return to the pan and continue as in the recipe.

Amount per portion
Energy 373 kcals, Protein 26.4g, Fat 2.9g, Saturated fat 0.5g, Carbohydrate 64.4g, Total sugars 5.3g, Salt 2.32g, Sodium 915mg

Fragrant Prawns with Hints of Fire

I love this Malaysian street food, cooked in an instant and yet packing a flavour punch. If prawns aren't your thing then try the same recipe with a white fish, but treat it a bit more delicately.

Serves 4

2 tablespoons sunflower oil
400g raw tiger prawns, shell off
    and deveined
100g seasoned flour
2 tablespoons ketchup
3 tablespoons sweet chilli sauce
2 tablespoons hot chilli sauce
1 tablespoon hot bean paste
1 teaspoon light soy sauce
1 teaspoon reduced-salt chicken stock
    granules
4 garlic cloves, chopped
2.5cm piece of fresh ginger, peeled
    and grated
1 bird's eye chilli, deseeded and
    finely chopped
1 mild green chilli, roughly chopped
½ green pepper, deseeded and diced
4 spring onions, sliced
salt and freshly ground black pepper
brown rice, to serve

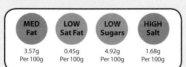

MED Fat	LOW Sat Fat	LOW Sugars	HIGH Salt
3.57g Per 100g	0.45g Per 100g	4.92g Per 100g	1.68g Per 100g

1 Heat the oil in a wok, toss the prawns in the seasoned flour then fry them in the oil until pink all over, about 2–3 minutes. Remove them from the wok and set aside to keep warm.

2 Drain the wok of most of the oil, then add the ketchup, chilli sauces, bean paste, soy sauce and stock granules. Heat until boiling then add the remaining ingredients except the prawns, and cook for 3 minutes. Fold in the prawns and warm through, then season to taste. Serve with a nutty brown rice.

Amount per portion
Energy 267 kcals, Protein 21.7g, Fat 7.1g, Saturated fat 0.9g, Carbohydrate 31.0g, Total sugars 9.8g, Salt 3.34g, Sodium 1318mg

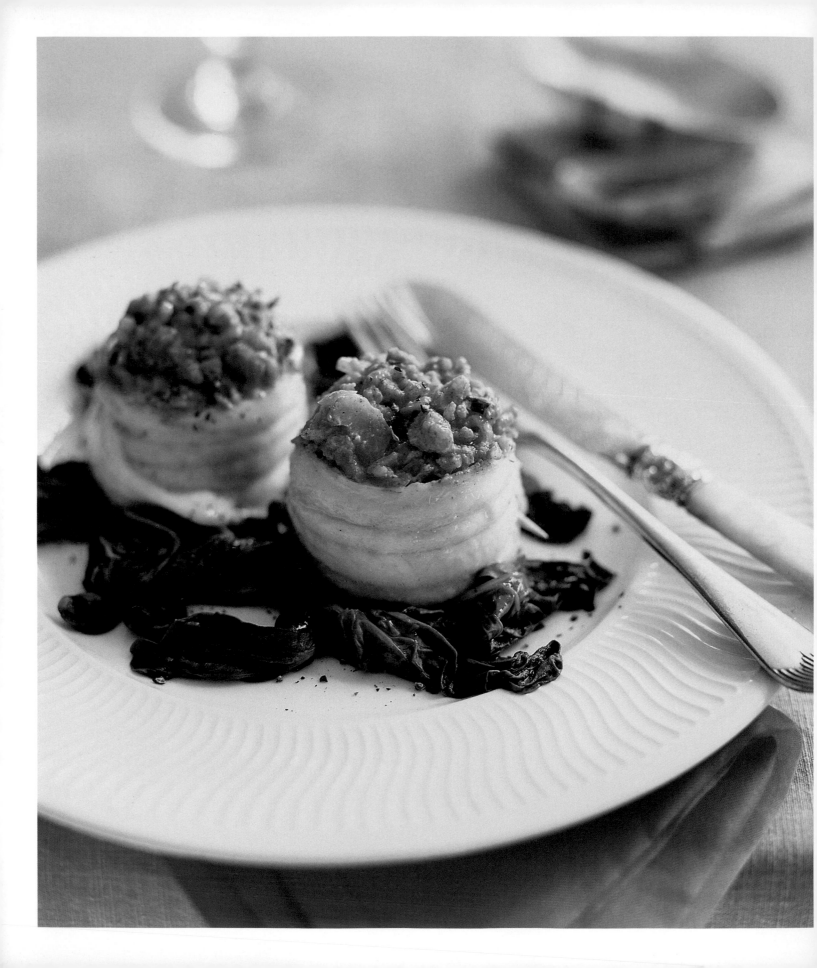

Lemon Sole with Lemon and Basil Stuffing

Let's be honest: it's quite hard to find indigenous American cuisine, it's usually been influenced by one country or another. This, however, is a dish I had in Boston, albeit made with another fish. It has wonderful flavours and can be prepared in advance and cooked just before serving.

Serves 4

1 tablespoon rapeseed oil
1 celery stalk, finely diced
1 garlic clove, chopped
½ onion, finely chopped
juice and zest of 1 lemon
1 teaspoon smoked paprika
225g cooked brown rice
4 tablespoon low-fat Greek natural yogurt
2 tablespoons chopped fresh basil
oil, for greasing
8 lemon sole fillets

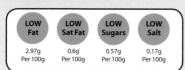

LOW Fat	LOW Sat Fat	LOW Sugars	LOW Salt
2.97g Per 100g	0.6g Per 100g	0.57g Per 100g	0.17g Per 100g

1 In a medium saucepan heat the oil over a medium heat and cook the celery, garlic and onion, stirring frequently, until softened without colouring – about 8 minutes. Add the lemon juice and zest, paprika and a couple of tablespoons of water, and bring to the boil. Add the rice, stir to combine, remove from the heat and leave to cool for 10 minutes. Add the yogurt and basil.

2 If you are preparing the dish for eating immediately, preheat the oven 180°C/350°F/gas mark 4. Lightly oil a baking tray. Roll each fillet, head to tail, slightly overlapping to form a hollow tube, secure with cocktail sticks, then place on their ends in the baking tray. With a tablespoon fill each cavity with the rice mix, slightly mounded. (At this point the dish can be set aside, lightly covered, ready to cook later.)

3 Pop the fish into the preheated oven for 12–15 minutes from room temperature or 20 minutes from refrigerated. Serve with greens.

Amount per portion
Energy 332 kcals, Protein 39.2g, Fat 9.4g, Saturated fat 1.9g, Carbohydrate 24.1g, Total sugars 1.8g, Salt 0.54g, Sodium 212mg

Paella

Paella is a wonderful one-pot dish but traditionally the shellfish has the texture of rubber so I am abusing tradition by cooking and adding the shellfish towards the end.

Serves 4
600ml chicken stock
pinch of saffron, soaked in
    a little warm water
2 tablespoons olive oil
50g chorizo sausage, cut into thin slices
50g pancetta, cut into small dice
4 skinless, boneless chicken thighs,
    each cut in half
2 garlic cloves, finely chopped, plus
    4 garlic cloves, unpeeled
1 Spanish onion, finely diced
1 small red pepper, deseeded and diced
1 teaspoon fresh thyme leaves
good pinch of dried red chilli flakes
300g Spanish short-grain rice (calasparra)
½ teaspoon paprika
4 tablespoons dry white wine
50g fresh or frozen peas
2 large tomatoes, peeled, deseeded
    and diced
325g small raw clams or mussels, cleaned
12 raw jumbo prawns, shell-on
225g squid, cleaned and chopped into
    bite-sized pieces
sprigs of flat-leaf parsley, to garnish
salt and freshly ground black pepper

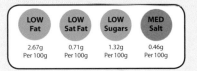

LOW Fat	LOW Sat Fat	LOW Sugars	MED Salt
2.67g Per 100g	0.71g Per 100g	1.32g Per 100g	0.46g Per 100g

1 Heat the stock and saffron together in a pan to boiling point and keep it hot. Heat half the olive oil in a paellera*, add the chorizo and pancetta and fry for a few minutes until crisp and lightly golden. Transfer to a plate and set aside. Add the chicken pieces to the pan and fry for a few minutes on each side until golden, then remove and set aside with the chorizo and pancetta.

2 Add the chopped garlic, onion and red pepper to the pan and cook for a few minutes until the vegetables have softened but not coloured, stirring occasionally. Add the thyme, chilli flakes and rice and stir for about 2 minutes or until all the rice grains are nicely coated and glossy. Stir in the paprika, then pour in the wine and allow it to bubble down a little, stirring. Pour in the hot chicken stock, add the cooked chorizo, pancetta and chicken, and cook for a further 5 minutes or so, stirring occasionally. Fold in the peas and tomatoes and season to taste.

3 Put the clams in the paella, with the edges that will open facing upwards, and continue to cook gently for a further 10–15 minutes or until the rice is just tender. Remove from the hob and leave to rest in a warm place for 10 minutes.

4 Meanwhile, heat the remaining oil in a separate large frying pan. Add the unpeeled garlic cloves and then quickly tip in the prawns. Stir-fry for a minute or two, then scatter the prawns over the paella, leaving the garlic in the pan. Add the squid to the pan and stir-fry for 1 minute or so until just tender, then scatter the squid over the paella; discard the garlic. Garnish with the parsley sprigs and serve immediately, straight from the pan, with a salad on the side.

Tip If you don't have a paellera, traditional paella dish, use a large heavy-based frying pan.

Amount per portion
Energy 678 kcals, Protein 62.2g, Fat 17.2g, Saturated fat 4.6g, Carbohydrate 72.0g, Total sugars 8.5g, Salt 2.97g, Sodium 1171mg

Asian Surf and Turf Balls in Sweet and Sour Sauce

A lovely Oriental combination of prawns and pork: sophisticated yet simple, and a perfect supper for hungry children.

Serves 4
For the balls
225g raw prawns, shell-off and finely chopped
225g minced pork
1 fresh red chilli, deseeded and finely diced
1.5cm piece of fresh ginger, peeled and grated
2 spring onions, finely chopped
1 tablespoon light soy sauce
1 tablespoon sesame oil
1 tablespoon chopped fresh coriander
½ tablespoon cornflour
2 tablespoons chopped water chestnuts
1 teaspoon sunflower oil

For the sauce
2 garlic cloves, finely chopped
2.5cm piece of fresh ginger, peeled and grated
1 fresh red chilli, deseeded and finely chopped
100ml pineapple juice
1 tablespoon light soy sauce
1 tablespoon white wine vinegar
1 tablespoon tomato purée
1 teaspoon dark brown soft sugar or low-calorie granulated sweetener
1 tablespoon cornflour, mixed to a paste with 2 tablespoons cold water

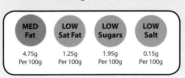

1 To make the balls, mix together all the ingredients except the water chestnuts and the oil. Combine well, then take about 40g of the mixture and roll into a ball. Repeat. Make an indentation in each ball and insert a little chopped water chestnut in the centre, then enclose within the balls.

2 Heat the oil in a wok and fry the balls until brown all over. Add the garlic, ginger and chilli from the sauce ingredients, reduce the heat and cook for 5 minutes. Add the remaining ingredients, except for the cornflour paste, bring to the boil and cook for 3 minutes. Add the cornflour paste and cook until thickened and glossy, about 2 minutes. To serve, place some steaming rice in individual warm bowls and top with the meatballs.

Tip If you find soy sauce too strong and salty, you can either dilute it with a little water or try a light soy sauce instead, as I have in this recipe; this is now widely available in larger supermarkets.

Amount per portion
Energy 217 kcals, Protein 21.6g, Fat 9.5g, Saturated fat 2.5g, Carbohydrate 11.1g, Total sugars 3.9g, Salt 0.3g, Sodium 340mg

New Potatoes and Smoked Mackerel with Avocado Horseradish Dressing

Smoked mackerel is a wonderfully nutritious standby, plus it's plentiful in the UK. The addition of new potatoes (good GI) and avocado (all the right fats), make this recipe a veritable superfood – so much goodness and tastiness in one plate!

Serves 4
500g new potatoes
1 tablespoon olive oil
4 bay leaves, broken
4 garlic cloves, smashed
juice and grated zest of 2 lemons
5cm-piece of fresh horseradish, grated, or 2 tablespoons from a jar
1 avocado, diced
4 tablespoons 0 per cent fat natural Greek yogurt
3 smoked peppered mackerel fillets, skin removed, flaked
handful of rocket leaves
salt and freshly ground black pepper

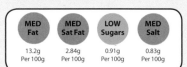

MED Fat	MED Sat Fat	LOW Sugars	MED Salt
13.2g Per 100g	2.84g Per 100g	0.91g Per 100g	0.83g Per 100g

1 Preheat the oven to 200°C/400°F/gas mark 6.

2 Put the potatoes in a bowl and toss with the olive oil, broken bay, garlic and half of the lemon juice and zest. Season with a little salt and a few grindings of pepper. Tip into a roasting tin and cook in the oven for about 40 minutes, tossing from time to time. When cooked, the potatoes will be tender, wrinkly and golden. Discard the bay leaves.

3 Combine the remaining lemon zest with the horseradish, avocado and yogurt. Mash with the back of a fork, retaining some texture. Gently fold in the mackerel flakes, leaving them as chunky as possible. If the mixture is very stiff, add a little of the remaining lemon juice. Season to taste.

4 Arrange the potatoes onto individual plates, top with the mackerel mix and scatter with rocket leaves, and serve.

Amount per portion
Energy 595 kcals, Protein 27g, Fat 45g, Saturated fat 9.7g, Carbohydrate 23g, Total sugars 3.1g, Salt 2.84g, Sodium 1118mg

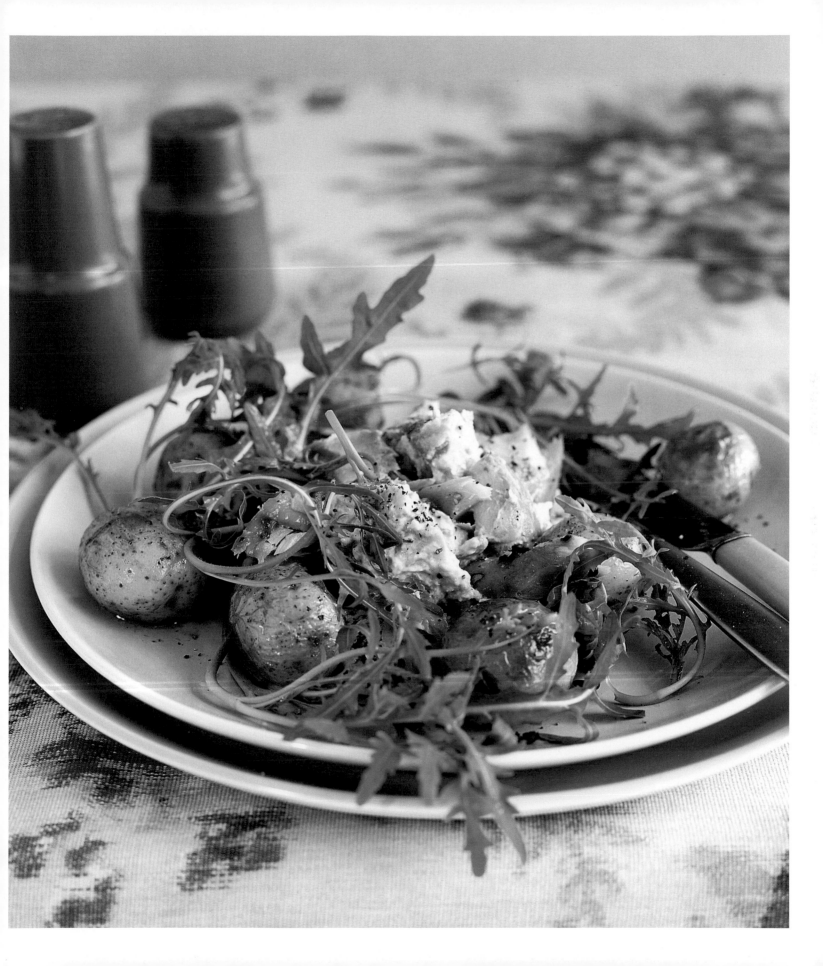

Poached Haddock with Eggs and Spinach

This classic combination, a firm British favourite, is wonderfully comforting. You could use smoked haddock, but beware of its salt content. You do need a certain amount of precise timing for this dish. Serve with some toasted granary bread.

Serves 4
600ml skimmed milk
2 bay leaves
1 onion, quartered
1 teaspoon black peppercorns
1kg fresh spinach, washed and tough
    stems removed
4 x 175g haddock fillets
2 tablespoons white wine vinegar
4 eggs
2 tablespoons white wine vinegar
salt and freshly ground black pepper

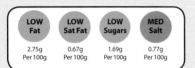

LOW Fat	LOW Sat Fat	LOW Sugars	MED Salt
2.75g Per 100g	0.67g Per 100g	1.69g Per 100g	0.77g Per 100g

1 In a frying pan over a low heat, heat the milk with the bay, onion and peppercorns, and simmer gently for 10 minutes.

2 Meanwhile, heat about 2.5cm of water in a large saucepan, add the spinach with a little pinch of salt and allow the heat to wilt and cook the leaves. Drain the spinach well, pressing down to release the water, return to the pan, loosen the leaves and keep warm. Season with pepper.

3 Put the haddock fillets in the simmering milk skin-side down and poach for 6 minutes, turning carefully once.

4 Meanwhile, bring about 10cm of water to the boil in a small pan, then add the vinegar. Break the eggs into separate coffee cups, then, one after the other, tip them into the roll of the boil and immediately reduce the heat slightly. Cook for 2 minutes 30 seconds and drain.

5 Arrange the spinach in the centre of a warmed plate, top with haddock and then a poached egg. Grind over some pepper and, if you like, spoon a little of the poaching milk around the spinach.

Tip For the best poached eggs with the best shape you'll need ultra-fresh eggs – if they are very fresh you won't even need any vinegar, which with older eggs helps coagulate the white so you don't get ugly strands. I'm lucky my chickens lay daily.

Amount per portion
Energy 312 kcals, Protein 48.6g, Fat 9.9g, Saturated fat 2.4g, Carbohydrate 7.5g, Total sugars 6.1g, Salt 2.78g, Sodium 804mg

Cotriade

Normally this fish and potato stew from Brittany uses floury potatoes but here I use new; it would also be served with a saffron mayonnaise or an aioli but you'll have to make do with a delicious saffron yogurt, unless, of course, you can be good and use only a scant amount of aioli.

Serves 4

For the saffron yogurt
small pinch of saffron, soaked in about
   2 tablespoons hot fish stock
120g 0 per cent fat natural Greek yogurt
50g leftover mashed potato
juice and zest of 1 lemon
2 garlic cloves, crushed
1 tablespoon extra virgin olive oil
freshly ground white pepper

For the stew
spray olive oil
4 shallots, thinly sliced
3 garlic cloves, thinly sliced
sprig of thyme
1 bay leaf
125ml dry white wine
600ml fish stock or dashi stock
225g new potatoes, halved
450g mixed fish fillets (cod, monkfish,
   mullet) cut into 2.5cm pieces
450g mussels, cleaned
115g peas, frozen or fresh and podded
225g leeks, chopped

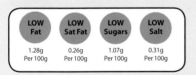

LOW Fat	LOW Sat Fat	LOW Sugars	LOW Salt
1.28g Per 100g	0.26g Per 100g	1.07g Per 100g	0.31g Per 100g

1 Whisk together all the saffron yogurt ingredients.

2 Heat a large saucepan and spray it with oil, add the shallots, garlic, thyme and bay leaf and cook for 5 minutes over a medium heat. Add the wine, stock and potatoes and cook gently until the potatoes are tender.

3 Add the fish, mussels, peas and leeks and cook vigorously for 5 minutes until the mussels have fully opened (discard any that have not). Serve, topping each individual bowl with a dollop of the saffron yogurt.

Variations Normally the solids are removed just before serving and kept warm while mayonnaise is whisked into the liquid to thicken it. For a healthier way to thicken your stew, make a cornflour paste and stir it in just before serving.

Amount per portion
Energy 282 kcals, Protein 32.5g, Fat 7.0g, Saturated fat 1.4g, Carbohydrate 21.1g, Total sugars 5.9g, Salt 1.72g, Sodium 675mg

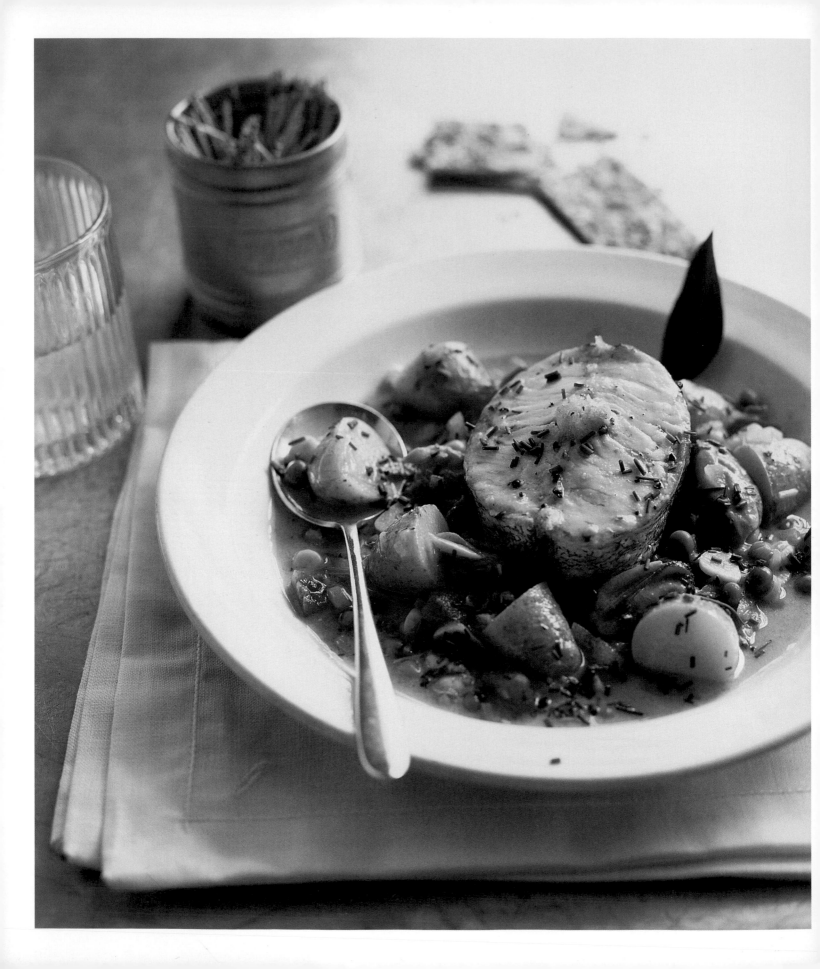

Roast Hake on a Chowder-style Broth

The broth that accompanies the hake could be served as a light soup but it goes very well with the roast fish. I've included more vegetables than there would be in a traditional North American chowder but, in essence, anything goes.

Serves 4
300ml dry white wine
1kg raw baby clams, washed
500g raw mussels, washed
1 tablespoon sunflower oil, plus sunflower oil spray
3 slices smoked streaky bacon, diced
1 large onion, finely chopped
2 garlic cloves, sliced
12 new potatoes, halved
2 bay leaves
sprig of thyme
300ml good-quality fish stock
300ml skimmed milk
115g canned sweetcorn
115g frozen peas
2 ripe tomatoes, deseeded and diced
4 x 175g hake steaks, skin and bone retained
1 tablespoon snipped fresh chives, to garnish
salt and freshly ground white pepper

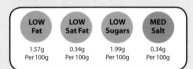

LOW Fat	LOW Sat Fat	LOW Sugars	MED Salt
1.57g Per 100g	0.34g Per 100g	1.99g Per 100g	0.34g Per 100g

1 Pour the wine into a large saucepan and bring to the boil. Add the clams, cover and cook for 2 minutes, then add the mussels, cover and cook for about 3 minutes or until the shellfish has opened, shaking the pan from time to time. Strain the shellfish in a colander, retaining the liquor, and discard any that have not opened. Set the shellfish aside.

2 Preheat the oven to 200°C/400°F/gas mark 6. Heat the sunflower oil in a large saucepan and fry the bacon until crispy. Drain any excess fat and discard. Add the onion and garlic to the bacon and fry for 6 minutes to soften them without colouring. Add the potatoes, bay leaves, thyme, stock and the shellfish cooking juices. Cook until the potatoes are tender, about 15–20 minutes. Add the milk, return to the boil and add the sweetcorn, peas and tomatoes. Cook for 5 minutes and season.

3 Spray the fish with sunflower oil, season with pepper and place on a baking tray. Transfer to the oven and cook for 12 minutes.

4 While the broth is cooking and the hake roasting, get shucking – remove the clams and mussels from their shells. When the broth is ready, add the shellfish to heat through but do not re-boil. Spoon the broth with its contents into individual warmed bowls, top with the hake and sprinkle with chives.

Variation If desired, the broth can be thickened with a paste of cornflour and water.

Amount per portion
Energy 511 kcals, Protein 53.3g, Fat 12.5g, Saturated fat 2.7g, Carbohydrate 43.2g, Total sugars 15.9g, Salt 2.73g, Sodium 1073mg

Barley Risotto with Greens and Prawns

Barley makes an interesting change to traditional Italian risotto rice – it produces a lovely nutty texture and taste and has a low GI. Give risotto your full attention, as it needs regular stirring and additions of stock. Once you've mastered the basic technique, you can add all sorts of flavourings.

Serves 4
1 tablespoon olive oil
2 shallots, finely chopped
2 garlic cloves, finely chopped
1 bay leaf
sprig of thyme
300g pearl barley
175ml dry white wine
1 litre fish or chicken stock, heated
   almost to boiling point
115g broad beans, frozen or fresh and
   podded, blanched
115g extra fine green beans, blanched
115g petit pois, frozen
handful of pea shoots
handful of baby spinach
225g raw shell-off tiger prawns
freshly ground black pepper

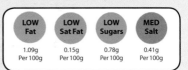

LOW Fat	LOW Sat Fat	LOW Sugars	MED Salt
1.09g Per 100g	0.15g Per 100g	0.78g Per 100g	0.41g Per 100g

1 Melt the butter in a large saucepan, add the shallots and garlic and cook gently for 5 minutes. Add the herbs and barley, and stir to combine. Add the wine and boil vigorously until the liquid has all but disappeared.

2 Now it's time to add the hot stock, only one ladle at a time and, just like with the wine, wait until the liquid has nearly disappeared before adding the next ladle. About 20 minutes or so into this process, test the barley to see whether it is cooked; it should be soft but still slightly nutty.

3 Add the vegetables and prawns, stir to combine and cook for 3 minutes (you may need a little extra stock). Season to taste and serve.

Tip Ensure the stock is almost boiling before you start the risotto process.

Amount per portion
Energy 427 kcals, Protein 23.0g, Fat 6.0g, Saturated fat 0.8g, Carbohydrate 72.0g, Total sugars 4.3g, Salt 2.26g, Sodium 892mg

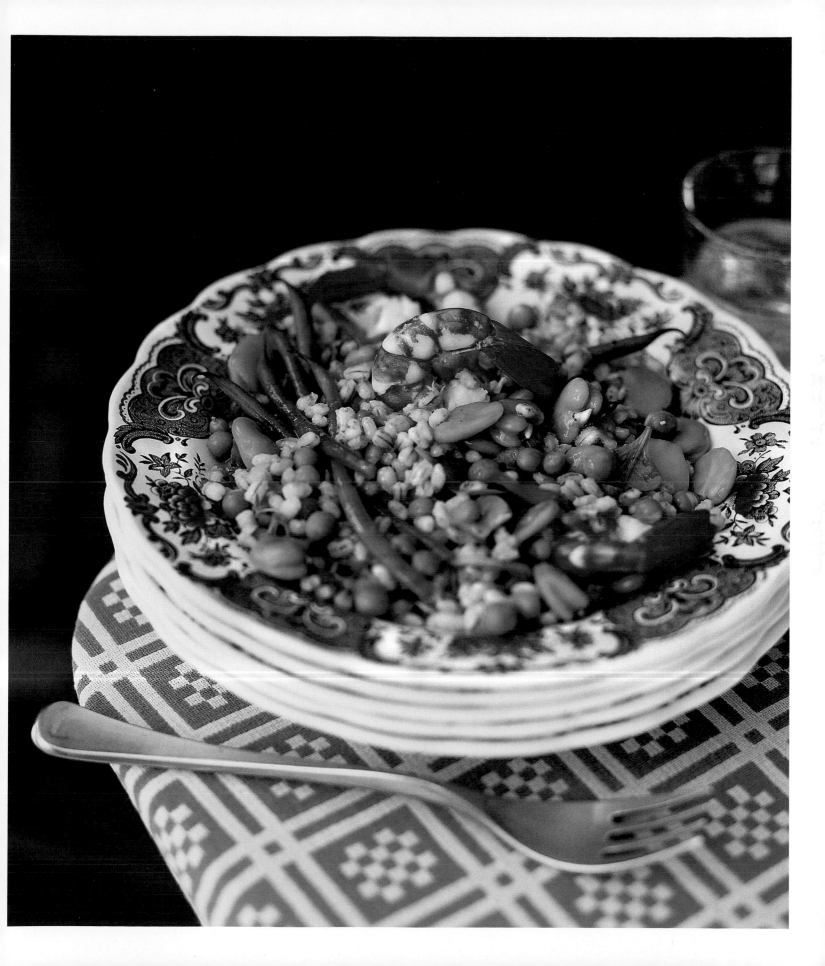

Meat and poultry

Casserole of Lamb and Loads of Spring Vegetables

The French have a dish called navarin of lamb on which this dish is loosely based. Spring offers loads of new vegetables but this casserole can be made any time of the year, just buy veg of the season. Great served with some crusty French bread to mop up all the juices.

Serves 4

1 tablespoon olive oil
675g lamb neck fillets, cut into 2.5cm pieces
4 garlic cloves, crushed
2 onions, roughly chopped
2 sprigs of fresh rosemary
175ml dry white wine
1 bay leaf
1 x 400g tin chopped tomatoes
1.25 litres lamb or chicken stock
8 carrots, topped (preferably Chantenais)
8 new potatoes, halved
115g extra fine French beans
115g broad beans, frozen or fresh and
    podded
½ spring cabbage, shredded
115g peas, frozen or fresh and podded
salt and freshly ground black pepper

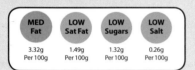

MED Fat	LOW Sat Fat	LOW Sugars	LOW Salt
3.32g Per 100g	1.49g Per 100g	1.32g Per 100g	0.26g Per 100g

1 Heat the oil in a deep casserole dish. Season the lamb pieces, then brown them all over on a fairly high heat. Remove and set aside, then discard any excess fat from the dish before adding the garlic, onion and rosemary. Reduce the heat and cook for 8 minutes, stirring occasionally, allowing the onions to go golden brown.

2 Add the wine, bay leaf, tomatoes and stock and bring to the boil. Return the meat to the dish, cover with a lid, reduce the heat and simmer gently for 1 hour 30 minutes.

3 Time now to stagger the introduction of the vegetables to the casserole: first add the carrots and potatoes and cook for 15 minutes. Add the French beans and broad beans and cook for a further 4 minutes. Add the cabbage and peas and cook for a final 3 minutes. All that remains is to check and adjust the seasoning, and dish up.

Tip Diced shoulder of lamb tends to have more flavour but it's fairly fatty so would need thorough trimming.

Amount per portion
Energy 623 kcals, Protein 43.7g, Fat 34.8g, Saturated fat 15.6g, Carbohydrate 32.5g, Total sugars 13.8g, Salt 2.67g, Sodium 1051mg

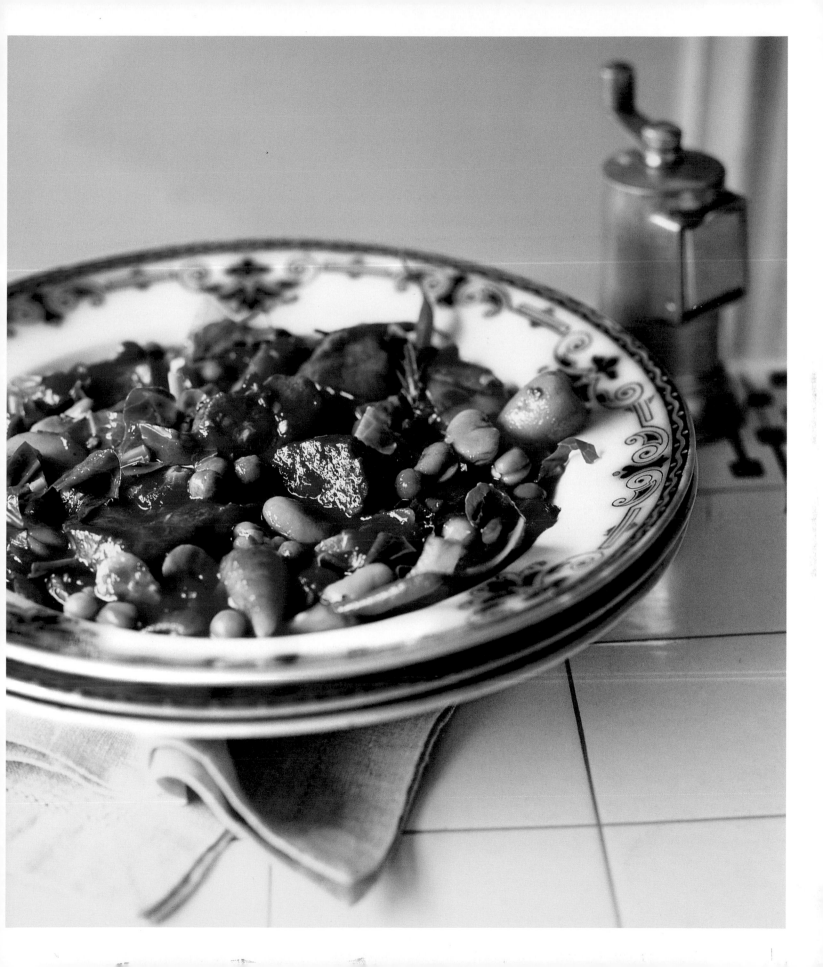

Chicken Tagine with Prunes, Almonds and Chickpeas

North African tagines are always a wonderful contrast of flavours and textures, in this one there's a lovely balance of sweet and savoury.

Serves 4

3 tablespoons olive or argan oil
6 boneless, skinless chicken thighs, each cut in 2
2 onions, 1 grated, 1 finely sliced
3 garlic cloves, crushed to a paste with a little salt
2 teaspoons ground coriander
1 teaspoon ground cinnamon
pinch of saffron
½ teaspoon each salt and freshly ground black pepper
500ml chicken stock
1 teaspoon orange flower water (optional)
1 tablespoon caster sugar
8 prunes, stoned and roughly chopped
50g raisins
1 x 400g tin chickpeas, drained and rinsed
50g toasted almond flakes
1 bunch of fresh coriander, leaves roughly chopped
1 tablespoon toasted sesame seeds
jewelled couscous, to serve

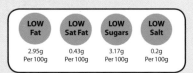

LOW Fat	LOW Sat Fat	LOW Sugars	LOW Salt
2.95g Per 100g	0.43g Per 100g	3.17g Per 100g	0.2g Per 100g

1 In a large, heavy saucepan heat 2 tablespoons of the oil then gently brown the chicken all over. Add the grated onion and cook over a medium heat for 10 minutes. Add the garlic, ground coriander, cinnamon, saffron, and the salt and pepper, and cook for a further 1 minute. Pour in enough stock to just cover the chicken and bring to the boil, then reduce the heat, cover and simmer for about 1 hour.

2 Meanwhile, in a frying pan heat the remaining oil. Add the sliced onion, orange flower water and sugar, cover and cook over a low heat, stirring from time to time, until the onions have collapsed and are becoming brown. Remove from the heat.

3 About 10 minutes before the chicken is cooked add the prunes, raisins, chickpeas, almond flakes, coriander and the caramelised onions. At the end of the cooking time transfer the solids to a serving dish and keep warm. Taste the sauce and adjust the seasoning to taste, and reduce by boiling if you like. Pour the sauce over the chicken and sprinkle with toasted sesame seeds. Serve with Jewelled Couscous.

Amount per portion
Energy 510 kcals, Protein 40.0g, Fat 23.1g, Saturated fat 3.4g, Carbohydrate 38.0g, Total sugars 24.8g, Salt 1.60g, Sodium 634mg

Turkey and Ham Meatballs with a Roasted Red Pepper and Bean Sauce

This has a very loose association with Italy as I don't think the Italians would ever have dreamed up a dish like this. Still, that's their loss and your gain.

Serves 4

For the sauce

1 tablespoon olive oil
1 onion, roughly chopped
2 garlic cloves, roughly chopped
1 hot red chilli, deseeded and
    roughly chopped
5 ready-roasted red peppers from a jar,
    drained and roughly chopped
2 tablespoons sweet chilli sauce
1 x 400g tin chopped tomatoes
1 x 400g tin cannellini beans, drained
    and rinsed
juice of 1 lemon
salt and freshly ground black pepper

For the meatballs

1 tablespoon olive oil
100g fresh or frozen sweetcorn niblets
3 slices seeded bread, crusts removed
25g prosciutto, Parma or serrano ham,
    chopped
1 small red onion, finely chopped
1 garlic clove, crushed to a paste with
    a little sea salt
1 teaspoon dried oregano
1 teaspoon ground cumin
1 tablespoon grated Parmesan cheese
1 egg, beaten
½ teaspoon each salt and freshly ground
    black pepper
400g minced turkey or chicken
spray oil, for frying
pasta and a leaf salad, to serve

1 To make the sauce, heat the olive oil in a saucepan and cook the onion over a gentle heat until soft but not browned, about 8–10 minutes. Add the garlic, chilli and roast peppers, and cook for a further 3 minutes. Blend in a food processor or with a hand-held blender.

2 Return the sauce to the pan and add the chilli sauce, tomatoes and beans, and cook gently until thick. Season with lemon juice, a pinch of salt and some pepper.

3 To make the meatballs, heat the oil in a small pan and fry the corn until lightly charred. Remove and set aside.

4 Soak the bread in a little cold water for a couple of minutes. Remove, squeeze dry and place in a bowl with the corn and the remaining meatball ingredients. With your hands, squidge the mixture for 2–3 minutes, making sure all the ingredients are evenly distributed. With wet hands, shape the mix into balls about 1.5cm diameter.

5 Lightly coat a frying pan with spray oil and brown the meatballs all over – you'll need to do this in batches. As they're ready, pop them in the red pepper and bean sauce and cook for 15 minutes. Serve with pasta and a leaf salad.

Amount per portion
Energy 498 kcals, Protein 40.0g, Fat 23.1g, Saturated fat 3.4g, Carbohydrate 34.6g, Total sugars 21.5g, Salt 1.60g, Sodium 633mg

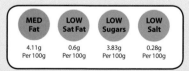

MED Fat	LOW Sat Fat	LOW Sugars	LOW Salt
4.11g Per 100g	0.6g Per 100g	3.83g Per 100g	0.28g Per 100g

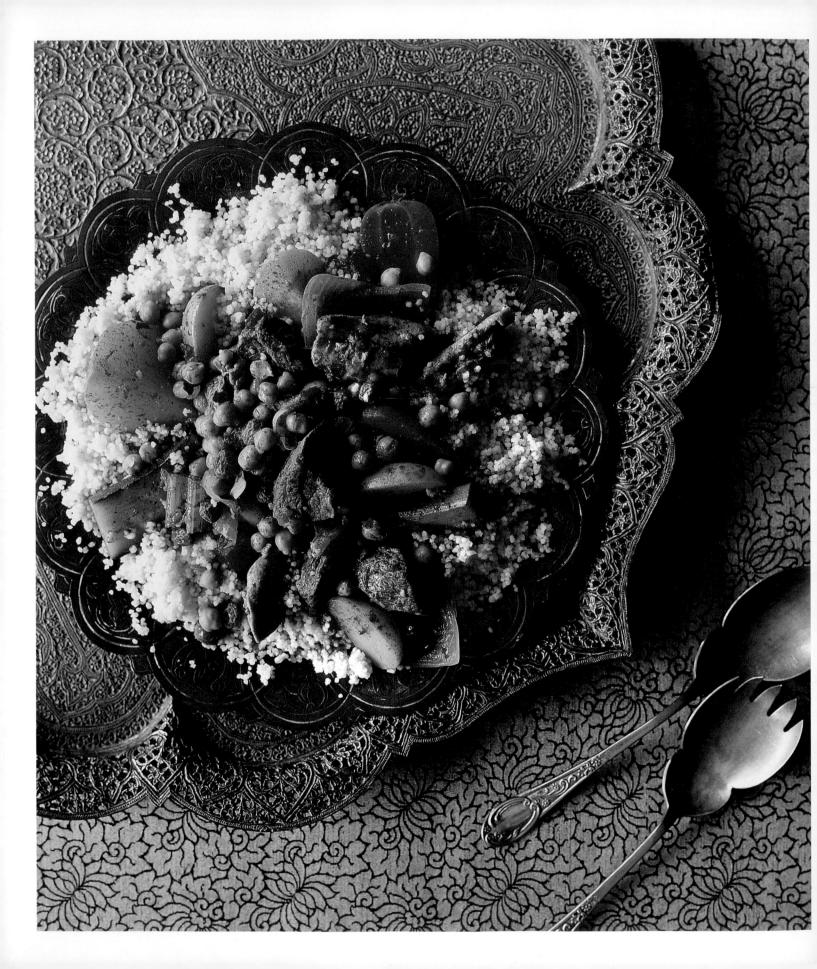

Couscous Royal

This is the giant of North African cooking: a meat and vegetable stew served with a big bowl of steaming couscous, which traditionally is cooked above the simmering stew. The stew would normally include merguez, a grilled spicy sausage, but in the interest of your health I've made it optional. To serve, present the broth, meat and vegetables together in one central serving dish and the couscous in another dish, and let everyone help themselves.

Serves 4

200g lean lamb, diced
3 boneless, skinless chicken thighs,
   each cut into 3 pieces
2 onions, cut in chunks
4 garlic cloves, crushed
2 litres chicken or lamb stock
2 Merguez sausages (optional)
pinch of salt
1 teaspoon freshly ground black pepper
pinch of saffron
1 teaspoon ground cinnamon
1 teaspoon ground coriander
½ teaspoon ground ginger
1 x 400g tin chopped tomatoes
12 new potatoes, halved
2 carrots, halved lengthways
2 turnips, quartered
1 x 400g tin chickpeas, drained
3 courgettes, each cut into 4 pieces
2 stalks celery, cut into 2cm pieces
30g sultanas
1 tablespoon harissa chilli paste
plain couscous, to serve

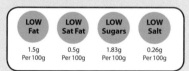

LOW Fat	LOW Sat Fat	LOW Sugars	LOW Salt
1.5g Per 100g	0.5g Per 100g	1.83g Per 100g	0.26g Per 100g

1 Put the lamb and chicken in a large saucepan and add the onions, garlic, stock, salt, pepper, saffron, cinnamon, coriander and ginger. Bring to the boil, cover, reduce the heat and simmer for 1 hour.

2 Add the tomatoes, potatoes, carrots, turnips and chickpeas, cover and simmer for 30 minutes.

3 Preheat the oven to 180°C/360°F/gas mark 4, then roast the merguez for 15 minutes, turning regularly until golden.

4 Then add the courgettes, celery and sultanas to the stew and cook for a further 20 minutes.

5 With a ladle, remove a little of the broth and combine with the harissa to make a hot liquid condiment, which is served separately. Check the seasoning of the stew and serve with plain couscous and the sausages cut into bite-sized pieces.

Amount per portion
Energy 574 kcals, Protein 54.7g, Fat 17.3g, Saturated fat 5.8g, Carbohydrate 53.7g, Total sugars 21.1g, Salt 2.97g, Sodium 1172mg

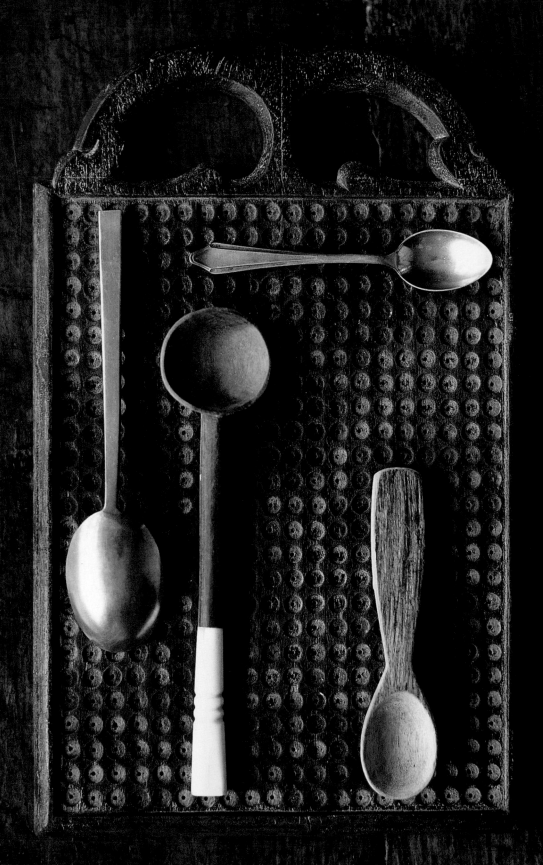

Supper in a Dash

I'm sure this fast and furious warm salad, loosely based on Middle Eastern and North African dishes, is the sort of thing they'd eat there if they'd thought of it first!

Serves 4
1 tablespoon olive oil
1 onion, chopped
2 garlic cloves, chopped
1 small aubergine, cut into 1cm dice
1 teaspoon ground coriander
½ teaspoon ground cumin
½ tablespoon tomato purée
½ tablespoon harissa chilli paste
1 x 400g tin chickpeas, drained with
    a tablespoon of the water retained
375g cooked chicken, cut into strips
2 teaspoons chopped fresh mint
2 tablespoons pomegranate seeds

1 Heat the oil in a frying pan and cook the onion and garlic over a moderate heat until golden, about 10 minutes. Add the aubergine, ground coriander and ground cumin, stir and cook for 6–7 minutes until the aubergine is well coloured.

2 Stir in the tomato purée and harissa, then the chickpeas with a little of their water to loosen the mixture. Add the chicken and warm through, then adjust the seasoning to taste. Tip into a bowl and scatter with mint and pomegranate seeds.

Amount per portion
Energy 293 kcals, Protein 31.4g, Fat 12.3g, Saturated fat 2.7g, Carbohydrate 15.1g, Total sugars 4.0g, Salt 0.58g, Sodium 227mg

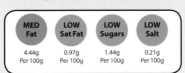

MED Fat	LOW Sat Fat	LOW Sugars	LOW Salt
4.44g Per 100g	0.97g Per 100g	1.44g Per 100g	0.21g Per 100g

Paprika Goulash

Paprika and caraway give this deliciously rich casserole a spicy sweetness. Serve it with rice noodles and a green vegetable such as cabbage, green beans or broccoli or with a dollop of yogurt sprinkled with paprika, and some rice or new potatoes.

Serves 4
2 tablespoons cornflour
450g chuck steak, brisket or silverside,
    cut into 4cm pieces
1 tablespoon sunflower oil
50g back bacon, chopped
3 garlic cloves, finely chopped
450g onions, grated
2 red peppers, cut into 1cm dice
1 tablespoon caraway seeds
1 tablespoon hot-smoked paprika, plus
    extra to garnish
600ml beef stock
2 tablespoons tomato purée
6 cornichons (baby gherkins), sliced
freshly ground black pepper
0 per cent fat Greek yogurt, to serve

1 Tip the cornflour and beef into a plastic bag, seal the top and shake well until all the beef pieces are lightly dusted.

2 Heat the oil in a casserole dish, add the bacon, garlic, onions, red peppers, caraway and paprika and cook for 3 minutes. Add the beef, followed by the stock and tomato purée and cornichons, and season with black pepper. Bring to a simmer, then cover and cook very gently for 2 hours, stirring occasionally, until the meat is tender and the sauce is reduced to a rich consistency.

Amount per portion
Energy 360 kcals, Protein 32.2g, Fat 16.2g, Saturated fat 5.4g, Carbohydrate 22.7g, Total sugars 12.1g, Salt 1.32g, Sodium 522mg

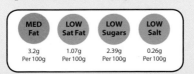

MED Fat	LOW Sat Fat	LOW Sugars	LOW Salt
3.2g Per 100g	1.07g Per 100g	2.39g Per 100g	0.26g Per 100g

Peruvian Chicken Kebabs with Garlic and Orange Salsa

Inspired by a recipe I found in a Peruvian cookbook. Simple, quick, tasty – what more do you need? Oh, and it's pretty good value for money, too, and perfect for the barbie.

Serves 4

6 garlic cloves
¼ teaspoon salt
1 teaspoon ground cumin
1 teaspoon ground coriander
1 teaspoon sweet paprika
4 tablespoons fresh coriander leaves,
    half of them chopped
juice and grated zest of 3 limes
2 large chicken breasts, skinned and
    cut into 2.5cm cubes
5 juicy oranges
1 red onion, thinly sliced
1 tablespoon toasted flaked almonds
spray olive oil
green salad and tortillas, to serve

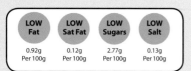

LOW Fat	LOW Sat Fat	LOW Sugars	LOW Salt
0.92g Per 100g	0.12g Per 100g	2.77g Per 100g	0.13g Per 100g

1 In a mini food processor, blitz the garlic and salt to a smooth paste. Remove half and set aside. To the remaining half in the food processor add the ground cumin, ground coriander, paprika, the whole coriander leaves and half the lime zest and juice, and blend to a paste.

2 Mix the chicken with the spicy garlic paste and allow to marinate for a couple of hours, or at least 30 minutes.

3 Meanwhile, grate the zest of 2 ½ oranges and juice 2 of them. Combine the orange zest and juice with the remaining lime zest and juice, the onion, the remaining chopped coriander leaves and the remaining garlic paste to make a salsa. Then remove the peel and pith from the remaining oranges, slice the flesh and combine with the garlic salsa.

4 Heat a griddle pan or barbecue. Thread the marinated chicken on to four wooden skewers. Spray the kebabs with olive oil then cook for 12–15 minutes, turning from time to time. Serve with the garlic and orange salsa and a green salad, and maybe some kind of tortilla/flat bread.

Variations If you're a leg person, try this recipe with boneless chicken thighs; you could also have a go with pork, lamb, salmon, tuna or halloumi cheese.

Amount per portion
Energy 154 kcals, Protein 20.5g, Fat 3.1g, Saturated fat 0.4g, Carbohydrate 11.8g, Total sugars 9.3g, Salt 0.44g, Sodium 175mg

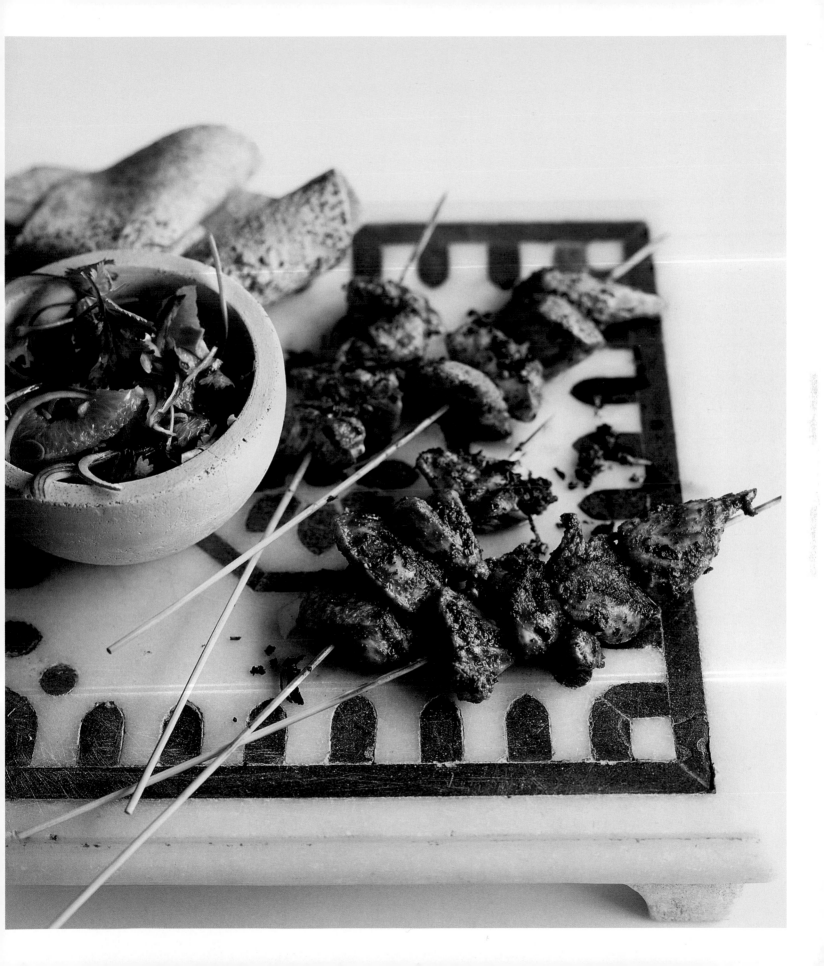

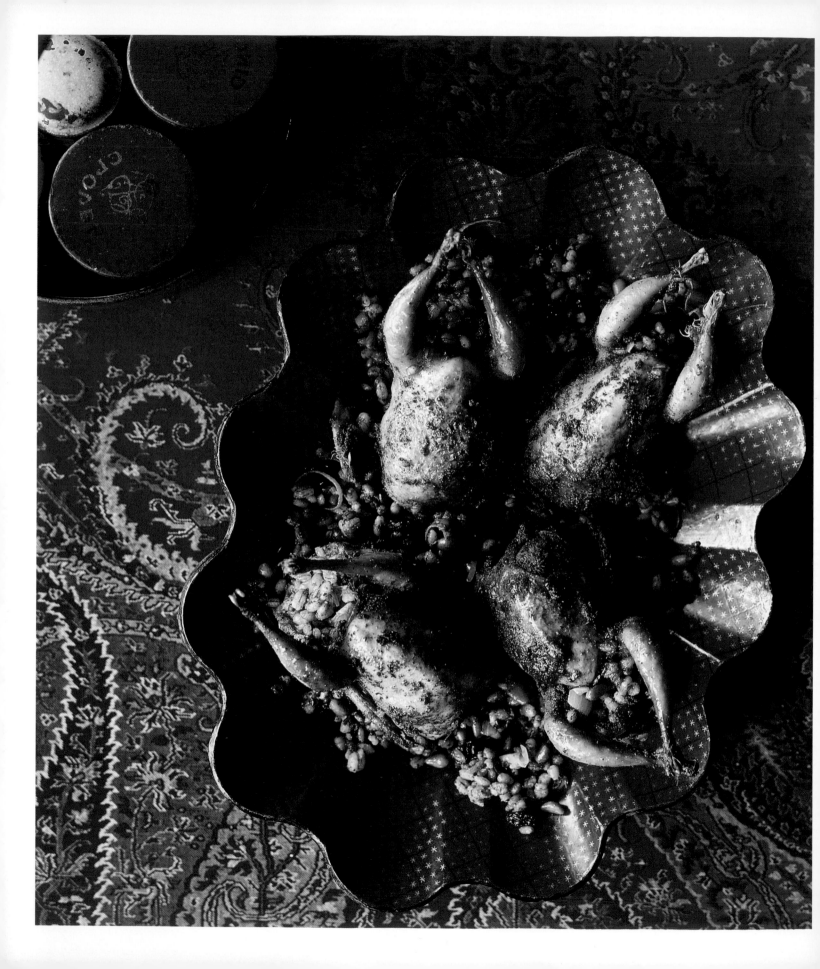

Barley-stuffed Quail with Indian Spices

'These little game birds' sweet-flavoured flesh has more depth than chicken and with these lovely Indian flavours, this recipe makes a great dinner party treat.'

Serves 4
4 quails

For the marinade
2 teaspoons ground coriander
½ teaspoon ground black pepper
½ teaspoon ground cardamom
½ teaspoon ground clove
½ teaspoon ground cumin
1 teaspoon curry powder
¼ teaspoon chilli powder
½ teaspoon ground turmeric
1 teaspoon grated fresh ginger
1 tablespoon sunflower oil

For the stuffing
15g unsalted butter
1 onion, finely chopped
1 teaspoon cumin seeds
grated zest and juice of 1 orange
85g sultanas
20g toasted pine nuts
175g quick-cook pearl barley, cooked
½ teaspoon salt
¼ teaspoon ground black pepper

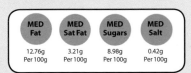

MED Fat	MED Sat Fat	MED Sugars	MED Salt
12.76g Per 100g	3.21g Per 100g	8.98g Per 100g	0.42g Per 100g

1 Mix together all the marinade ingredients to form a paste. Gently lift the skin of each quail, trying not to puncture the skin, and work a little of the paste under the skin. Rub some paste inside the cavity of each bird and over the outside. Leave to marinate for as long as possible (ideally overnight or for at least 1 hour).

2 Meanwhile, preheat the oven to 180°C/350°F/gas mark 4, and make the stuffing. Heat the butter in a pan and gently cook the onion until soft and translucent, about 8 minutes. Add the cumin seeds, orange zest and juice, sultanas and pine nuts and mix well. Stir in the pearl barley and season to taste. Use the mixture to stuff the cavity of each marinated quail.

3 Place the birds in a roasting tin and cook in the preheated oven for 20–25 minutes. Serve with plenty of steamed vegetables.

Amount per portion
Energy 550 kcals, Protein 28g, Fat 25g, Saturated fat 6.3g, Carbohydrate 57g, Total sugars 17.6g, Salt 0.82g, Sodium 324mg

Involtini in Ragu

In Italian *involtini* means 'little birds'. These stuffed meat parcels are usually served with pasta, but here I've used cannellini beans to boost the slow-release carbohydrates.

Serves 4
4 very thin sirloin steaks, about 85–115g each, fat removed
2 tablespoons drained cannellini beans (from the sauce ingredients, see below)
15g grated Parmesan cheese
2 garlic cloves, roughly chopped
1 tablespoon chopped fresh parsley
½ tablespoon snipped fresh chives
freshly ground black pepper

For the sauce
spray olive oil
1 onion, finely chopped
3 garlic cloves, crushed to a paste with a little salt
1 teaspoon chopped fresh oregano
1 carrot, diced
1 celery stalk, finely sliced
2 fresh red chillies, deseeded and finely chopped
90ml red wine
200ml tomato passata
200ml chicken stock
2 teaspoons sugar or low-calorie granulated sweetener
1 x 400g tin chopped tomatoes
1 x 400g tin cannellini beans, drained and rinsed
handful of fresh basil leaves, ripped
salt and freshly ground black pepper

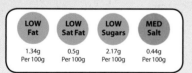

LOW Fat	LOW Sat Fat	LOW Sugars	MED Salt
1.34g Per 100g	0.5g Per 100g	2.17g Per 100g	0.44g Per 100g

1 Beat the steaks flat with a meat mallet or a rolling pin, taking care not to tear the meat. Season with black pepper. In a mini food processor blend the beans with the Parmesan, garlic, parsley and chives and season with pepper. Spread this mixture over the steaks then roll each slice tightly, securing each involtini with a cocktail stick.

2 Spray a little oil in the bottom of a large ovenproof lidded pan or casserole dish, then over a medium heat fry the involtini all over to brown. Remove from the pan and set aside. Into the pan add the onion, garlic, oregano, carrot, celery and chillies. Cook over a moderate heat until the onions have softened and are starting to brown, about 12–15 minutes.

3 Meanwhile, preheat the oven to 160°C/325°F/gas mark 3. When the onions in the pan have softened, pour in the wine and boil vigorously until the liquid has all but disappeared. Add the passata, chicken stock, sugar or sweetener and chopped tomatoes. Return the involtini to the sauce and bring to the boil, cover and place in the preheated oven. Cook for 2 hours, stirring from time to time.

4 Remove the involtini from the sauce and keep them warm, then add the beans and basil to the pan and cook over a medium heat for 5 minutes. Season to taste, then return the involtini to the dish. Serve hot.

Variation Italians will often eat the sauce with pasta first, and then serve the involtini with a salad or a green vegetable such as broccoli or spinach.

Amount per portion (low-calorie sweetener)
Energy 274 kcals, Protein 30.7g, Fat 6.2g, Saturated fat 2.3g, Carbohydrate 23.7g, Total sugars 10.0g, Salt 2.04g, Sodium 804mg

Amount per portion (Ssugar)
Energy 283 kcals, Protein 30.7g, Fat 6.2g, Saturated fat 2.3g, Carbohydrate 26.1g, Total sugars 12.4g, Salt 2.04g, Sodium 804mg

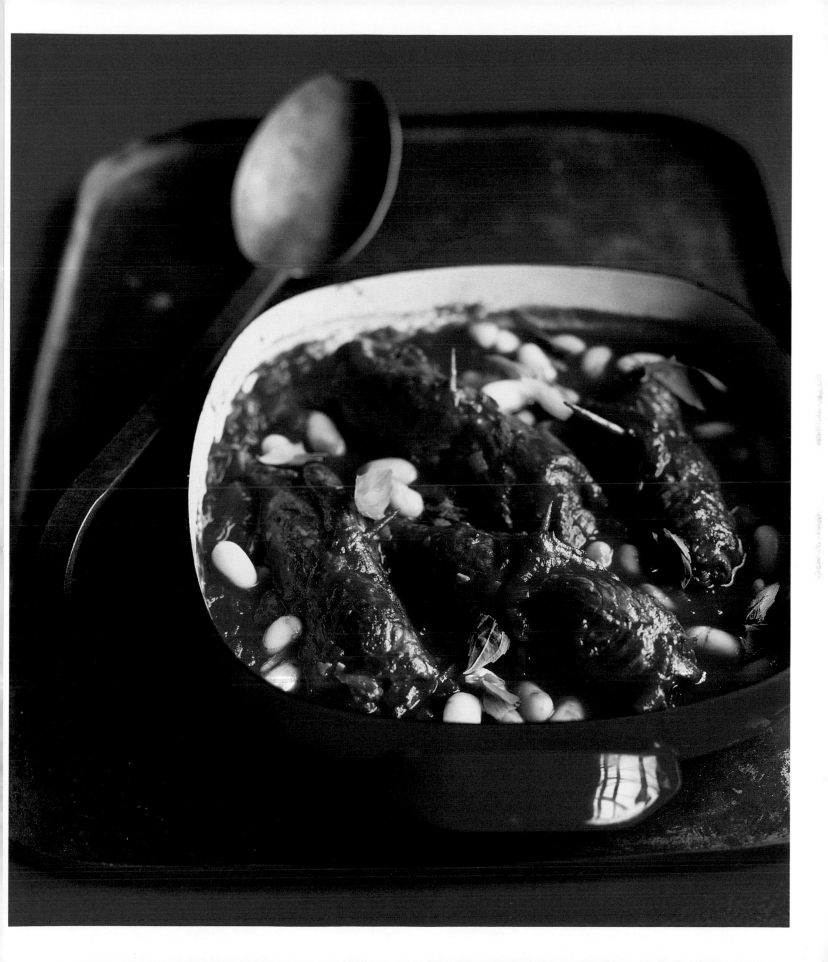

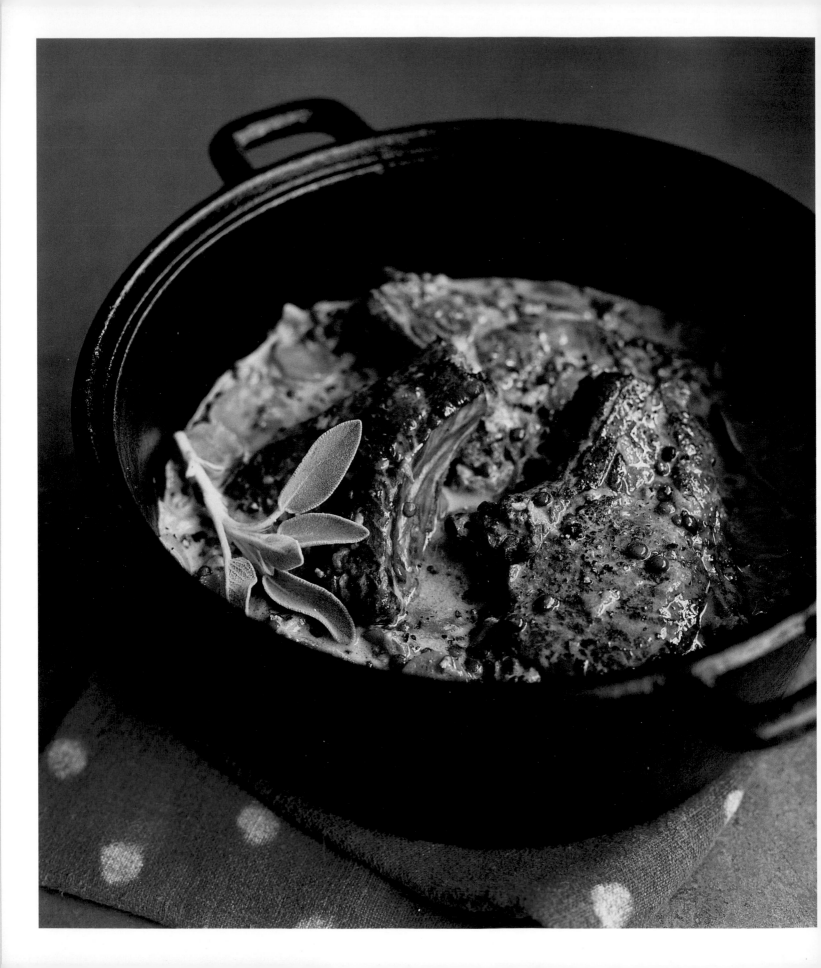

Slow-cooked Pork Chops with Lentils and Cider

Pork, sage and apple are a great partnership. Try to get an old British breed such as a Middle White or a Gloucester Old Spot if you can: old breeds, more flavour.

Serves 4

1 tablespoon olive oil
4 pork chops, about 175g each, rind and most of the fat removed
1 onion, chopped
1 carrot, sliced
2 crunchy eating apples, unpeeled and grated
2 sprigs of fresh sage
175g puy lentils
300ml good-quality dry cider
420ml chicken stock
1 tablespoon Dijon mustard
splash of Worcestershire sauce
100g 0 per cent fat natural Greek yogurt
freshly ground black pepper

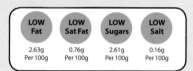

LOW Fat	LOW Sat Fat	LOW Sugars	LOW Salt
2.63g Per 100g	0.76g Per 100g	2.61g Per 100g	0.16g Per 100g

1 Heat the oil in a large casserole dish, add the chops and brown them all over. Remove the meat from the dish and set aside, and discard any excess fat in the bottom of the pan. Add the onion, carrot, apple and sage and cook over a moderate heat for 8 minutes.

2 Add the lentils, stir to combine then add the cider and stock and bring to the boil. Return the chops to the dish, reduce the heat, cover and cook gently for 1 hour. Remove the chops, cover with foil and set aside to rest.

3 Increase the heat under the casserole dish and boil the sauce to reduce it. Meanwhile, whisk together the mustard, Worcestershire sauce and yogurt, and season with pepper. When the sauce has reduced by half, fold in the flavoured yogurt, then return the chops, turn off the heat and check the seasoning before serving.

Variation This works really well with whole pheasant; reduce the cooking time from 1 hour to 30 minutes.

Amount per portion
Energy 491 kcals, Protein 54.3g, Fat 14.2g, Saturated fat 4.1g, Carbohydrate 36.4g, Total sugars 14.1g, Salt 0.87g, Sodium 344mg

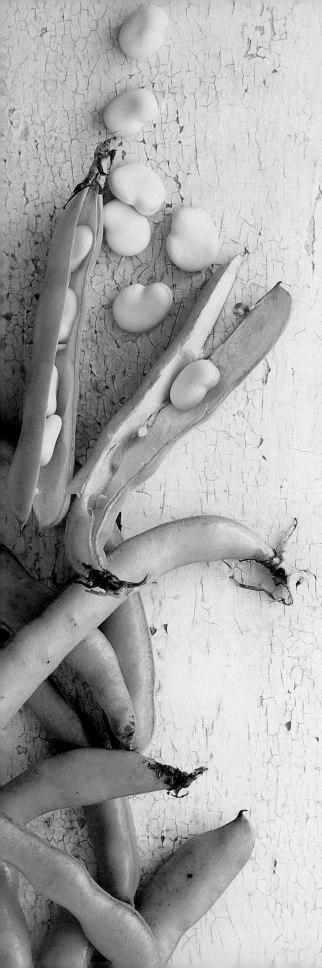

Roast Pork with Potatoes in Retsina Wine

Called *hirino yiouvetsi* in Greece, this delicious roast pork dish is dead simple to make.

Serves 4–6
spray olive oil
1kg loin of pork, rind and most of the fat
    removed, boned and rolled
450g potatoes, halved
2 onions, sliced
2 teaspoons chopped fresh oregano
225g broad beans, frozen or fresh and
    podded
2 celery stalks, sliced
1 x 400g tin chopped tomatoes
225ml retsina white wine
leaf salad, to serve

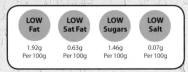

LOW Fat	LOW Sat Fat	LOW Sugars	LOW Salt
1.92g Per 100g	0.63g Per 100g	1.46g Per 100g	0.07g Per 100g

1 Preheat the oven to 180°C/350°F/gas mark 4. Spray some oil over the base of a heavy-based pan and fry the pork until brown all over.

2 Toss together the potatoes, onions, oregano, broad beans and celery. Oil a baking dish and spread the potato mix at the bottom, then spoon over the tinned tomatoes and their juice. Set the pork on top, transfer to the preheated oven and cook for 1 hour 20 minutes.

3 Remove the baking dish from the oven, set the pork aside, cover the meat with foil and allow to rest. Meanwhile, add the retsina wine to the potatoes in the baking dish and boil on the hob, without stirring, until the liquid has reduced by half. Slice the pork and serve with the potatoes and sauce. A leaf salad is the only extra you will need.

Tip If you can't find retsina or another resinated white wine, use a gewürztraminer-style white.

Amount per portion
Energy 495 kcals, Protein 58.9g, Fat 12.8g, Saturated fat 4.2g,
Carbohydrate 33.6g, Total sugars 9.7g,
Salt 0.45g, Sodium 178mg

Garbure

This hearty French soup is a meal in itself, made with a profusion of vegetables and several meats, including the fabulous duck confit.

Serves 4

85g lean smoked bacon, cut into lardons
2 leeks, roughly chopped
225g new potatoes, halved
3 celery stalks, thinly sliced
4 baby turnips
115g cooked ham, roughly chopped
4 garlic cloves, finely chopped
2 sprigs of thyme
1 onion, thinly sliced
2 carrots, sliced
2 bay leaves
2 litres reduced-salt chicken stock
1 x 400g tin white haricot beans, drained
　　and rinsed
½ Savoy cabbage, shredded
2 legs duck confit, shop-bought, skin
　　removed, picked off the bone
salt and freshly ground black pepper
chopped flat-leaf parsley, to garnish

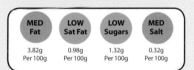

MED Fat	LOW Sat Fat	LOW Sugars	MED Salt
3.82g Per 100g	0.98g Per 100g	1.32g Per 100g	0.32g Per 100g

1 Put the bacon in a large saucepan, add the leeks, potatoes, celery, turnips, ham, garlic, thyme, onion, carrots, bay leaves and stock, and cook gently for 45 minutes.

2 Add the beans, cabbage and duck confit and cook for a further 15 minutes. Remove the bacon and ham, blend them in a food processor until smooth, and add back to the soup. Season to taste and garnish with parsley.

Amount per portion
Energy 629 kcals, Protein 34.0g, Fat 40.0g, Saturated fat 10.3g, Carbohydrate 35.5g, Total sugars 13.8g, Salt 3.35g, Sodium 1322mg

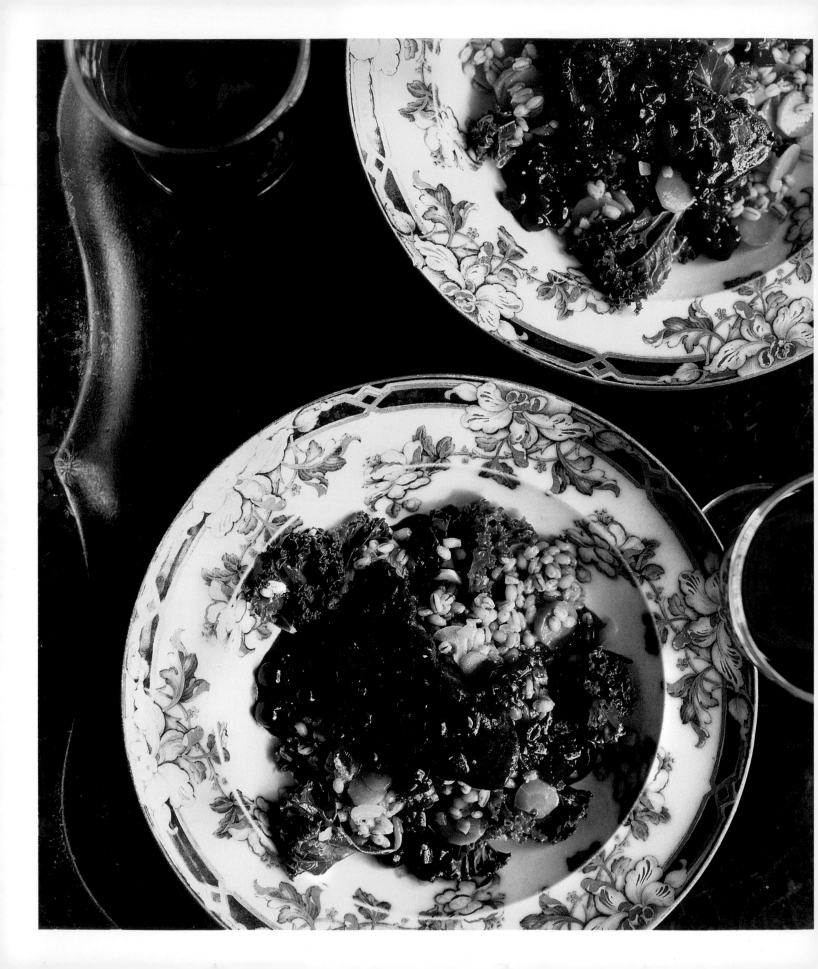

Venison with Blackcurrants, Kale and Barley

Venison takes to red fruits perfectly. In Britain I've often seen it cooked with redcurrants but when I had it with blackcurrants, I thought, yes, this is really good.

Serves 4

450g blackcurrants
175ml 'robust' red wine
4 venison loin or haunch steaks,
    about 150g each
1 tablespoon olive oil
3 garlic cloves, sliced
1 onion, finely chopped
2 carrots, finely sliced
175g pearl barley
900ml game or beef stock
325g curly kale, coarse stems
    removed, shredded
salt and freshly ground black pepper

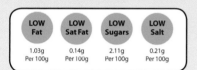

LOW Fat	LOW Sat Fat	LOW Sugars	LOW Salt
1.03g Per 100g	0.14g Per 100g	2.11g Per 100g	0.21g Per 100g

1 In a food processor blend half the blackcurrants with the wine until smooth, then pass through a sieve. Transfer to a large non-metallic dish and add the remaining blackcurrants and the venison steaks, cover and leave to marinate overnight in the refrigerator, or for a minimum of two hours.

2 Before cooking the venison, heat half the olive oil in a saucepan and cook half the garlic, three quarters of the onion and all the carrot for about 10 minutes until the vegetables start to colour. Add the barley and stir well to mix in, then pour in just over three quarters of the stock, setting aside the remainder for the sauce. Bring to the boil, then reduce the heat and simmer for 20 minutes. Add the kale and cook for a further 10 minutes. Season to taste.

3 Meanwhile, remove the venison from the marinade, wipe dry with kitchen paper, and reserve the marinade. Heat the remaining oil in a frying pan over a high heat, sear the venison on both sides then reduce the heat and cook for a further 2 minutes each side. Remove, cover to keep warm and set aside.

4 In the pan used for cooking the venison, fry the remaining onion and garlic gently until soft, about 6 minutes. Add the marinade with the blackcurrants and boil over a high heat until reduced by half, then add the remaining stock and continue boiling until reduced by a third. Check the seasoning and adjust to taste.

5 Spoon the barley and kale mix on to individual warmed plates, top with the venison and spoon the sauce around.

Variation This recipe works very well with pork steaks, turning them slightly gamey.

Amount per portion
Energy 467 kcals, Protein 45.7g, Fat 7.6g, Saturated fat 1.0g, Carbohydrate 53.8g, Total sugars 15.6g, Salt 1.54g, Sodium 606mg

Chicken Pot in the style of Cacciatore

One pot that goes in the middle of the table, everyone happy, very little washing up and an Italian-influenced dish that explodes with flavour.

Serves 4

2 x 400g tins chopped tomatoes
100ml red wine
8 chicken thighs, skin off, bone in
4 sprigs of fresh rosemary
2 bay leaves
2 onions, finely chopped
6 garlic cloves, crushed to
    a paste with a little salt
1 teaspoon dried oregano
6 anchovy fillets, roughly chopped
2 tablespoons capers
225g new potatoes, thinly sliced
20 kalamata olives, stoned
2 handfuls of baby spinach
salt and freshly ground black pepper
leaf salad or green vegetables, to serve

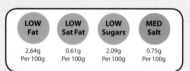

LOW Fat	LOW Sat Fat	LOW Sugars	MED Salt
2.64g Per 100g	0.61g Per 100g	2.09g Per 100g	0.75g Per 100g

1 Preheat the oven to 180°C/350°F/gas mark 4. In a large bowl, put all the ingredients except the spinach and salt and pepper, and stir to blend well. If possible leave for a couple of hours for the flavours to develop, if not don't worry. Tip everything into a large casserole dish, pop on the lid and cook for 1 hour 15 minutes, checking after 45 minutes to see whether it is drying out – if so add a little water.
2 At the end of the cooking, remove the chicken pieces and keep warm. Check the sauce for seasoning then fold in the spinach and stir until wilted. Return the chicken to the pot. Serve with a leaf salad or steamed green vegetables.

Amount per portion
Energy 392 kcals, Protein 44.4g, Fat 13.5g, Saturated fat 3.1g, Carbohydrate 22.8g, Total sugars 10.7g, Salt 3.83g, Sodium 1511mg

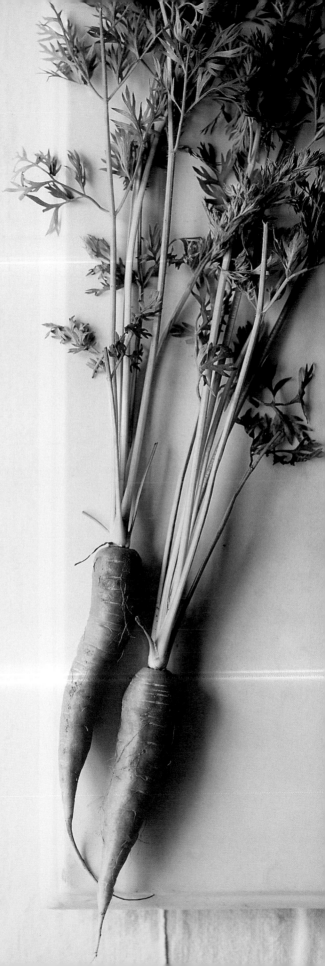

Pot Roast Rabbit with Tomato and White Beans

The Northern Italians love a good stew, and this one is really gutsy, with strong flavours. Ask your butcher to joint the rabbit for you. If bunny is not your thing then use skinless chicken thighs instead.

Serves 4

1 rabbit, jointed (legs, shoulders, belly flaps cut into strips, the saddle and neck cut into 4)
1 tablespoon olive oil
1 bunch baby carrots, about 12
4 shallots, cut in half through the root
50g smoked back bacon, cut into lardons
8 garlic cloves
100ml dry white wine

600ml chicken stock
2 bay leaves
4 sprigs of fresh thyme
grated zest and juice of 1 orange
325g cherry tomatoes, halved
1 x 400g tin cannellini beans, drained and rinsed
1 tablespoon anchovy essence
2 tablespoons chopped fresh parsley
freshly ground black pepper

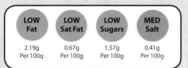

LOW Fat	LOW Sat Fat	LOW Sugars	MED Salt
2.19g Per 100g	0.67g Per 100g	1.57g Per 100g	0.41g Per 100g

1 Preheat the oven to 180°C/350°F/gas mark 4. Season the rabbit pieces with ground black pepper. In a casserole dish heat the olive oil over a medium heat and brown the rabbit pieces all over. Remove the meat and set aside.

2 Put the carrots into the casserole, add the shallots, bacon and whole garlic cloves and cook for about 10 minutes, stirring occasionally, until everything has a golden colour.

3 Pour in the wine, scrape the bottom of the casserole to remove any residue then add the stock, bay leaves, thyme and orange juice. Return the rabbit to the dish and stir. Cover, transfer to the preheated oven and cook for 40 minutes, stirring occasionally.

4 With a slotted spoon, transfer the meat and vegetables to a serving platter and keep warm. To the juices in the pan add the cherry tomatoes, cannellini beans and anchovy essence. Bring to the boil and reduce the juices by one third. Meanwhile, combine the orange zest with the parsley.

5 Spoon the tomato and bean sauce over the rabbit and vegetables, and sprinkle with the orange parsley.

Amount per portion
Energy 356 kcals, Protein 38.1g, Fat 13.0g, Saturated fat 4.0g, Carbohydrate 21.1g, Total sugars 9.3g, Salt 2.43g, Sodium 955mg

Lamb Tagine

A lovely dish packed full of flavour, perfect for cold winter nights, plus it's full of good GI foods too.

Serves 4

1 tablespoon ground ginger
1 tablespoon paprika
2 teaspoons ground turmeric
1 teaspoon ground cinnamon
1 teaspoon cayenne pepper
1 teaspoon freshly ground black pepper
450g lean lamb, cut into 2.5cm pieces
1 tablespoon olive oil
½ head of garlic, peeled and crushed
    with ¼ teaspoon salt
325g onion, grated
55g dried apricots, halved and soaked
    in a little water
25g flaked almonds
25g sultanas
½ teaspoon saffron, soaked in
    1 teaspoon cold water
150ml lamb stock
150ml tomato juice
1 x 400g tin tomatoes, roughly chopped
1 x 400g tin chickpeas, drained and rinsed
fresh coriander leaves, to garnish
couscous, to serve

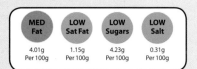

MED Fat	LOW Sat Fat	LOW Sugars	LOW Salt
4.01g Per 100g	1.15g Per 100g	4.23g Per 100g	0.31g Per 100g

1 Combine all the spices. Put half the mix into a bowl and stir in the lamb, ensuring all the pieces are well coated. Leave for a few hours, or overnight if possible.

2 Preheat the oven to 160°C/325°F/gas mark 3. Heat half the oil in a large heavy-based ovenproof lidded pan or casserole dish over a high heat and brown the lamb pieces, then remove the meat and set aside. In the same pan, fry the remaining spices, crushed garlic and grated onion using the remaining oil, over a low to medium heat. Allow the onion to soften without browning.

3 Add the apricots and their soaking water, the almonds, sultanas, saffron, stock, tomato juice, tinned tomatoes, chickpeas and the browned meat. Bring to the boil, cover, place in the preheated oven and cook for 1 hour 30 minutes to 2 hours.

4 Remove from the oven. If you like, remove the meat pieces and boil the sauce over a high heat until reduced and thickened, then return the meat to the pan. Garnish the tagine with coriander leaves, and serve with couscous.

Tip The fresh coriander leaves scattered over the cooked dish are vital to a truly authentic tagine.

Amount per portion
Energy 439 kcals, Protein 33.6g, Fat 18.4g, Saturated fat 5.3g, Carbohydrate 37.2g, Total sugars 19.4g, Salt 1.43g, Sodium 562mg

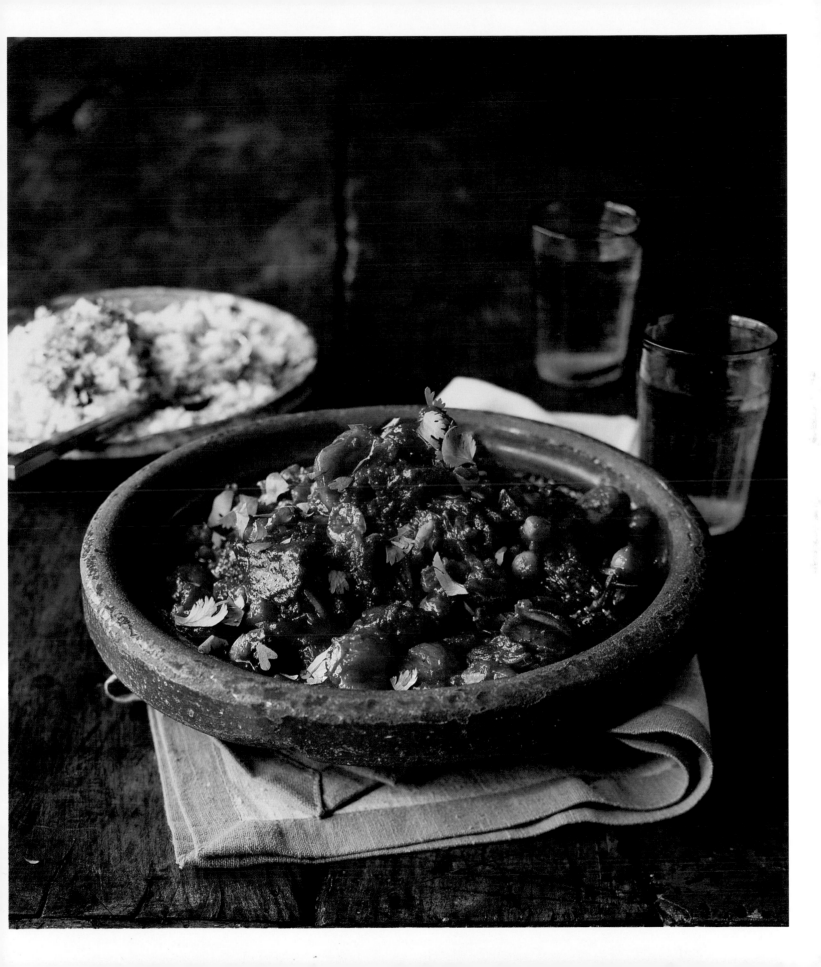

Barley with Greens, Sausage and Ham

A bowl of this Australian-inspired dish will nourish you in every way.

Serves 4

1 tablespoon sunflower oil
2 onions, finely chopped
2 garlic cloves, finely chopped
½ teaspoon fresh thyme leaves
2 handfuls of mixed spinach and
    rocket, roughly chopped
225g pearl barley
50g Parma ham, chopped
½ teaspoon cayenne pepper
900ml chicken stock
110g chorizo sausage, diced
10g freshly grated Parmesan cheese
4 tablespoons chopped fresh flat-leaf
    parsley
2 tablespoons snipped fresh chives
2 tablespoons toasted pine nuts

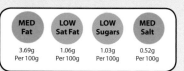

MED Fat	LOW Sat Fat	LOW Sugars	MED Salt
3.69g Per 100g	1.06g Per 100g	1.03g Per 100g	0.52g Per 100g

1 Melt the butter in a saucepan over a medium heat, then add the onions, garlic and thyme and cook for 8 minutes until the onions have started to soften.

2 Stir in the chopped greens, then the barley, Parma ham, cayenne and stock. Bring to the boil, then cover, reduce the heat and simmer until the liquid has been absorbed and the barley is tender.

3 Add the chorizo, Parmesan, parsley, chive and pine nuts. Mix well and heat through.

Amount per portion

Energy 448 kcals, Protein 24.2g, Fat 16.4g, Saturated fat 4.7g, Carbohydrate 54.4g, Total sugars 4.6g, Salt 2.30g, Sodium 909mg

Chickpeas with Chicken and Black Pudding

This is the sort of dish you might get as a tapa when visiting Spain. Chicken wouldn't necessarily feature, but I've added it to reduce the potency of the black pudding.

Serves 4

spray olive oil
1 onion, finely chopped
2 garlic cloves, finely chopped
1 chicken breast, skinned and cut into
   1cm cubes
50g good-quality black pudding,
   skinned and cut into 1cm cubes
25g shelled hazelnuts, roughly chopped
25g toasted pine nuts
25g sultanas
1 teaspoon ground coriander
½ teaspoon dried chilli flakes
1 x 400g tin chickpeas, drained and rinsed
1 tablespoon chopped fresh parsley
1 tablespoon sherry or red wine vinegar
freshly ground black pepper
leaf salad, to serve

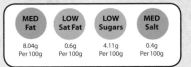

MED Fat	LOW Sat Fat	LOW Sugars	MED Salt
8.04g Per 100g	0.6g Per 100g	4.11g Per 100g	0.4g Per 100g

1 Spray a large frying pan with olive oil and warm up over a moderate heat, add the onion and garlic and cook for 10 minutes until the onions have softened and slightly browned.
2 Add the chicken pieces, increase the heat and cook for 5 minutes, then add the black pudding and cook for a further 2 minutes. Fold in the hazelnuts and pine nuts, sultanas, coriander, chilli and chickpeas. Cook for about 5 minutes more until the chickpeas have heated through. Fold in the parsley, stir in the vinegar and add pepper to taste. Serve with a leaf salad.

Variation If black pudding is not to your liking, then omit it and use a small amount of your favourite sausage, skin removed.

Amount per portion
Energy 265 kcals, Protein 17.3g, Fat 13.5g, Saturated fat 1.0g, Carbohydrate 19.8g, Total sugars 6.9g, Salt 0.67g, Sodium 263mg

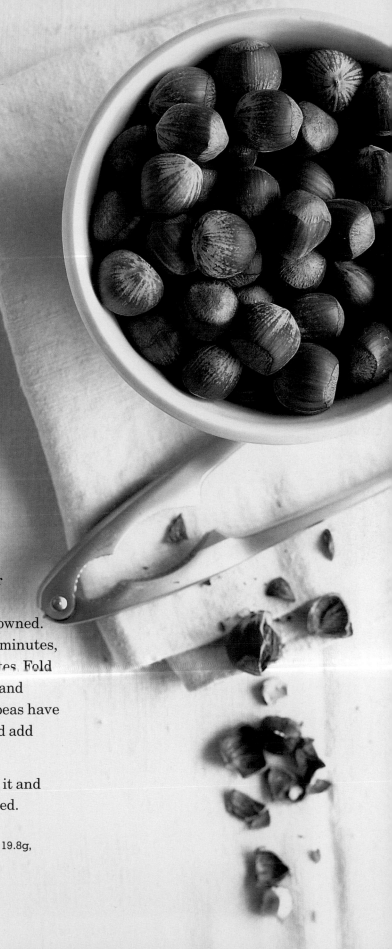

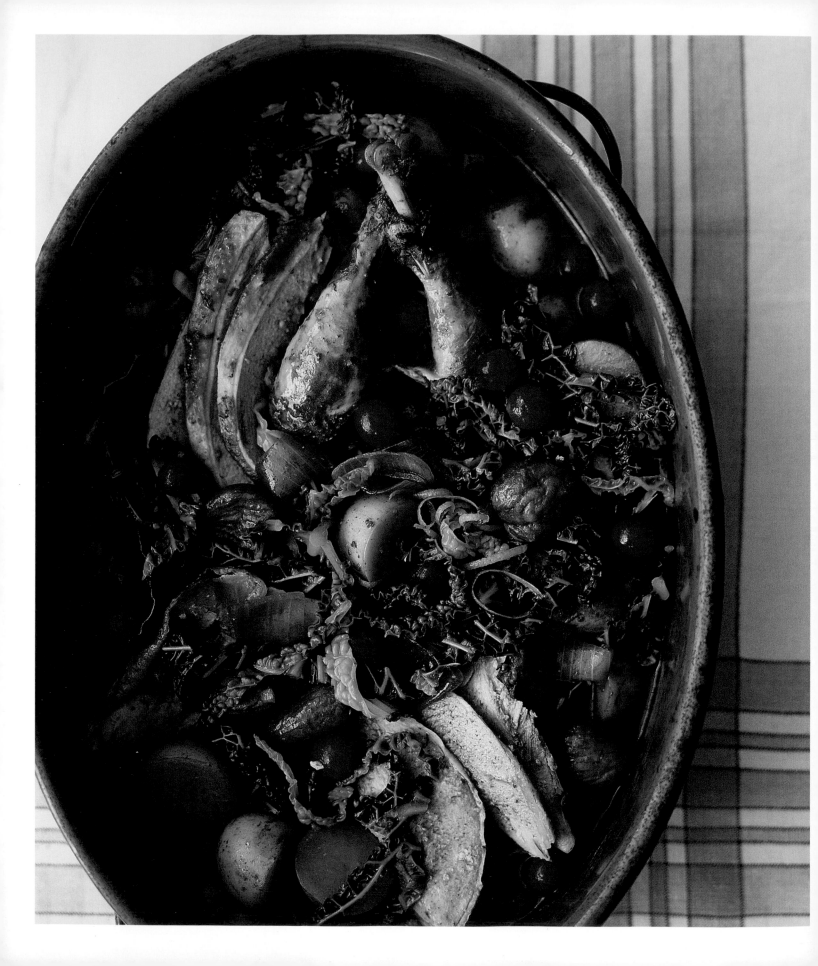

Pot Roast Pheasant with Chestnuts, New Potatoes and Cabbage

It's a shame that game birds are so under-utilised in Britain, despite being readily available in season. They are raised in the wild, are good value and are lower in fat and thus healthier to eat than most other meats. There are loads of flavours going on here, perfect for autumn and winter.

Serves 4
1 tablespoon olive oil
2 pheasants
2 onions, roughly chopped
1 bay leaf
sprig of thyme
6 juniper berries
12 new potatoes, halved
175g pre-cooked and peeled chestnuts
450ml game or beef stock
150ml 'robust' red wine
115g cranberries
175g Savoy cabbage, shredded
grated rind and juice of 1 orange
salt and freshly grated black pepper

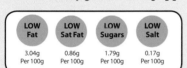

LOW Fat	LOW Sat Fat	LOW Sugars	LOW Salt
3.04g Per 100g	0.86g Per 100g	1.79g Per 100g	0.17g Per 100g

1 Preheat the oven to 200°C/400°F/gas mark 6. Heat the olive oil in a casserole dish, then add the pheasants and brown them all over. Remove and set aside. Put the onions in the casserole and cook until softened and golden, about 8 minutes.

2 Add the bay leaf, thyme, juniper, new potatoes and chestnuts, and stir to combine. Return the pheasants to the dish, breast side up. Pour the stock and wine around the pheasants, cover the casserole and bring to the boil. Transfer to the preheated oven and cook for 25 minutes.

3 Remove the pheasants and set aside to rest. Transfer the casserole to the hob. Add the cranberries, cabbage and orange zest and juice. Cook over a medium heat for 10 minutes.

4 Carve the pheasants and return the meat to the casserole. Season to taste and serve in warmed bowls.

Tip The pheasant carcasses and drumsticks are excellent for soup. If you prefer a thicker sauce, add a little cornflour thinned with cold water and simmer gently for a few minutes to thicken.

Amount per portion
Energy 570 kcals, Protein 46.8g, Fat 21.1g, Saturated fat 6.0g, Carbohydrate 45.0g, Total sugars 12.4g, Salt 1.15g, Sodium 454mg

Pot Roast Chicken with Leeks, Green Beans and Peas

You see this delicious simple stew on many menus of unpretentious restaurants in France. It's just what you want on a winter's evening.

Serves 4

8 new potatoes, halved
spray olive oil
55g pancetta or smoked streaky bacon lardons
6 boneless and skinless chicken thighs, halved
750g leeks, cut in 2.5cm pieces
8 garlic cloves, crushed
sprig of fresh rosemary
2 bay leaves
2 tablespoons soy sauce
120ml dry white wine
4 anchovy fillets
115g extra fine French beans, topped and cut into 2.5cm pieces
115g petit pois, frozen
12 cherry tomatoes
juice of ½ lemon
freshly ground black pepper
warm seeded bread, to serve

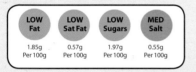

LOW Fat	LOW Sat Fat	LOW Sugars	MED Salt
1.85g Per 100g	0.57g Per 100g	1.97g Per 100g	0.55g Per 100g

1 Put the new potatoes in a pan of lightly salted water, bring to the boil and cook for 10 minutes. Drain and set aside.

2 Lightly spray a large saucepan with olive oil and heat, add the lardons and cook for 5–6 minutes over a medium heat, stirring occasionally until golden. Discard excess fat then add the chicken and brown all over.

3 Add the leeks and garlic and cook for a further 3 minutes, stirring regularly, then add the rosemary, bay leaves, soy sauce, white wine, anchovies and partly cooked potatoes. Cover and cook gently for 15 minutes.

4 Add the beans, peas and cherry tomatoes and cook, uncovered, for 8 minutes. Stir in the lemon juice and pepper to taste. Spoon into warmed bowls and serve with warm seeded bread.

Variation I'm a leg man, but feel free to use chicken breasts if you prefer them, although I don't believe they will be as juicy.

Amount per portion
Energy 345 kcals, Protein 38.2g, Fat 9.4g, Saturated fat 2.9g, Carbohydrate 26.4g, Total sugars 10.0g, Salt 2.77g, Sodium 1090mg

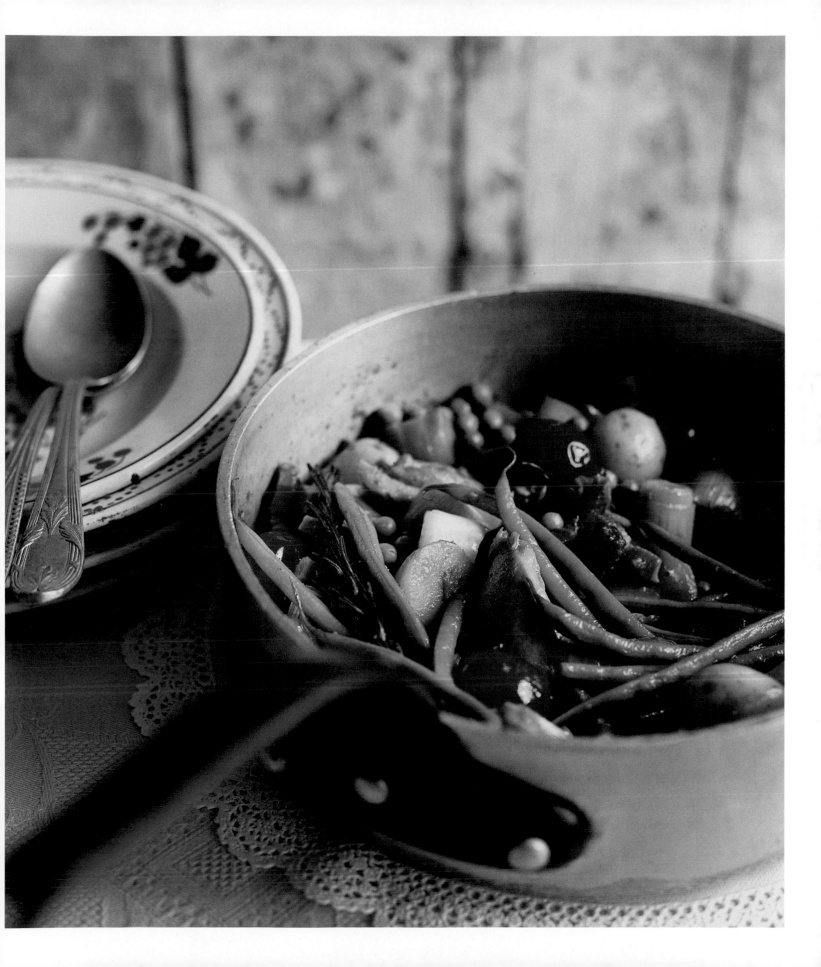

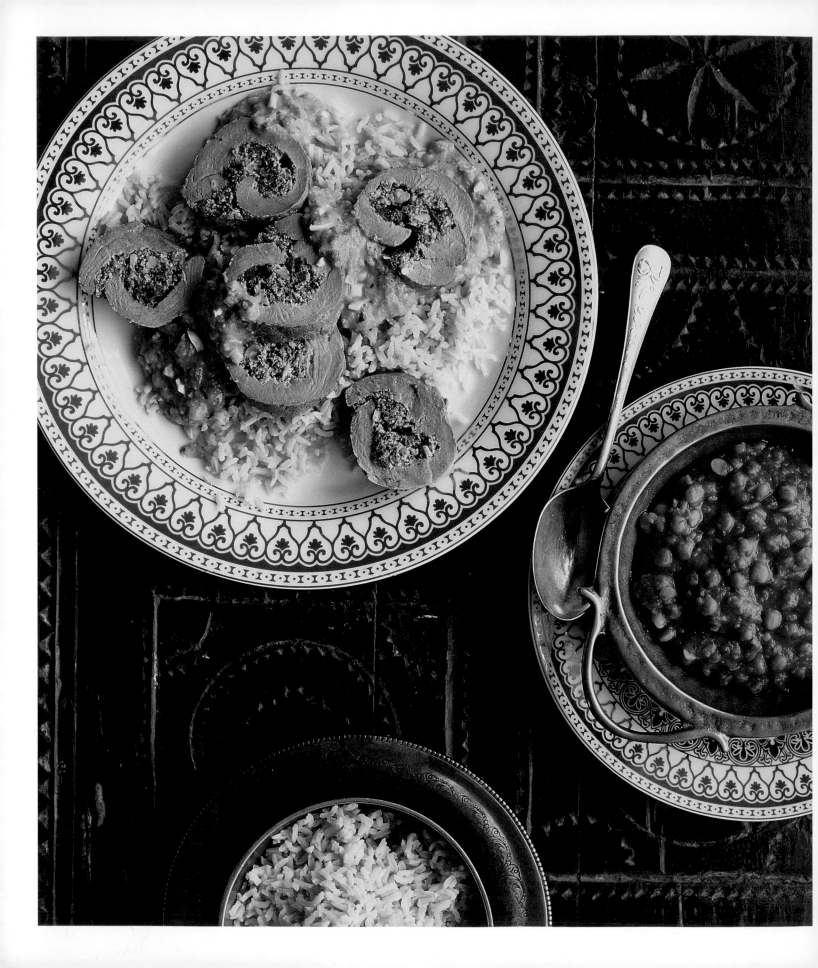

Duck Breast with a Nutty Filling

This is a dish for a dinner party – it's got lots of ingredients, as you'd expect with Indian food, but it's relatively simple to make. Serve it with some dhal and rice.

Serves 4

1 litre chicken stock, or duck stock if you can find it
4 duck breasts, skin removed
1 tablespoon each flaked almonds and chopped cashews
rice and dhal, to serve

For the stuffing

100g low-fat ricotta or cream cheese
1 tablespoon ground almonds
1 tablespoon chopped pistachios
100g cooked spinach, squeezed dry and chopped
1 tablespoon dried cherries
¼ teaspoon ground cardamom
1 teaspoon chopped fresh mint
¼ teaspoon chilli powder
¼ teaspoon salt

For the sauce

1 teaspoon sunflower oil
2 onions, finely sliced
2 teaspoons chopped garlic
1 teaspoon grated ginger
½ teaspoon ground turmeric
½ teaspoon ground cumin
½ teaspoon ground coriander
1 teaspoon garam masala
3-cm piece of cinnamon stick
3 cardamom pods
5 curry leaves
50g ground almonds
300ml chicken stock, or duck stock from poaching the duck
1 tablespoon chopped cashew nuts
2 tablespoons chopped fresh coriander
salt and freshly ground pepper

1 In a saucepan, gently heat the stock. Meanwhile, with a sharp knife make a horizontal slice through the duck breasts, leaving each joined at the side so you can open it up like a book – this is called butterflying. Cover each open breast with clingfilm and beat flat with a mallet or rolling pin.

2 Mix together all the stuffing ingredients, then spread a quarter of the mix over each breast, leaving a small border all around. Roll up the breasts then wrap in clingfilm to create tight sausages. Place them in the hot stock and poach gently for 20 minutes. Leave them in the stock to keep warm until ready to serve.

3 Meanwhile, make the sauce. Heat the oil in a frying pan and cook the onions gently until soft, about 8 minutes. Add the garlic, ginger, spices and ground almonds and cook for a further 5 minutes, stirring frequently. Add the sauce stock and simmer gently for 15 minutes. Discard the cinnamon stick and allow the sauce to cool slightly. Liquidise or purée the sauce, return it to the heat and stir in the cashews and coriander. Adjust the seasoning to taste.

4 Remove the clingfilm from the duck and slice each 'sausage' into 6 pieces, arrange on to individual plates and spoon over the sauce. Sprinkle with 'slivered' almonds and chopped cashews and serve with rice and dhal.

Amount per portion

Energy 510 kcals, Protein 51.1g, Fat 28.2g, Saturated fat 5.2g, Carbohydrate 14.2g, Total sugars 8.2g, Salt 2.43g, Sodium 959mg

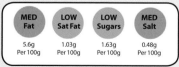

MED Fat	LOW Sat Fat	LOW Sugars	MED Salt
5.6g Per 100g	1.03g Per 100g	1.63g Per 100g	0.48g Per 100g

Souvlakia

This brings back memories of being in a Greek port snacking on this delicious lamb stuffed in pitta with salad and a yogurt dressing.

Serves 4
2 tablespoons extra virgin olive oil
1 tablespoon lemon juice
1 tablespoon grated onion and juice
1 tablespoon finely chopped fresh oregano
450g lamb (from leg), fat removed and cut
   into 1.5cm cubes
salt and freshly ground black pepper
salad and pitta bread, to serve

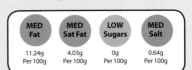

MED Fat	MED Sat Fat	LOW Sugars	MED Salt
11.24g Per 100g	4.03g Per 100g	0g Per 100g	0.64g Per 100g

1 In a large bowl, mix together the oil, lemon juice, onion and oregano to make a marinade. Stir in the meat and let it stand at room temperature for 1 hour, or preferably overnight.

2 Preheat the grill or barbecue. Drain the marinade off the lamb and thread the meat pieces on to metal skewers. Cook for 5–10 minutes, depending on how rare you like your lamb. Season and serve with salad and warm pitta bread.

Tip The meat is best when nicely brown on the outside but still pink on the inside.

Amount per portion
Energy 225 kcals, Protein 22.8g, Fat 14.5g, Saturated fat 5.2g, Carbohydrate 0.6g, Total sugars 0.3g, Salt 0.82g, Sodium 325mg

Lamb and Lentil Burgers

We know that meat burgers can often be high in fat, but the lentils make these a healthier choice and the Indian flavourings will certainly make them enjoyable.

Serves 4
2 tablespoons sunflower oil
2 onions, finely chopped
1 teaspoon lazy garlic (see Tip on page 144)
1 teaspoon lazy ginger (see Tip on page 144)
1 medium-heat green chilli, deseeded
    and finely chopped
1 teaspoon ground turmeric
1 teaspoon hot curry paste
300g lamb mince
175g split red lentils, washed and drained
2 tablespoons brown breadcrumbs
1 tablespoon chopped fresh mint
1 tablespoon chopped pine nuts
3 eggs, beaten
spray oil, for frying
salad and seeded bread, to serve

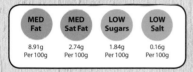

MED Fat	MED Sat Fat	LOW Sugars	LOW Salt
8.91g Per 100g	2.74g Per 100g	1.84g Per 100g	0.16g Per 100g

1 Heat the oil in a large frying pan and gently fry the onions for 6–8 minutes. Add the garlic, ginger and chilli and fry for a further 2 minutes, then add the mince and cook until brown.
2 Add the lentils, turmeric and curry paste and fry this mixture until the mince and lentils are cooked (about 20 minutes), making sure the mixture is completely dry. Drain off any liquid fat and leave the mixture to cool. (The burger mixture can be made in advance up to this point.)
3 Mix together the cooled burger mixture with the breadcrumbs, mint and pine nuts, then add a third of the beaten egg and mix well to bind. Divide the mixture into 4 patties, and refrigerate for about an hour, or as long as possible, to firm up.
4 Spray a frying pan with oil, then dip the burgers into the remaining egg and fry for 3 minutes each side until golden. Serve with salad and seeded bread.

Amount per portion
Energy 464 kcals, Protein 32.1g, Fat 23.7g, Saturated fat 7.3g, Carbohydrate 32.6g, Total sugars 4.9g, Salt 0.43g, Sodium 172mg

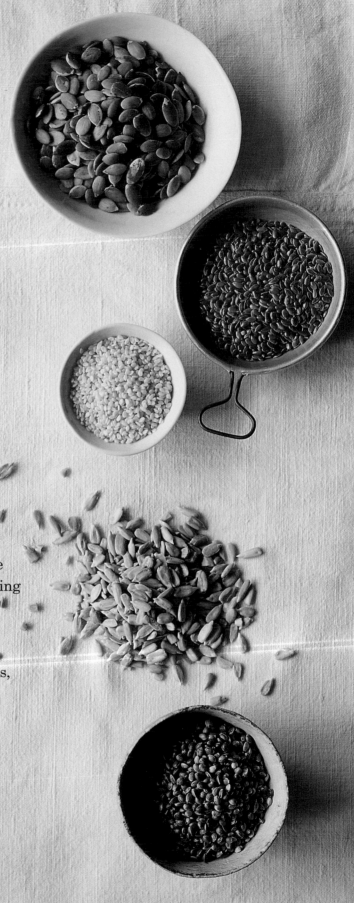

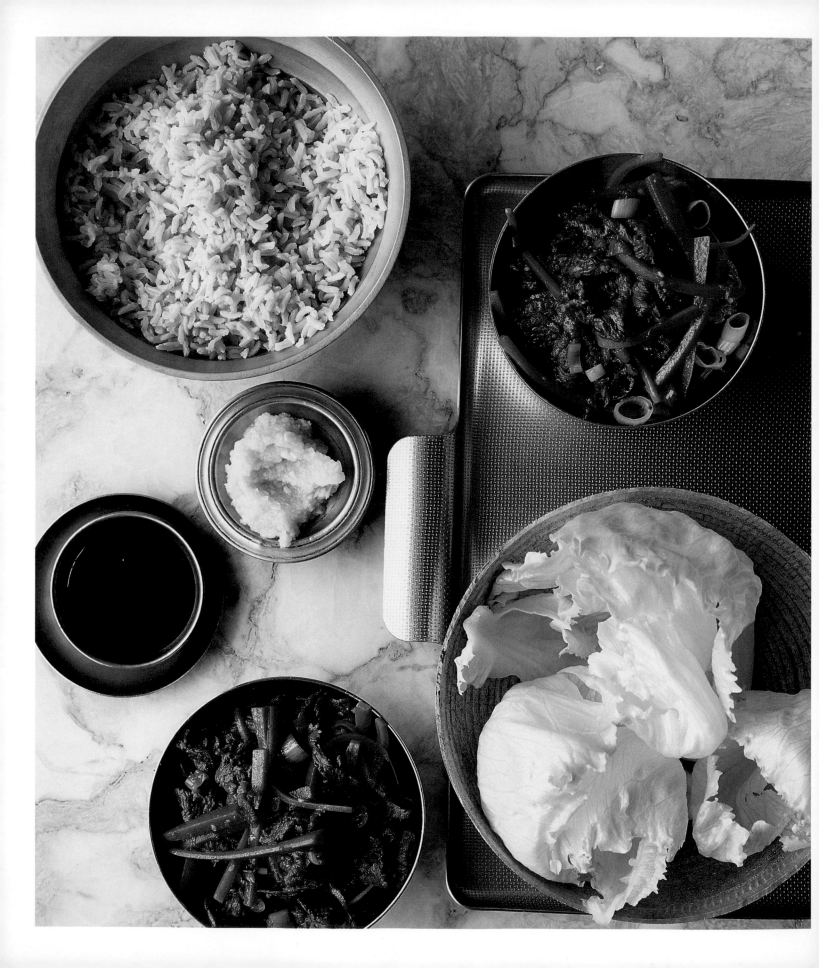

Bulgogi – Marinated Beef and Lettuce Parcels

One of Korea's best-known dishes, this combination of salty and sweet has great depth of flavour and a lovely crunch from the iceberg lettuce. It's not difficult to make, but allow plenty of time before cooking for all the flavours to develop. In this adaptation I've substituted brown rice for the usual sticky white rice.

Serves 4

375g beef (sirloin or rump), fat removed, frozen for 1hr 30mins to firm up
1 medium Bramley apple, cored and peeled
1 large conference pear, cored and peeled
1 onion, grated
2 garlic cloves, grated
2 large carrots, cut into matchsticks
4 spring onions, thinly sliced
2 green chillies, deseeded and thinly sliced
½ head of iceberg lettuce, leaves separated
375g cooked and cooled brown rice
1½ tablespoons soybean paste
2 teaspoons garlic purée

For the marinade

1½ tablespoons ketjap manis (Indonesian sweet soy sauce)
1 tablespoon sesame oil
2 tablespoons low-calorie sweetener
4 garlic cloves, crushed to a paste with a little salt
2 tablespoons sesame seeds

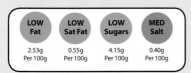

LOW Fat	LOW Sat Fat	LOW Sugars	MED Salt
2.53g Per 100g	0.55g Per 100g	4.15g Per 100g	0.40g Per 100g

1 Mix together all the marinade ingredients in a bowl. Set aside for the flavours to develop.

2 Meanwhile, slice the frozen piece of beef into very thin strips, then put them into a large bowl. Grate the apple and pear on to the meat and mix, along with the onion and garlic. Set aside for 20 minutes for the beef to take in the different flavours.

3 Pour the marinade over the beef and mix well, then mix in the carrots, spring onions and chillies. Leave to marinate, ideally overnight but at least for 1 hour.

4 When ready to cook, heat a wok over a high heat then add the beef mix with its marinade, and stir-fry for 3 minutes. To eat, take a lettuce leaf, place some rice in it and add a whisper of soybean paste and a dab of garlic purée. Top with hot beef, then enjoy the contrast of hot and cold, silky and crunchy.

Amount per portion
Energy 428 kcals, Protein 28.8g, Fat 12.3g, Saturated fat 2.7g, Carbohydrate 54.0g, Total sugars 20.2g, Salt 1.93g, Sodium 764mg

Tofu, Pork and Shellfish Hot Pot

And you thought healthy food had to be boring ... not so! This Korean winter warmer smacks you in the mouth, rolls you over and challenges you to have more.

Serves 4

1 teaspoon sunflower oil
4 garlic cloves, crushed to a paste
1 teaspoon grated ginger
3 teaspoons chilli powder
2 teaspoons sesame oil
115g pork fillet or tenderloin, cut into strips
1 tablespoon ketjap manis (Indonesian
    sweet soy sauce)
1 litre reduced-salt fish or chicken stock
225g fresh mussels, cleaned and any open
    mussels discarded
4 spring onions, sliced
115g sugarsnap peas
225g silken tofu, cut into bite-sized pieces
115g raw tiger prawns, shell-on
1 tablespoon chopped fresh coriander
salt and freshly ground black pepper
lime wedges and brown rice, to serve

1 Heat the oil in a frying pan and cook the garlic, ginger and chilli powder for 1–2 minutes. Add the sesame oil and increase the heat, then add the pork and cook for 4 minutes until browned. Stir in the ketjap manis and set aside.

2 In a separate deep pan, bring the stock to the boil. Tip in the mussels, cover and cook for 3 minutes until all the shells have opened – discard any that have not. Add the pork mix, the spring onions, sugarsnaps, tofu and prawns, bring back to the boil and cook for 1 minute. Adjust the seasoning to taste and stir in the coriander. Serve with lime wedges and some brown rice.

Amount per portion
Energy 189 kcals, Protein 19.9g, Fat 8.8g, Saturated fat 1.5g, Carbohydrate 8.2g, Total sugars 2.0g, Salt 2.12g, Sodium 837mg

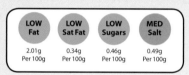

LOW Fat	LOW Sat Fat	LOW Sugars	MED Salt
2.01g Per 100g	0.34g Per 100g	0.46g Per 100g	0.49g Per 100g

Malaysian Lamb Biryani

One-pot dining at its best. I've given the classic Asian flavours little twists such as adding puy lentils to make the meal much more beneficial.

Serves 4
2 tablespoons sunflower oil
300g diced leg of lamb, cut into 1cm pieces
1 large onion, finely diced
2 garlic cloves, finely chopped
2cm piece of cinnamon stick
1 teaspoon ground turmeric
1 teaspoon ground cardamom
1 star anise, broken
2 tablespoons curry paste
200g brown rice, rinsed
100g puy lentils
8 new potatoes, cut into 1cm dice
40g raisins
1 carrot, cut into 1cm dice
1 litre lamb stock
50g frozen peas
½ red pepper, deseeded and cut into 1cm dice
2 tomatoes, deseeded and diced
40g chopped cashew nuts, to garnish
1 tablespoon chopped fresh coriander, to garnish

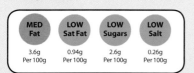

MED Fat	LOW Sat Fat	LOW Sugars	LOW Salt
3.6g Per 100g	0.94g Per 100g	2.6g Per 100g	0.26g Per 100g

1 Preheat the oven to 180°C/350°F/gas mark 4. Heat the oil in a casserole dish and, when very hot, add the lamb and cook briefly (maximum 2 minutes) to seal the meat. Remove and set aside.

2 Cook the onion in the same casserole dish for 6 minutes. Add the garlic, cinnamon, turmeric, cardamom, star anise and curry paste, and cook gently for a further 3 minutes. Add the rice and lentils and stir to coat. Add the potatoes, raisins and carrots, return the meat to the casserole, pour in the stock and stir. Cover, transfer to the preheated oven and cook for 30 minutes.

3 Check that the rice is cooked. Add the peas, red pepper and tomatoes, and return to the oven for 3 minutes. Divide the biryani between individual warmed bowls and scatter with the chopped cashews and coriander.

Amount per portion
Energy 669 kcals, Protein 32.8g, Fat 24.5g, Saturated fat 6.4g, Carbohydrate 84.6g, Total sugars 17.7g, Salt 1.75g, Sodium 690mg

Pot Noodle It's Not . . .

This rustic dish is heart-warming, perfect for winter, with loads of flavour and so very British. Here I've used pot barley (also known as Scotch barley or milled barley), which still contains the bran – a good source of fibre. You may have to go to a wholefood or health food store to obtain it.

Serves 6

1 tablespoon sunflower oil
1kg lamb shanks or neck chops
   (flavourwise, mutton would be even
   better but can be too fatty)
2 onions, roughly chopped
2 celery stalks, thinly sliced
2 carrots, thickly sliced
2 bay leaves
2 sprigs of thyme
1 tablespoon tomato purée
1 litre lamb or chicken stock
8 tablespoons pot barley
1 small sweet potato, cut into 1cm dice
¼ Savoy cabbage, shredded
115g peas, frozen or fresh and podded
salt and freshly ground black pepper
seeded bread, to serve

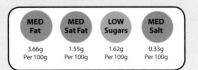

MED Fat	MED Sat Fat	LOW Sugars	MED Salt
3.66g Per 100g	1.55g Per 100g	1.62g Per 100g	0.33g Per 100g

1 Heat the oil in a large casserole dish and brown the meat all over, then remove and set aside. Put the onions in the casserole, and the celery, carrots, bay leaves and thyme, and cook for 6 minutes until the onions have browned slightly.

2 Stir in the tomato purée, then add the stock, cover and simmer gently for 2 hours. Remove the meat and allow it to cool enough for you to pick the meat off the bone.

3 While the meat is cooling, add the barley and sweet potato to the casserole and simmer for a further 20 minutes. Add the cabbage and peas, cook for a further 3 minutes, then mix the meat back in and continue cooking just long enough to heat through. Season with a touch of salt and plenty of black pepper. Serve piping hot, with chunks of seeded bread.

Tip If you're worried about the dish containing too much fat, make it the day before you want to eat it, allow to cool, then refrigerate. When cold, the fat will have solidified on the surface and can be skimmed off.

Amount per portion
Energy 381 kcals, Protein 32.2g, Fat 17.3g, Saturated fat 7.4g, Carbohydrate 25.5g, Total sugars 7.7g, Salt 1.56g, Sodium 615mg

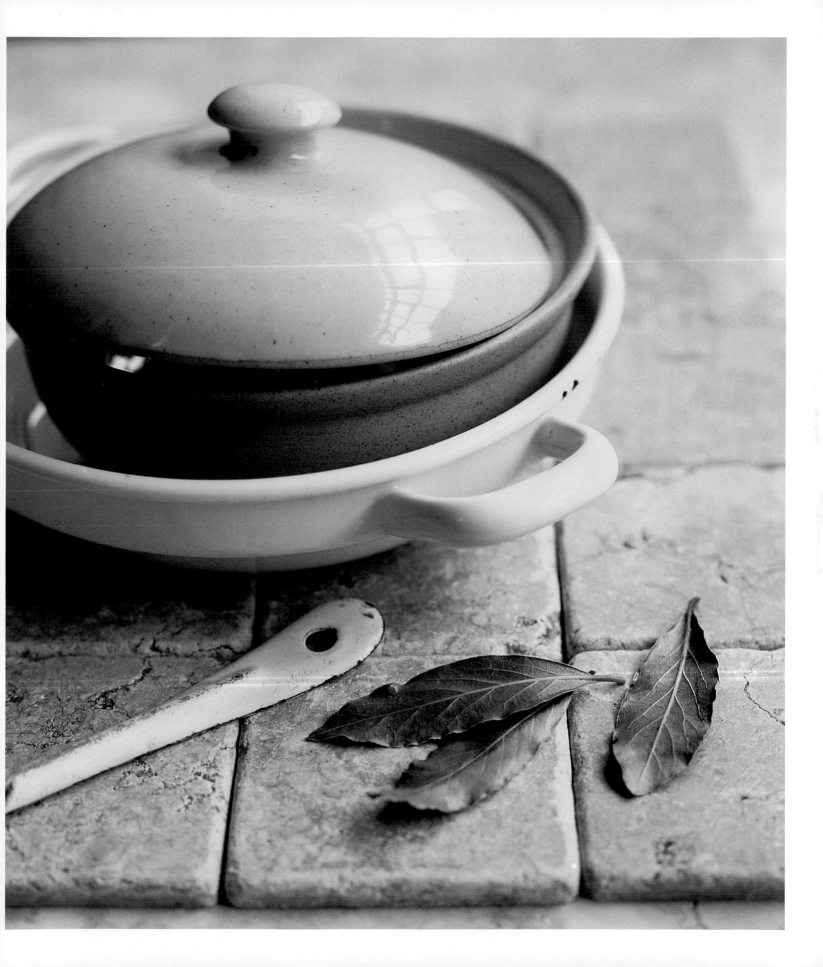

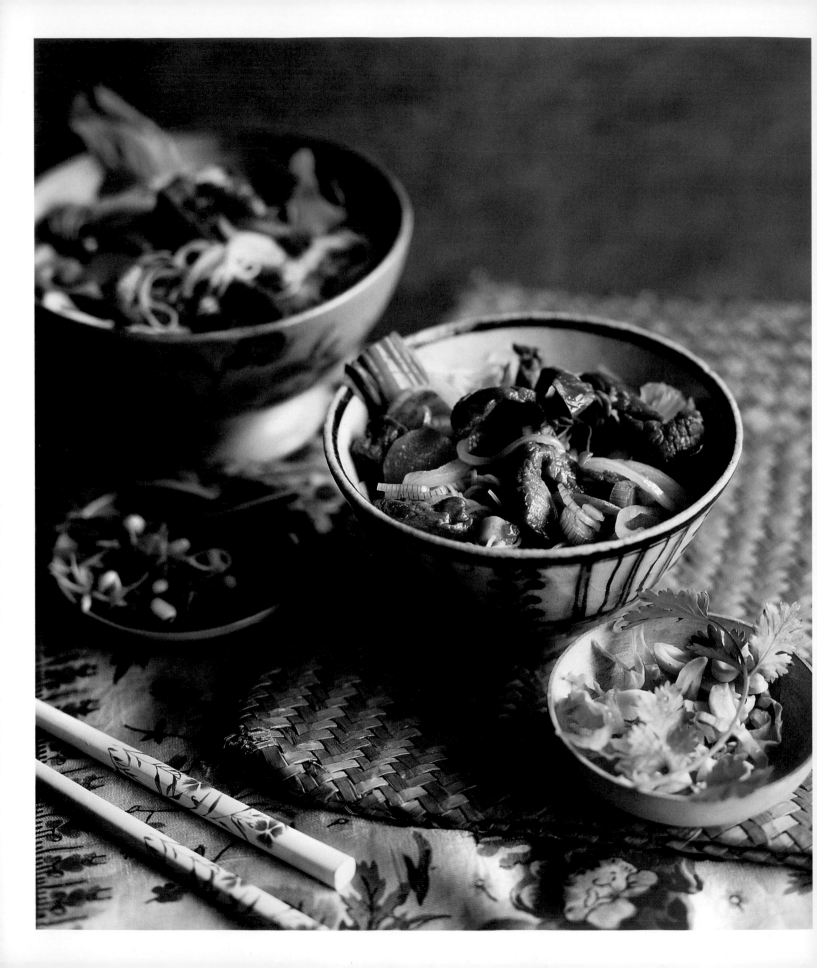

Bo Bun – Vietnamese Beef and Noodles

Really this is like a warm salad, with classic Asian flavours, offering both protein and carbs. Serve it with a few extra vegetables, as I've suggested here, for a more complete meal.

Serves 4

450g rump or sirloin steak, fat removed and cut into 5cm-wide strips, then sliced very thinly crossways
2 garlic cloves, crushed to a paste with a little salt
4 spring onions, sliced
1 stick of lemongrass, outer leaves removed, very finely chopped
2 tablespoons fish sauce (nuoc mam, nam pla)
½ teaspoon granulated low-calorie sweetener
175g rice vermicelli
2 tablespoons sunflower oil
¼ teaspoon dried chilli flakes
1 onion, thinly sliced
1 carrot, finely sliced
2 tablespoons diced water chestnuts
2 heads of bok choi, roughly chopped
salt and freshly ground black pepper

To serve

Mung bean sprouts
shredded lettuce
cucumber sticks
carrot strips
fresh coriander leaves
crushed peanuts

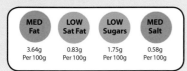

MED Fat	LOW Sat Fat	LOW Sugars	MED Salt
3.64g Per 100g	0.83g Per 100g	1.75g Per 100g	0.58g Per 100g

1 In a bowl, mix together the beef, garlic, spring onion, lemongrass, fish sauce and sugar, and leave to marinate for at least 30 minutes.

2 Bring a large pot of salted water to the boil, add the rice vermicelli and cook for approximately 2 minutes until the noodles are white but still firm. Drain and rinse in cold water. (This can be done ahead of time.)

3 Just before serving, drain the beef and reserve the marinade. Heat a wok, add the oil and when nearly smoking, add the beef and stir-fry for about 1 minute until brown. Remove and set aside.

4 Add the chilli flakes and the onion to the wok and cook for about 5 minutes, then add the carrot and stir-fry for 3 minutes. Add the water chestnuts and bok choi, along with a splash of water, and cook until the bok choi starts to wilt, about 2 minutes.

5 Add the beef, reserved marinade and noodles and stir-fry for 1 minute, and season to taste. Serve with the accompaniments suggested.

Amount per portion

Energy 373 kcals, Protein 31g, Fat 11g, Saturated fat 2.5g, Carbohydrate 41g, Total sugars 5.3g, Salt 1.74g, Sodium 684mg

Singapore Fried Noodles

A good bowl of noodles makes an excellent lunch or light supper. As you would expect from an Asian dish, this has loads of flavour.

Serves 4

400g rice noodles
2 tablespoons sunflower oil
100g raw tiger prawns, shells removed
    and deveined
100g chicken breast, skin removed,
    thinly sliced
2 eggs, well beaten
1 large onion, sliced
2 carrots, sliced
85g sugar snap peas, thinly sliced
2 teaspoons chopped garlic
100g bean sprouts
100g water chestnuts, chopped
½ red pepper, deseeded and thinly sliced
2 teaspoons fish sauce (nam pla)
1 tablespoon light soy sauce
1 tablespoon ketjap manis (Indonesian
    sweet soy sauce)
1 tablespoon Worcestershire sauce
3 red chillies, deseeded and thinly sliced
handful of watercress sprigs, large stems
    removed
handful of baby spinach leaves

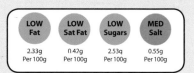

LOW Fat	LOW Sat Fat	LOW Sugars	MED Salt
2.33g Per 100g	0.42g Per 100g	2.53g Per 100g	0.55g Per 100g

1 Bring a pan of lightly salted water to the boil, tip in the noodles and cook for 1–3 minutes depending on their thickness. Drain and leave in a colander.

2 Heat half the oil in a wok, add the prawns and chicken and cook for 2 minutes, stirring regularly. Remove and set aside. Pour the beaten eggs into the wok and stir-fry for 1 minute, then remove and set aside.

3 Heat the remaining oil in the wok, then add the onion and carrots and stir-fry for 5 minutes. Add the sugarsnaps, garlic, bean sprouts, water chestnuts and red pepper, and cook for 2 minutes.

4 Return the noodles, prawns, chicken and eggs to the wok, then add the fish sauce, soy sauce, ketjap manis and Worcestershire sauce. Stir well then add the chillies, watercress and spinach, and stir until wilted. Serve hot.

Amount per portion
Energy 544 kcals, Protein 23g, Fat 10g, Saturated fat 1.8g, Carbohydrate 96g, Total sugars 10.9g, Salt 2.36g, Sodium 928mg

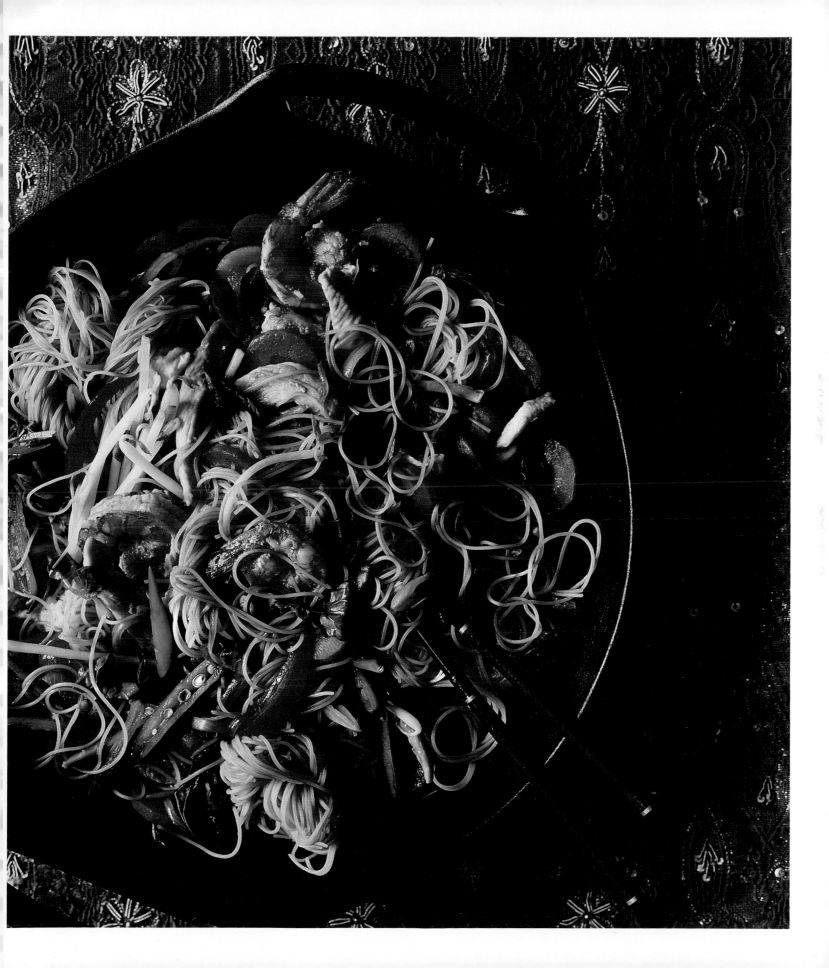

Desserts and drinks

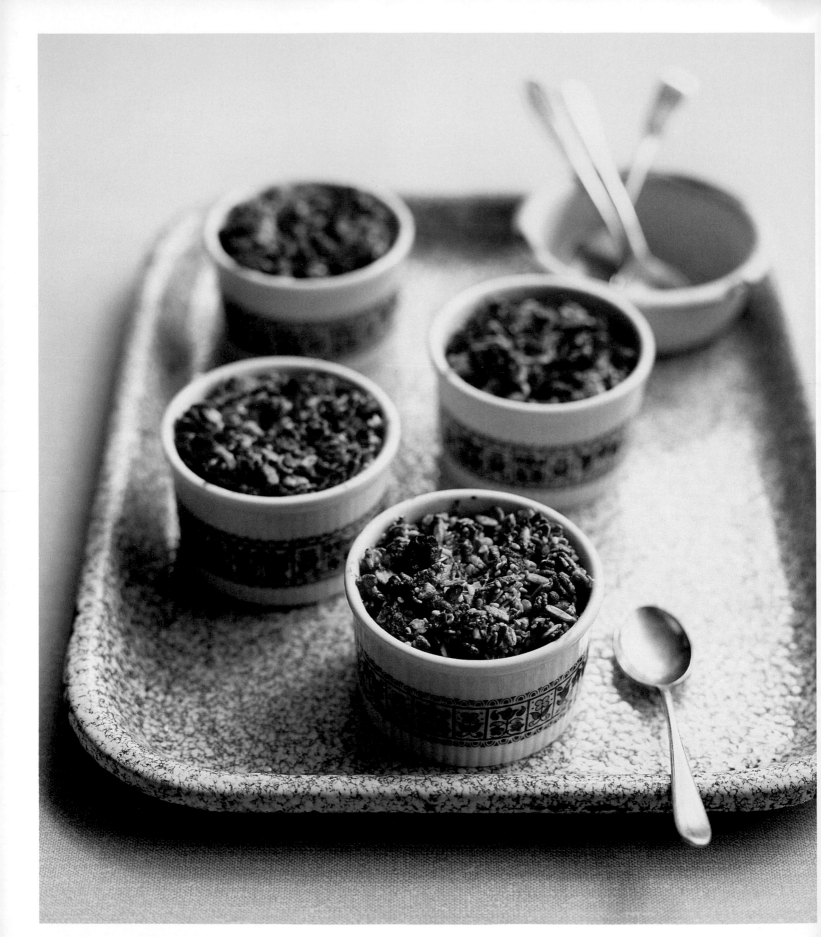

Crumble in a Flash

What could be more comforting than a homemade crumble? This version using sunflower seeds and sesame seeds is much healthier for you than traditional recipes.

Serves 4
2 x 227g tins pineapple, drained and
    lightly crushed
1 conference pear, diced
1 dessert apple (Cox, Granny Smith), diced
110g unsweetened muesli or granola
2 tablespoons sunflower seeds
2 teaspoons sesame seeds
100g low-fat Greek yogurt
2 tablespoons runny honey

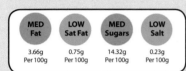

MED Fat	LOW Sat Fat	MED Sugars	LOW Salt
3.66g Per 100g	0.75g Per 100g	14.32g Per 100g	0.23g Per 100g

1 Preheat the oven to 180°C/350°F/gas mark 4.

2 Mix together the pineapple, pear and apple then spoon the mixture into four medium-sized ramekins. Crumble the muesli or granola into a bowl, stir in the seeds, then mix in the yogurt and honey. Spoon on to the fruit.

3 Bake, uncovered, for 20–25 minutes or until golden brown. Serve with a little extra yogurt if you like.

Amount per portion (granola)
Energy 261 kcals, Protein 5.9g, Fat 7.8g, Saturated fat 1.6g, Carbohydrate g 44.5g, Total sugars g 30.5g, Sodium 35mg

Amount per portion (muesli, no added sugar)
Energy 254 kcals, Protein 6.4g, Fat 7.5g, Saturated fat 1.6g, Carbohydrate 42.9g, Total sugars 27.7g, Sodium 35mg

Citrus and Honey Cheesecake with Plum Compote

Come on, spoil yourself. Not every day, mind, but as they say, a little of what you enjoy does you good.

Serves 12

For the crust
325g walnut pieces, toasted and cooled
    to room temperature
2 tablespoons sugar
½ teaspoon ground cinnamon

For the filling
900g low-fat cottage cheese
60g 0 per cent fat natural yogurt
1 tablespoon acacia honey
1 tablespoon sugar
4 large eggs
grated zest of 1 lemon
grated zest of 1 orange
1 teaspoon vanilla extract

For the plum compote
150ml red wine
25g caster sugar
25g low calorie sweetener
sprig of fresh rosemary
1 bay leaf
1 strip each lemon and orange zest
2 cloves
5cm piece of cinnamon stick
300g red plums, halved and stoned
butter, for greasing

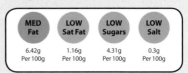

MED Fat	LOW Sat Fat	LOW Sugars	LOW Salt
6.42g Per 100g	1.16g Per 100g	4.31g Per 100g	0.3g Per 100g

1 Preheat the oven to 180°C/350°F/gas mark 4. Grease a 20cm flan dish or loose-bottomed cake tin and line with greaseproof paper. Make the crust by mixing together in a food processor the toasted walnut pieces, sugar and ground cinnamon, and processing until finely ground. Spread the mixture into the bottom of the prepared dish and press well to compact it.

2 Ensure all the filling ingredients are at room temperature. In the bowl of an electric mixer, combine the cream cheese and yogurt. Beat at a medium speed with the paddle attachment, scraping the sides of the bowl and the paddle often, until smooth. Add the honey and sugar and continue beating until there are no lumps. Add the eggs one at a time, beating between each addition. Then add the lemon and orange zest and the vanilla, and mix well. Pour the mixture over the crust in the prepared tin – do not scrape the sides of the bowl as this will add lumps to the mixture.

3 Set the flan dish or cake tin in a large roasting tin and add enough water to come halfway up the side of the cheesecake dish. Bake for about 25 minutes until just barely set. Turn off the oven, leave the cake in it with the door ajar, and leave to cool gently for 1–2 hours; this will prevent the cake from splitting on the top. When cold, cover in clingfilm and refrigerate overnight.

4 To make the compote, bring all the ingredients, except the plums, to the boil and simmer until the sugar has dissolved. Add the plums, cover and cook gently until the plums are just tender, about 10 minutes. Remove the plums and set aside. If wished, boil the juices to reduce slightly, and discard the rosemary sprig, bay leaf, zests, clove and cinnamon stick. Set aside to cool before using.

5 To serve, remove the cheesecake from its dish: first line a baking tray with clingfilm then dip the cheesecake dish in a hot-water bath and turn the cake out on to the prepared baking tray. Then invert the cake on to a serving dish – the cake should be just barely set in the centre. Serve at room temperature, topped with juicy plum compote.

Amount per portion
Energy 246 kcals, Protein 15.3g, Fat 14.9g, Saturated fat 2.7g, Carbohydrate 10.1g, Total sugars 10g, Salt 0.7g, Sodium 258mg

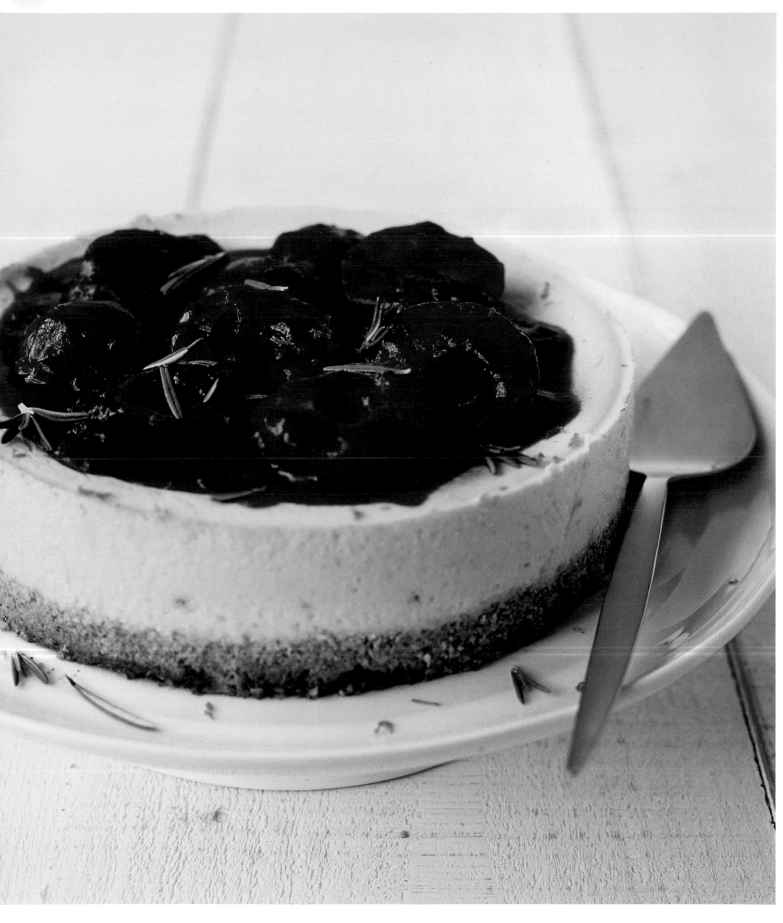

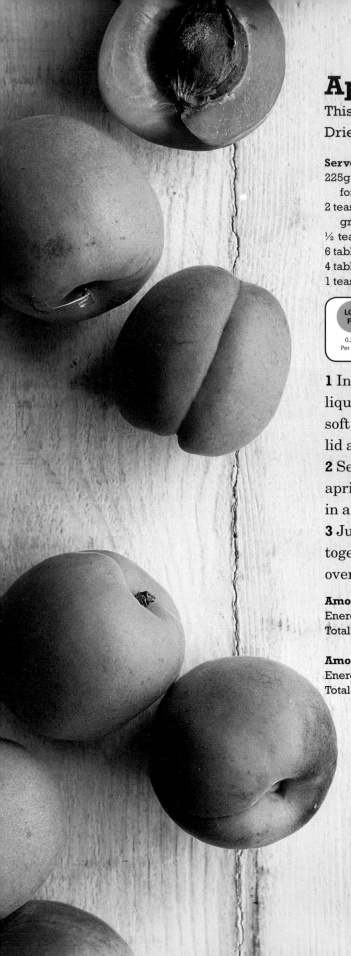

Apricot Fool

This is a pud for those in need of a little sweetness.
Dried apricots have a more intense flavour than fresh.

Serves 4
225g dried apricots, soaked in 600ml water
    for 1 hour
2 teaspoons caster sugar or low-calorie
    granulated sweetener
½ teaspoon vanilla extract
6 tablespoons 0 per cent fat Greek yogurt
4 tablespoons fresh pomegranate seeds
1 teaspoon chopped fresh mint leaves

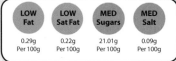

LOW Fat	LOW Sat Fat	MED Sugars	MED Salt
0.29g Per 100g	0.22g Per 100g	21.01g Per 100g	0.09g Per 100g

1 In a covered saucepan, cook the apricots and their soaking
liquor together with the sugar or sweetener until the fruit are
soft, about 30 minutes. Towards the end of cooking, remove the
lid and boil until you are left with about 3 tablespoons of liquid.
2 Set aside a quarter of the apricots. Blend together the remaining
apricots, all the poaching liquor, the vanilla extract and the yogurt
in a food processor. Spoon into glasses and refrigerate until chilled.
3 Just before serving, chop the remaining apricots, then mix
together with the pomegranate and the mint. Scatter the mixture
over the chilled fools and serve.

Amount per portion (low-calorie sweetener)
Energy 126 kcals, Protein 5.1g, Fat 0.4g, Saturated fat 0.3g, Carbohydrate 27.1g,
Total sugars 26.8g, Salt 0.12g, Sodium 48mg

Amount per portion (sugar)
Energy 135 kcals, Protein 5.1g, Fat 0.4g, Saturated fat 0.3g, Carbohydrate 29.5g,
Total sugars 29.2g, Salt 0.12g, Sodium 48mg

Gooseberry Fool Crunch

Along with rhubarb, gooseberries epitomise the UK for me, with their short seasons of fab tart fruit that demand you do something with them. A fool may be a slight cop-out but it's delicious, so go for it.

Serves 4
400g gooseberries, stalks removed
85g golden caster sugar, plus 3 tablespoons
    sugar or low calorie granulated
    sweetener
3 vanilla pods, split lengthways or
    2 teaspoons vanilla extract
500ml 0 per cent fat natural Greek yogurt
4 tablespoons unsweetened muesli

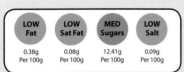

LOW Fat	LOW Sat Fat	MED Sugars	LOW Salt
0.38g Per 100g	0.08g Per 100g	12.41g Per 100g	0.09g Per 100g

1 Put the gooseberries and 85g of sugar in a saucepan and cook over a gentle heat for about 10 minutes until the gooseberries have softened. Scrape out the seeds from the split vanilla and stir them into the gooseberries, retaining the pods for another use. Stir to combine. Leave the gooseberries to cool and put 4 empty glasses (wine or tumbler) to chill.

2 Set aside half the stewed gooseberries. To the remaining half, add the additional sweetener and yogurt and mix well to blend.

3 In each of the four glasses, spoon in a layer of stewed gooseberries followed by some gooseberry yogurt and then the crunchy muesli, then add a layer of gooseberry yogurt and finish off with some stewed gooseberries. Chill until ready to eat.

Amount per portion (sugar)
Energy 265 kcals, Protein 15 g, Fat 1 g, Saturated fat 0.2 g, Carbohydrate 52g, Total sugars 44.1g, Salt 0.25g, Sodium 100mg

Amount per portion (low-calorie sweetener)
Energy 225 kcals, Protein 15g, Fat 1g, Saturated fat 0.2g, Carbohydrate 41g, Total sugars 33.4g, Salt 0.25g, Sodium 99mg

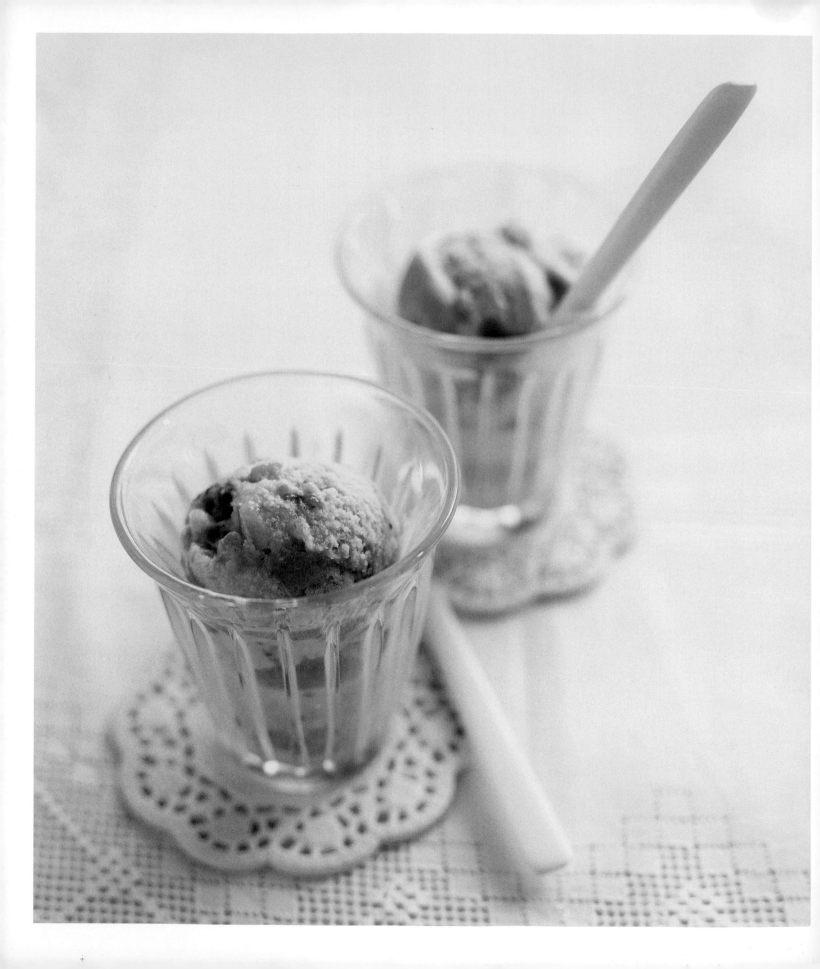

Peaches and Cream Ice Cream

A little treat is essential from time to time and this luscious American-themed ice cream fits the bill. If you're freezing ahead, ensure you remove it from the freezer well in advance to allow it to soften.

Serves 6
50g low calorie sweetener
4 ripe peaches, cut into 1cm cubes
1 tablespoon peach schnapps, brandy
   or orange-flavoured liqueur
4 tablespoons double cream
200g 0 per cent fat natural Greek yogurt
2 tablespoons chopped toasted hazelnuts

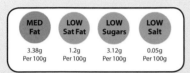

MED Fat	LOW Sat Fat	LOW Sugars	LOW Salt
3.38g Per 100g	1.2g Per 100g	3.12g Per 100g	0.05g Per 100g

1 Put 300ml of water into a saucepan, add the sweetener and bring to the boil, stirring occasionally, and continue to boil to a clear syrup. Pour the syrup over the peaches while hot, stir in the alcohol and leave to cool.

2 Set aside half the fruit. In a blender or food processor, blend together the remaining peaches with all of the syrup liquor, the cream and the yogurt.

3 If using an ice-cream maker, pour the mixture into the machine and follow the manufacturer's instructions; alternatively, pour the mixture into containers and chill in the freezer, whisking every 30 minutes as it freezes. Towards the end of the freezing process, fold in the remaining diced fruit and the hazelnuts. Enjoy immediately or freeze until needed.

Amount per portion
Energy 122 kcals, Protein 3.6g, Fat 7.9g, Saturated fat 2.8g, Carbohydrate 7.5g, Total sugars 7.3g, Salt 0.1g, Sodium 30mg

Pomegranate and Red Berry Jelly

I always think of jellies as a British experience but I'm sure a whole host of countries have their own versions, so I've experimented with a Middle Eastern ingredient. There's no added sugar in this recipe and it is low-calorie pudding so no need to go easy.

Serves 6
12 sheets gelatine
1.5 litres unsweetened pomegranate juice
3 tablespoons pomegranate seeds
100g blueberries
100g raspberries

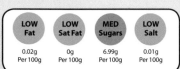

LOW Fat	LOW Sat Fat	MED Sugars	LOW Salt
0.02g Per 100g	0g Per 100g	6.99g Per 100g	0.01g Per 100g

1 Put a jelly mould in the freezer to chill. Soak the gelatine leaves in a small bowl of cold water for 8–10 minutes. Heat 500ml of the pomegranate juice in a saucepan over a low heat. Squeeze any excess water from the gelatine sheets then add it to the warm juice, and stir to dissolve and combine. Add the remaining juice and leave to cool to room temperature.

2 Remove the jelly mould from the freezer, scatter in the pomegranate seeds and pour in 2.5cm of the liquid jelly. Pop into the fridge to lightly set, about 30 minutes.

3 Remove from the fridge and scatter the blueberries over the set jelly. Pour on half the remaining liquid jelly, then return to the fridge to set.

4 Finally finish off with raspberries and the remaining jelly. Chill for about 4 hours to set properly, or preferably overnight.

Tip If you want to be a touch more professional, swirl the jelly around the chilled mould before putting in the fruit to coat the mould with jelly all over; this gives the jelly a better look.

Amount per portion
Energy 130 kcals, Protein 2.6g, Fat 0.1g, Saturated fat 0.0g, Carbohydrate 31.6g, Total sugars 31.6g, Salt 0.03g, Sodium 10mg

Fruity Cream Cheese Cup

I wanted to include a trifle in this book so I opted for this fab-tasting American version that is lower in calories than a traditional trifle.

Serves 4
100g raspberries
100g blueberries
150g strawberries, quartered
juice and zest of 1 orange
225g low-fat cream cheese
3 teaspoons sugar or low-calorie
   granulated sweetener
6 mini whole wheat cereal, crumbled
1 tablespoon maple syrup
1 tablespoon toasted almonds, to garnish

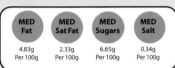

MED Fat	MED Sat Fat	MED Sugars	MED Salt
4.83g Per 100g	2.33g Per 100g	6.65g Per 100g	0.34g Per 100g

1 Mix together all the berries, stir in half the orange juice and set aside. Combine the cream cheese with the remaining orange juice, the zest and the sugar or sweetener.

2 Put four large wine glasses or tumblers on your work surface. Put a spoonful of the berry mix in the bottom of each, followed by a spoonful of cream cheese, and then sprinkle on some of the cereal. Repeat all the layers then drizzle with maple syrup and sprinkle with almonds.

Amount per portion (low-calorie sweetener)
Energy 166 kcals, Protein 6.8g, Fat 8.5g, Saturated fat 4.1g, Carbohydrate 16.2g, Total sugars 11.7g, Salt 0.59g, Sodium 230mg

Amount per portion (sugar)
Energy 180 kcals, Protein 6.8g, Fat 8.5g, Saturated fat 4.1g, Carbohydrate 19.8g, Total sugars 15.2g, Salt 0.59g, Sodium 231mg

Rhubarb and Yogurt Crunch Pots

This great British favourite is equally good for breakfast, but it does require a bit of preparation.

Serves 4
4 rhubarb stalks, destrung and cut
   into 2.5cm pieces
2 teaspoons sugar or low-calorie
   granulated sweetener
150ml fresh orange juice
360g 0 per cent fat Greek-style yogurt
100g unsweetened muesli
2 teaspoons runny honey

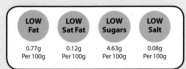

LOW Fat	LOW Sat Fat	LOW Sugars	LOW Salt
0.77g Per 100g	0.12g Per 100g	4.63g Per 100g	0.08g Per 100g

1 Preheat the oven to 200°C/400°F/gas mark 6.

2 Spread out the rhubarb on a roasting tray, sprinkle with the sweetener and pour over the orange juice. Bake for 15 minutes, without stirring or you will break up the rhubarb. Leave to cool.

3 Spoon a little yogurt into the bottom of four glass tumblers or wine glasses, cover with a layer of muesli and then top with some rhubarb pieces. Repeat the layers, finishing with rhubarb, then drizzle with a little honey.

Amount per portion (low-calorie sweetener & no added sugar muesli)
Energy 164 kcals, Protein 12.2g, Fat 2.0g, Saturated fat 0.3g, Carbohydrate 25.9g, Total sugars 12.1g, Salt 0.2g, Sodium 78mg

Amount per portion (sugar & no added sugar muesli)
Energy 173 kcals, Protein 12.2g, Fat 2.0g, Saturated fat 0.3g, Carbohydrate 28.3g, Total sugars 14.5g, Salt 0.2g, Sodium 78mg

Carrot and Pineapple Cake

This moist, luscious cake is a real treat, filled with carrots, nuts and spices. It also freezes well.

Serves 12
450g wholemeal self-raising flour
2 teaspoons baking powder
½ tablespoon ground cinnamon
½ teaspoon grated nutmeg
½ teaspoon ground allspice
110g dark muscovado sugar
125ml light olive oil
2 eggs, lightly beaten
350g carrots, grated
50g walnut pieces
110g raisins
25g desiccated coconut
250g pineapple, crushed, in natural juice
icing sugar, for dusting

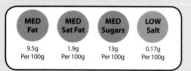

MED Fat	MED Sat Fat	MED Sugars	LOW Salt
9.5g Per 100g	1.9g Per 100g	13g Per 100g	0.17g Per 100g

1 Preheat the oven to 180°C/350°F/gas mark 4. Grease a 23cm spring-release tin and line its base with greaseproof paper.
2 Mix all the dry ingredients together in a large bowl. Add the remaining ingredients and mix well until evenly combined.
3 Transfer the mixture to the prepared tin and level the surface. Bake in the centre of the preheated oven for about 1 hour until risen and golden and a fine metal skewer comes out clean when inserted in the cake.
4 Cool in the tin for 15 minutes then transfer to a wire rack until completely cold. Dust with icing sugar and serve.

Amount per portion
Energy 343 kcals, Protein 7.3g, Fat 15.8g, Saturated fat 3.2g, Carbohydrate 45.7g, Total sugars 21.7g, Salt 0.27g, Sodium 108mg

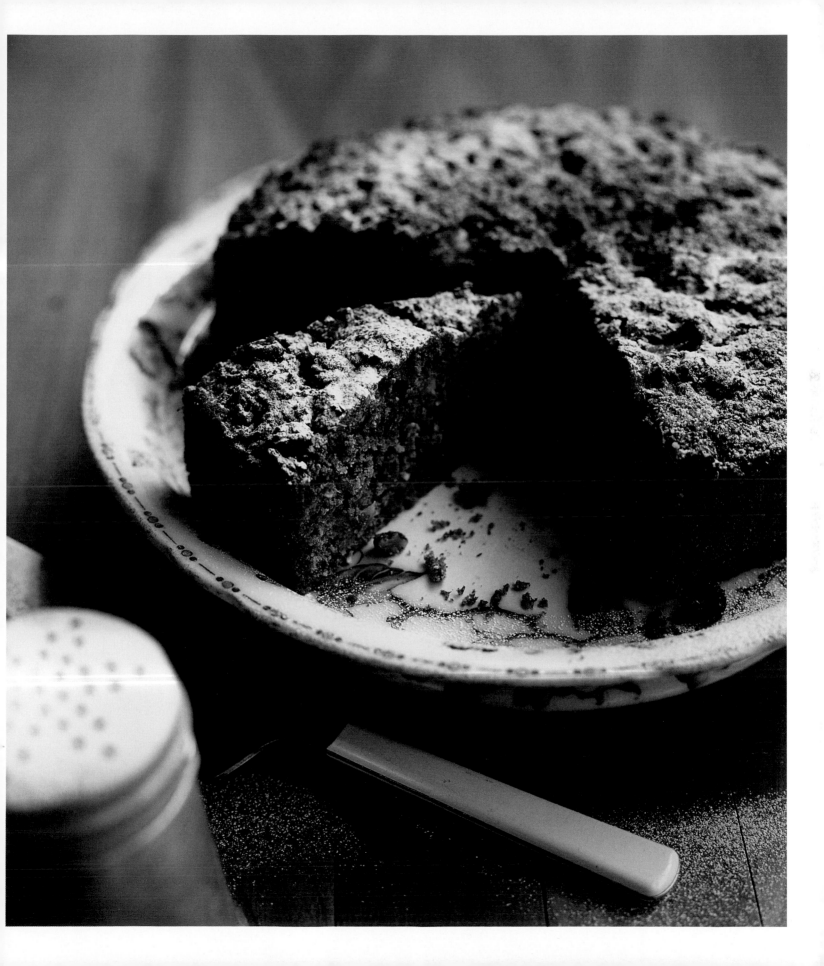

Summer Pudding

Berries are one of the best low GI fruit so by using a seeded bread and a low-calorie sweetener this version of the traditional British pudding makes a perfect fruity treat. If you need an accompaniment low-fat yogurt or low-fat ice cream is better than cream.

Serves 4

sunflower oil, for greasing
85g redcurrants, stripped from their stalks
85g blackcurrants, stripped from their stalks
450g raspberries
4 tablespoons low-calorie granulated sweetener
1 loaf of seeded bread, thinly sliced, crusts removed and discarded, cut into triangles

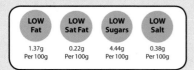

LOW Fat	LOW Sat Fat	LOW Sugars	LOW Salt
1.37g Per 100g	0.22g Per 100g	4.44g Per 100g	0.38g Per 100g

1 Lightly oil a 1-litre pudding basin, then line it with clingfilm, leaving plenty overhanging.

2 Put the fruit and sweetener in a saucepan and add 120ml of water. Bring to the boil, then remove from the heat. Tip the fruit into a sieve placed over a bowl to catch some juices – only remove the excess juice as you need the fruit to be quite wet.

3 Dip the bread triangles into the saved juice then use to line the prepared pudding basin, overlapping each piece of bread slightly. There will be some bread left, which will be needed later.

4 Set the pudding basin on a tray to catch any juices. Spoon the fruit to the top of the basin, pour in a little juice, then cover with the remaining bread. Cover the top with the overhanging clingfilm, then with a saucer or plate that fits inside the rim of the bowl, and set a heavy weight such as a few filled tins on top. Refrigerate for up to 2 days to completely set.

5 Remove the weight and saucer and peel back the clingfilm. Invert the pudding on to a plate. To serve, cut into wedges.

Amount per portion
Energy 284 kcals, Protein 10.2g, Fat 3.7g, Saturated fat 0.6g, Carbohydrate 56.0g, Total sugars 12.0g, Salt 1.02g, Sodium 405mg

Strawberry and Mint Tea Jelly

This is one for the adults, or perhaps the sophisticated child. I've chosen mint tea because the flavour goes well with the strawberries, a classic British combination, but there are loads of different teas you could try, such as jasmine and lapsung souchong.

Serves 8
1 litre mint tea, hot
4 teaspoons sugar or low-calorie
   granulated sweetener
juice of 2 limes
9 gelatine leaves, soaked for 6–8 minutes
   in a small bowl of cold water to soften
   and bloom
150g strawberries, sliced or diced

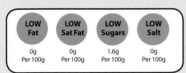

1 Put a jelly mould in the freezer to chill. Combine the tea with the sugar or sweetener and lime juice. Remove the gelatine from the water and squeeze out any excess moisture, then stir it into the tea to dissolve and blend.

2 Now you've got two options in how you prepare the set jelly. You can go all cheffy and pour a little jelly into the frozen mould, swirl it around to give a thin coating, and then stick slices of strawberry to the set jelly; pour in a bit more jelly with some strawberries and allow to set, then repeat 2 or 3 times until the mould is full. This way you get strawberries throughout the jelly. Or, you can simply spoon strawberries into the mould then pour on the jelly – the strawberries will float up, not as professionally pretty as with the cheffy method but it has the same fantastic taste. Chill in the fridge for a few hours to set.

3 Turn the set jelly out by dipping the mould in warm water for a few seconds, then turn it out on to a serving dish.

Variation Make individual jellies that you don't have to turn out at all, by filling wine glasses or tumblers that you can bring straight to the table.

Amount per portion (low-calorie sweetener)
Energy 11 kcals, Protein 1.1g, Fat 0.0g, Saturated fat 0.0g, Carbohydrate 1.7g, Total sugars 1.7g, Salt 0.01g, Sodium 5mg

Amount per portion (sugar)
Energy 20 kcals, Protein 1.1g, Fat 0.0g, Saturated fat 0.0g, Carbohydrate 4.1g, Total sugars 4.1g, Salt 0.01g, Sodium 5mg

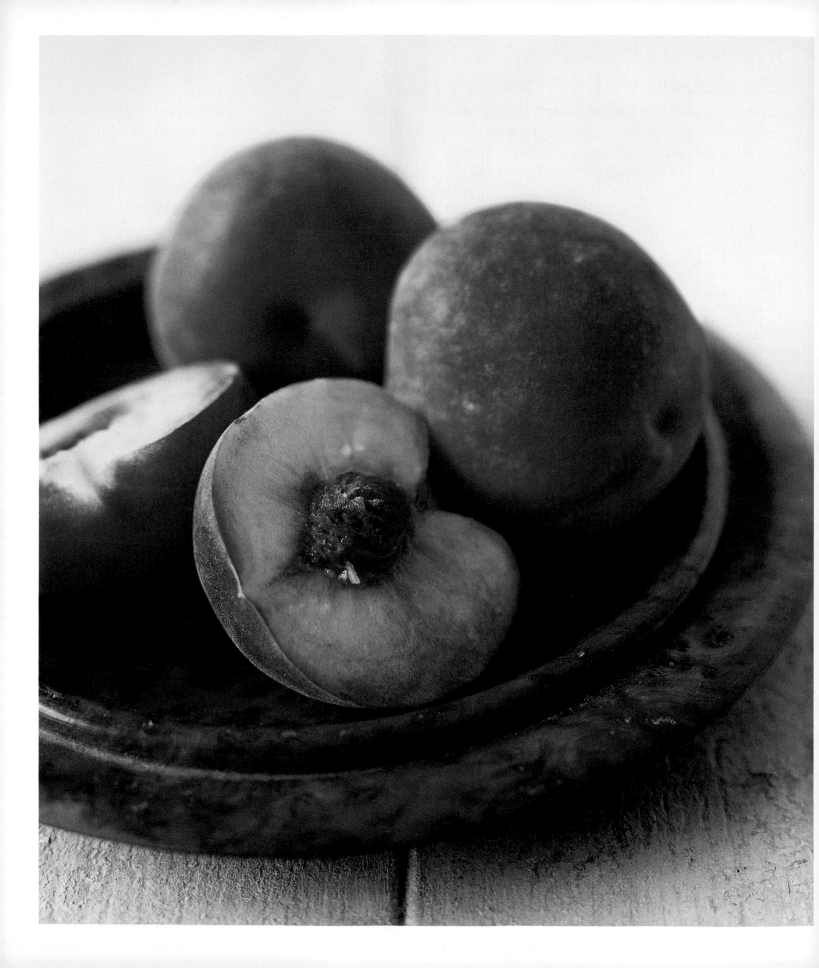

Melon Pudding

If you are going to choose a pudding, try and opt for a fruit based one. This Italian pud should add a little twist to your normal repertoire as the infusion of spice with jasmine tea and orange flower water is a beautiful combination with chocolate, fruit and nut.

Serves 4

1 Galia or Cantaloupe melon, rind and
    seeds removed
4 tablespoons low-calorie sweetener
15g cornflour
pinch of grated nutmeg
90ml brewed Jasmine tea, leaves strained
½ teaspoon orange flower water
40g dark chocolate, grated or finely
    chopped, plus extra shavings to serve
2 teaspoons chopped pistachio nuts, plus
    extra to serve
40g candied lemon peel, finely chopped

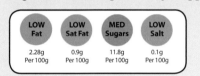

LOW Fat	LOW Sat Fat	MED Sugars	LOW Salt
2.28g Per 100g	0.9g Per 100g	11.8g Per 100g	0.1g Per 100g

1 Cut the melon into chunks and process to a fine purée in a liquidiser or food processor. Pass through a sieve into a bowl.

2 Whisk a little of the melon juice with the sweetener and cornflour to a smooth paste, then place in a saucepan over a low heat and stir in the remaining juice little by little. Slowly bring to the boil, stirring regularly, then remove from the heat. Stir in the nutmeg, jasmine tea and orange flower water. Leave to cool.

3 When the mixture is hand-hot, fold in the chocolate, pistachios and candied peel and divide between individual glass bowls or tumblers. Refrigerate until ready to serve. Just before serving, decorate with chocolate shavings and chopped pistachios.

Amount per portion
Energy 150 kcals, Protein 1.6g, Fat 4.3g, Saturated fat 1.7g, Carbohydrate 27.8g, Total sugars 22.3g, Salt 0.19g, Sodium 76mg

Minty Melon and Strawberries

Keep it simple, keep it fresh, as the Australians do; the mint adds a refreshing point of difference. I've chosen Charentais melon, but feel free to mix and match: a combination of watermelon, Charentais and honeydew makes for great colour.

Serves 6

2 teaspoons sugar or low-calorie
    granulated sweetener
leaves from 1 small bunch mint
2 Charentais or Galia melons, deseeded
150g strawberries, hulled and halved

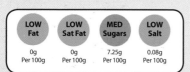

LOW Fat	LOW Sat Fat	MED Sugars	LOW Salt
0g Per 100g	0g Per 100g	7.25g Per 100g	0.08g Per 100g

1 Heat 250ml of water with the sugar or sweetener and half the mint, stir to dissolve the sweetener and simmer for 10 minutes. Strain and leave the syrup to cool. Chop the remaining mint leaves and add them to the syrup.

2 If you have a melon baller, scoop out balls from the melon flesh, otherwise dice the melon into bite-size pieces. Mix together with the strawberries. Chill the fruit salad, then pour over the mint syrup and stir to coat the fruit.

Variations Mint goes well with all sorts of fruit, such as peaches, pears and nectarines, so experiment with different combinations.

Amount per portion (low-calorie sweetener)
Energy 55 kcals, Protein 1.2g, Fat 0.3g, Saturated fat 0.0g, Carbohydrate 12.5g, Total sugars 12.5g, Salt 0.16g, Sodium 62mg

Amount per portion (sugar)
Energy kcals 61, Protein 1.2g, Fat 0.3g, Saturated fat 0.0g, Carbohydrate 14.1g, Total sugars 14.0g, Salt 0.16g, Sodium 62mg

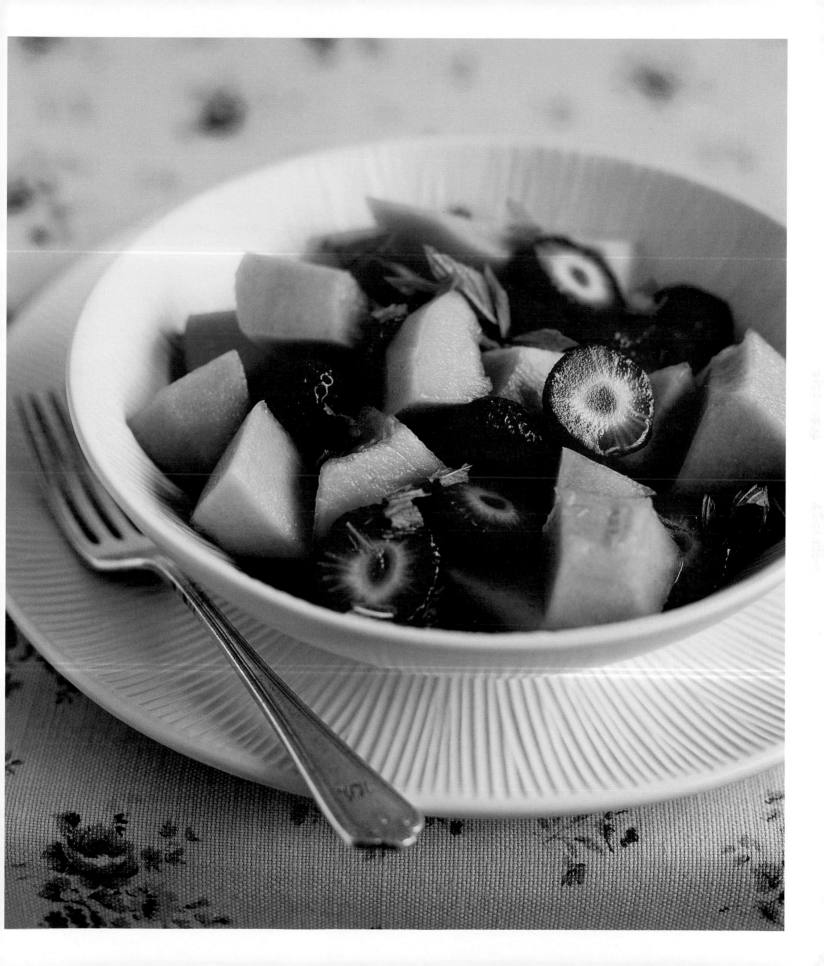

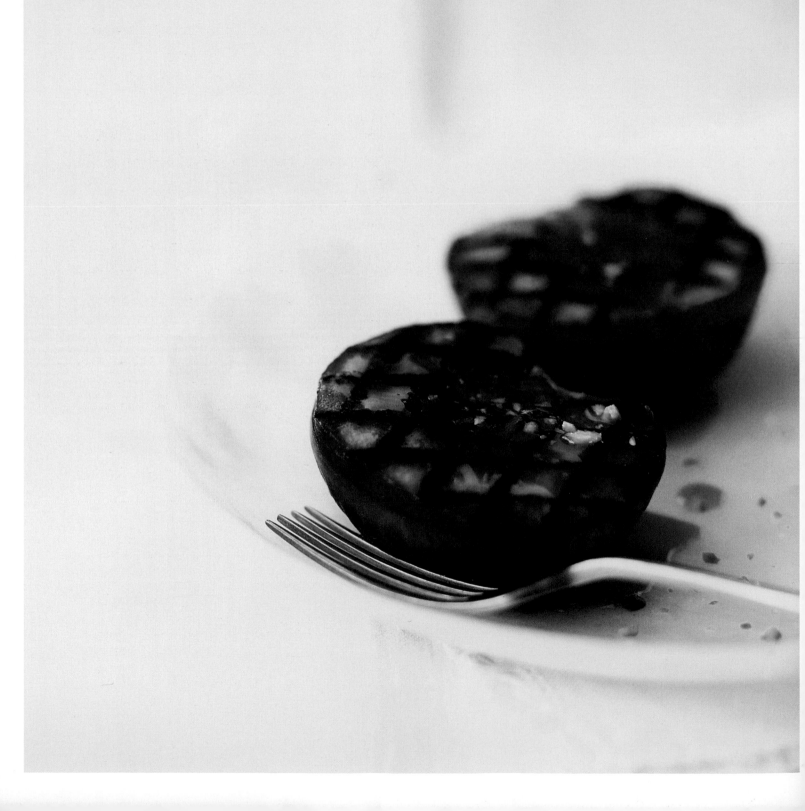

Char-grilled Peaches with Honey and Vanilla Yogurt

I love cooked peaches, as in this Italian dessert, but it's getting increasingly hard to find sweet-tasting ripe peaches, with most having a cardboardy texture; the same goes for nectarines and apricots. At least when you cook these fruit, you intensify the natural sweetness they do have.

Serves 4
spray sunflower oil
4 ripe peaches, halved and stoned
120ml fresh orange juice
1 tablespoon runny honey
180ml 0 per cent fat natural yogurt
1 teaspoon vanilla extract
1 teaspoon sugar
40g chopped pistachios, to garnish

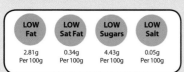

LOW Fat	LOW Sat Fat	LOW Sugars	LOW Salt
2.81g Per 100g	0.34g Per 100g	4.43g Per 100g	0.05g Per 100g

1 Preheat the oven to 200°C/400°F/gas mark 6. Spray oil in the bottom of a griddle pan or frying pan, heat, then add the peaches cut-side down and cook for 5 minutes over a fierce heat. If using a griddle pan turn the peaches sideways by 45° halfway through cooking to create patchwork markings.

2 Set the peach halves cut-side up in a roasting tin, pour the orange juice around them then drizzle the cut surfaces with the honey. Roast for 10–15 minutes, depending on their ripeness – you want the peaches soft but not collapsed.

3 Meanwhile, combine the yogurt with the vanilla and sugar. Place the peach halves into individual warmed bowls cut-side up, spoon on a dollop of yogurt and scatter with the pistachios.

Tip If possible buy 'freestone' peaches rather than 'clingstone' ones. Your greengrocer may not know what on earth you are talking about, and I'm sure the supermarket won't have a clue, but freestone, as the name suggests, are much easier when trying to remove the stone. Basically, if the peach twists easily it's freestone, if you have to cut the flesh from the stone it's not.

Amount per portion
Energy 147 kcals, Protein 5.8g, Fat 5.7g, Saturated fat 0.7g, Carbohydrate 19.5g, Total sugars 19.0g, Salt 0.1g, Sodium 38mg

Mango Lassi

In India, variations on this yogurt drink are popular for any time of the day. Over here, this version should be a regular on your breakfast menu.

Serves 4
600g 0 per cent fat natural yogurt
2 mangoes, roughly diced
2 tablespoons bran
3 tablespoons pomegranate seeds
1 tablespoon runny honey
12 ice cubes

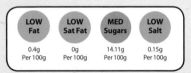

LOW Fat	LOW Sat Fat	MED Sugars	LOW Salt
0.4g Per 100g	0g Per 100g	14.11g Per 100g	0.15g Per 100g

1 In a smoothie machine or food processor, whizz all the ingredients (except the ice) together until well blended. Pour into 4 glasses and serve immediately over ice.

Amount per portion
Energy 195 kcals, Protein 10g, Fat 1g, Saturated fat 0g, Carbohydrate 40g, Total sugars 35.7g, Salt 0.37g, Sodium 146mg

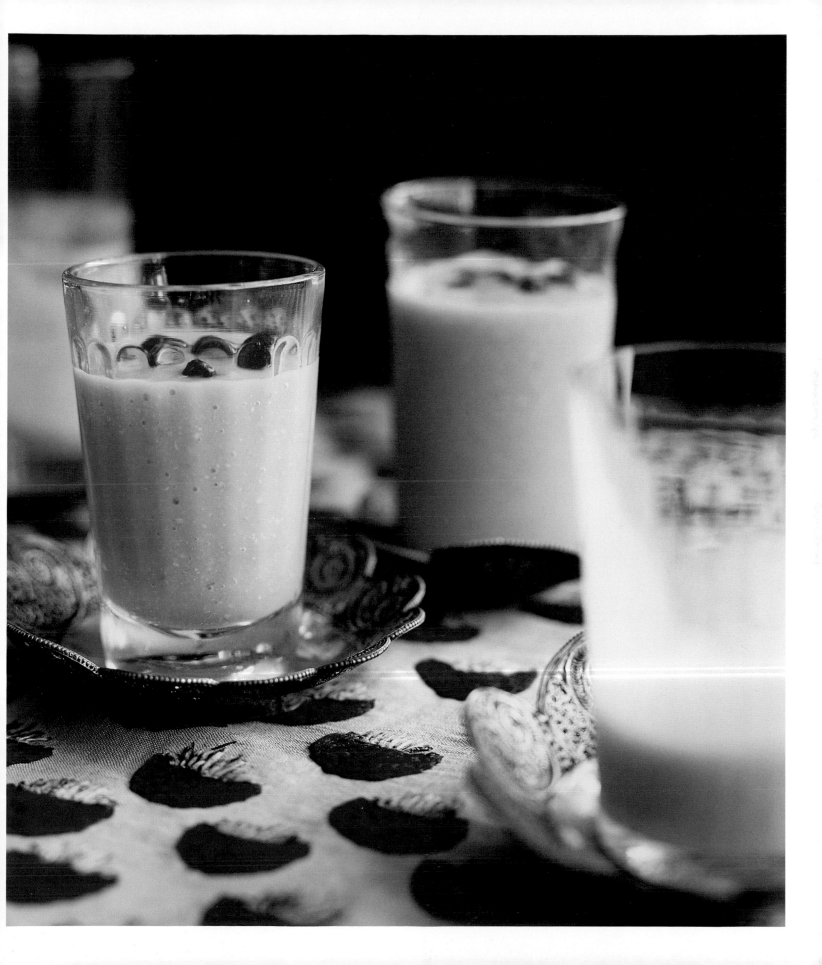

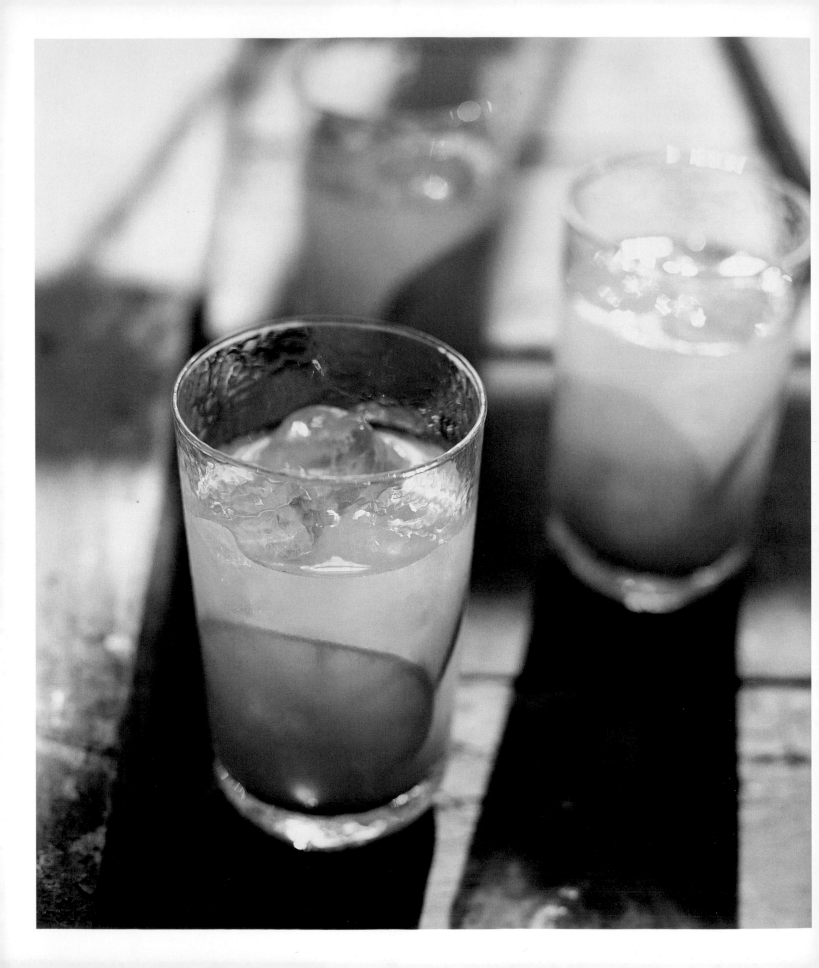

Old-Fashioned Barley Water

When I saw the recipe for this traditional British drink in one of the cookbooks my aunt put together a long time ago, I had to put it in this book. As long as you use low-calorie sweetener, the rest of the drink is nothing but health.

Serves 4
300g pearl barley, washed
grated zest and juice of 6 oranges
grated zest and juice of 3 lemons
low-calorie sweetener

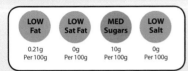

LOW Fat	LOW Sat Fat	MED Sugars	LOW Salt
0.21g Per 100g	0g Per 100g	10g Per 100g	0g Per 100g

1 Tip the barley into a saucepan, add 2.5 litres of water and the orange and lemon zests. Bring to the boil, reduce the heat and simmer for 1 hour. Strain the liquid and leave to cool.

2 Stir in the citrus juices and sweeten to taste. Decant the barley water into bottles or a jug and refrigerate. Drink within 3 days.

Tip Think thrifty – the discarded barley would be useful added to another dish, such as a soup.

Amount per portion
Energy 85 kcals, Protein 1.9g, Fat 0.2g, Saturated fat 0.0g, Carbohydrate 20.2g, Total sugars 9.7g, Salt 0.01g, Sodium 4mg

Index

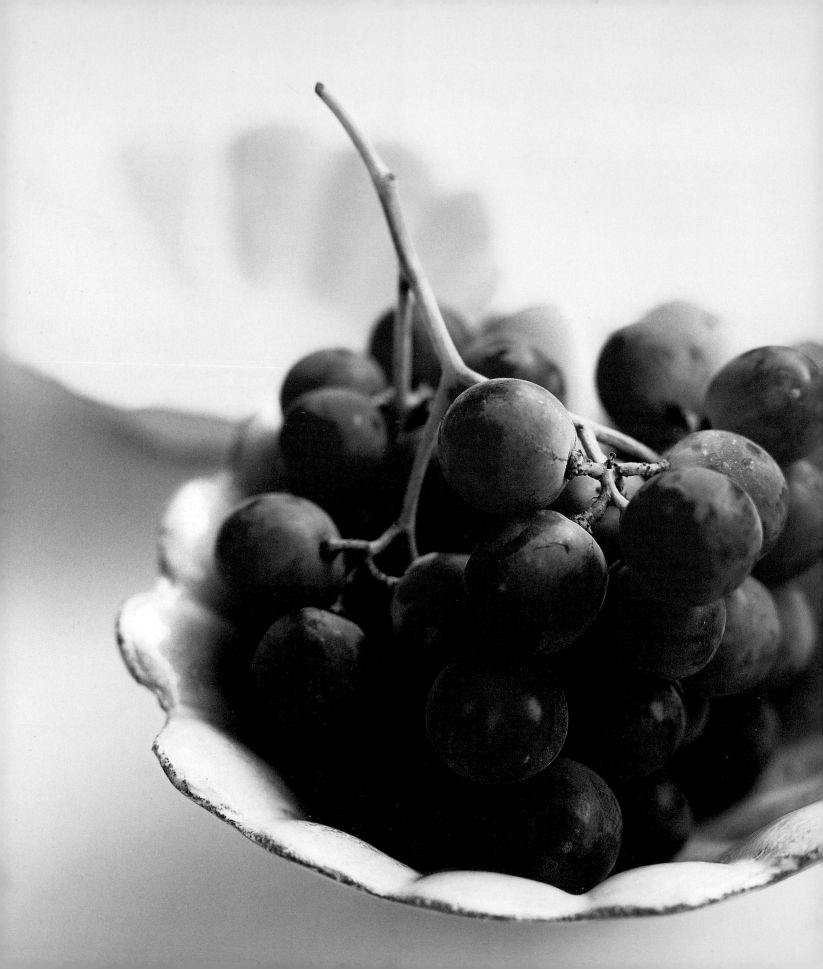